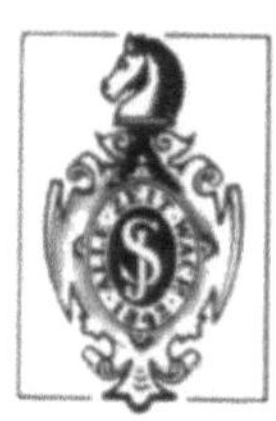

Erich Rügheimer (Editor)

New Aspects on Respiratory Failure

Editorial Assistants:
Harald Mang, Klaus Tschaikowsky

With 150 Figures and 27 Tables

Springer-Verlag
Berlin Heidelberg New York
London Paris Tokyo
Hong Kong Barcelona Budapest

Editor:

Prof. Dr. med. Erich Rügheimer
Institut für Anaesthesiologie
Universität Erlangen-Nürnberg
Krankenhausstrasse 12, D-8520 Erlangen, FRG

Editorial Assistants:

Dr. med. Harald Mang
Dr. med. Klaus Tschaikowsky
Institut für Anaesthesiologie
Universität Erlangen-Nürnberg
Krankenhausstrasse 12, D-8520 Erlangen, FRG

Proceedings of the 4th International Symposium on Anaesthesia in Erlangen, FRG, 15–17 June 1989

ISBN-13: 978-3-642-74945-2 e-ISBN-13: 978-3-642-74943-8
DOI: 10.1007/978-3-642-74943-8

Library of Congress Cataloging-in-Publication Data.
International Symposium on Anaesthesia (4th: 1989: Erlangen, Germany) New aspects on respiratory failure/Erich Rügheimer (editor): Harald Mang, Klaus Tschaikowsky (editorial assistants). "Proceedings of the 4th International Symposium on Anaesthesia in Erlangen, R.R.G., 15–17 June 1989" – T.p. verso.

1. Respiratory insufficiency – Congresses. 2. Respiratory distress syndrome. Adult – Congresses. 3. Anesthesia – Complications and sequelae – Congresses. I. Rügheimer, E. (Erich) II. Mang, Harald. III. Tschaikowsky, Klaus. IV. Title. [DNLM: 1. Respiratory Insufficiency – diagnosis – congresses. 2. Respiratory Insufficiency – physiopathology – congresses. 3. Respiratory Insufficiency – therapy – congresses. WF 140 1608n 1989]

Softcover reprint of the hardcover 1st edition 1992

Typesetting; Macmillan India Ltd., Bangalore-25
19/3020-543210-Printed on acid-free paper

Preface

Surgical intervention and anaesthetic, including patient positioning and mechanical ventilation, result in changes to the mechanics of breathing and gas exchange, even in otherwise healthy patients, and often lead to postoperative bronchopulmonary complications. As numerous investigations have shown, the risk of complications developing can be up to six times greater in patients with pre-existing pulmonary pathology. The patients at greatest risk are those with severe post-traumatic or haemorrhagic shock, sepsis and prior burns, or a rejection crisis following transplantation. Such patients may develop ARDS, which is still associated with a high mortality rate. Thus, respiratory insufficiency is, and will remain, a central problem for the anaesthetist, both during the anaesthetic and in the postoperative phase.

The program of our 4th International Anaesthesia Symposium held in Erlangen was intended to present genuinely new aspects of pathophysiology, diagnostic evaluation and treatment of respiratory insufficiency. When selecting the topics and speakers, we attached considerable importance to ensuring that all those disciplines would be represented which could be expected to contribute to future improvements in the optimal treatment of severely-ill patients with respiratory insufficiency. The result of this interdisciplinary synopsis is reflected in the papers published in this volume, which it is hoped will provide the physician with a particular interest in anaesthesia and intensive care medicine with an overview of the present state of our knowledge in terms of its therapeutic usefulness, and to indicate the direction further developments can be expected to take.

We would like to thank all the authors for their patience in the face of the unexpected difficulties that delayed the publication of this volume. Thanks are also due to the publishers for their usual good cooperation that has resulted in the production of this well-appointed book. A special vote of thanks are due to Drs. Mang and Tschaikowsky for their unstinting help with the editorial work.

Erlangen, March 1991 E. Rügheimer

List of Contributors

Adolph, M., Dr. med.
Institut für Anästhesiologie und Operative Intensivmedizin, Zentralklinikum, Stenglinstrasse 2, D-8900 Augsburg, FRG

Ailion, D.C., M.D.
Division of Respiratory, Critical Care and Occupational Pulmonary Medicine, University of Utah Medical Center, 50 North Medical Drive, Salt Lake City, UT 84132, USA

Baum, M., Ing.
Univ.-Klinik für Anästhesiologie und Allgemeine Intensivmedizin, Anichstrasse 35, A-6020 Innsbruck, AUSTRIA

Beger, H.G., Prof. Dr. med.
Abteilung für Allgemeine Chirurgie, Klinikum der Universität Ulm, Steinhövelstrasse 9, D-7900 Ulm, FRG

Benzer, H., Prof. Dr. med.
Univ.-Klinik für Anästhesiologie und Allgemeine Intensivmedizin, Anichstrasse 35, A-6020 Innsbruck, AUSTRIA

Blümel, G., Dr. med.
Institut für Anästhesiologie und Operative Intensivmedizin, Zentralklinikum, Stenglinstrasse 2, D-8900 Augsburg, FRG

Bos, J.A.H., Dr.
Erasmus Universiteit, Department of Anaesthesiology, Postbus 1738, NL-3000 DR Rotterdam, THE NETHERLANDS

Brain, J.D., M.D.
Department of Environmental Science and Physiology, Harvard University, School of Public Health, 665 Huntington Ave, Boston, MA 02115, USA

Braquet, P., M.D.
Institut Henri Beaufour, 17, avenue Descartes, F-92350 Le plessis Robinson, FRANCE

Burchardi, H., Prof. Dr. med.
Institut für Anästhesiologie, Universität Göttingen, Robert-Koch-Strasse 40, D-3400 Göttingen, FRG

Chang, S., M.D.
Cardiovascular Pulmonary Laboratory, University of Colorado, Health Sciences Center, Denver, Colorado 80262, USA

Chen, C., M.D.
Cardiovascular Pulmonary Laboratory, University of Colorado, Health Sciences Center, Denver, Colorado 80262, USA

Cohen, H., M.D.
Respiratory Care Department – COX-3, Massachusetts General Hospital, Fruitstreet, Boston, MA 02114, USA

Criée, C.-P., Prof. Dr. med.
Kreiskrankenhaus Lenglern, Universität Göttingen, D-3406 Bovenden, FRG

Cutillo, A.G., M.D.
Division of Respiratory, Critical Care and Occupational Pulmonary Medicine, University of Utah Medical Center, 50 North Medical Drive, Salt Lake City, UT 84132, USA

Czartolomna, J., M.D.
Cardiovascular Pulmonary Laboratory, University of Colorado, Health Sciences Center, Denver, Colorado 80262, USA

Dugas, B., M.D.
Institut Henri Beaufour, 1, avenue des Tropiques, F-91952 Les Ulis, FRANCE

Durney, C.H., M.D.
Division of Respiratory, Critical Care and Occupational Pulmonary Medicine, University of Utah Medical Center, 50 North Medical Drive, Salt Lake City, UT 84132, USA

Eberhard, L., Dr. med.
Institut für Anästhesiologie und Operative Intensivmedizin, Zentralklinikum, Stenglinstrasse 2, D-8900 Augsburg, FRG

Eckart, J., Prof. Dr. med.
Institut für Anästhesiologie und Operative Intensivmedizin, Zentralklinikum, Stenglinstrasse 2, D-8900 Augsburg, FRG

Falke, K.J., Prof. Dr. med.
Institut für Anästhesiologie, FU Berlin, Klinikum Charlottenburg, Spandauer Damm 130, D-1000 Berlin, FRG

Fritz, H., Prof. Dr. rer. nat.
Institut für Klinische Chemie und Klinische Biochemie, Universität München, Nußbaumstrasse 20, D-8000 München 2, FRG

Fung, Y.C., Ph.D.
Department of Applied Mechanics and Engineering Sciences, Bioengineering, University of California, San Diego, La Jolla, CA 92093, USA

Ganesan, K., M.D.
Division of Respiratory, Critical Care and Occupational Pulmonary Medicine, University of Utah Medical Center, 50 North Medical Drive, Salt Lake City, UT 84132, USA

Gebhardt, P., Dr.
Drägerwerk AG, Moislinger Allee 53–55, D-2400 Lübeck, FRG

Georgieff, M., Prof. Dr. med.
Institut für Anaesthesiologie, Universität Erlangen-Nürnberg, Krankenhausstrasse 12, D-8520 Erlangen, FRG

Goulet, R.L., M.D.
Respiratory Care Department – COX-3, Massachusetts General Hospital, Fruitstreet, Boston, MA 02114, USA

Grimminger, F., Dr. med.
Zentrum Innere Medizin, Universität Gießen, Klinikstrasse 36, D-6300 Gießen, FRG

Guttmann, J., Dr. med.
Institut für Anästhesiologie und Operative Intensivmedizin, Zentralklinikum, Stenglinstrasse 2, D-8900 Augsburg, FRG

Hawgood, S., M.D.
University of California at San Francisco – Cardiovascular Research Institute, M 1327, San Francisco, CA 94143-0130, USA

Hecker, E., Dr. rer. nat.
Drägerwerk AG, Moislinger Allee 53–55, D-2400 Lübeck, FRG

Heinze, R., Dr. med.
1. Medizinische Klinik, TU München, Ismaninger Strasse 22, D-8000 München 8, FRG

Hinshaw, L.B., Ph.D.
Professor of Physiology and Biophysics, Veterans Administration, Medical Center, Research (151C), 921 N.E. 13th Street, Oklahoma City, OK 73104, USA

Hörmann, Ch., Dr. med.
Univ.-Klinik für Anästhesiologie und Allgemeine Intensivmedizin, Anichstrasse 35, A-6020 Innsbruck, AUSTRIA

Hosford, D., M.D.
Institut Henri Beaufour, 1, avenue des Tropiques, F-91952 Les Ulis, FRANCE

Jaegers, A., Dr. med.
Institut für Anaesthesiologie, Universität Erlangen-Nürnberg, Krankenhausstrasse 12, D-8520 Erlangen, FRG

Kacmarek, R.M., Ph.D., RRT
Respiratory Care Department – COX-3, Massachusetts General Hospital, Fruitstreet, Boston, A 02114, USA

Koller, W., Dr. med.
Univ.-Klinik für Anästhesiologie und Allgemeine Intensivmedizin, Anichstrasse 35, A-6020 Innsbruck, AUSTRIA

Konrad, J., Dr. med.
Institut für Anästhesiologie, Universität Düsseldorf, Moorenstrasse 5, D-4000 Düsseldorf, FRG

Krayer, S., Dr. med.
Institut für Anästhesiologie, Universitätsspital, Rämistrasse 100, CH-8091 Zürich, SWITZERLAND

Lachmann, B., Prof. Dr. med.
Erasmus Universiteit, Department of Anaesthesiology, Postbus 1738, NL-3000 DR Rotterdam, THE NETHERLANDS

Lagente, V., M.D.
Institut Henri Beaufour, 1, avenue des Tropiques, F-91952 Les Ulis, FRANCE

Laule, M., Dr. med.
1. Medizinische Klinik, TU München, Ismaninger Strasse 22,
D-8000 München 8, FRG

Layer-Groeneveld, G., Dr. med.
Kreiskrankenhaus an der Lieth, Pneumologische Klinik Lengern,
Pappelnweg 5, D-3406 Bovenden, FRG

Lee, P.A., Ph.D.
Pediatric Critical Care Research, Humana Hospital, Medical City-Dallas,
7777 Forest Lane, Suite C-740, Dallas, Texas 75230, USA

Lichtwarek-Aschoff, M., Dr. med.
Institut für Anästhesiologie und Operative Intensivmedizin,
Zentralklinikum, Stenglinstrasse 2, D-8900 Augsburg, FRG

Loring, S.H., M.D.
Department of Environmental Science and Physiology, Harvard University,
School of Public Health, 665 Huntington Ave, Boston, MA 02115, USA

Luger, Th., Dr. med.
Univ.-Klinik für Anästhesiologie und Allgemeine Intensivmedizin,
Anichstrasse 35, A-6020 Innsbruck, AUSTRIA

Mang, H., Dr. med.
Institut für Anaesthesiologie, Universität Erlangen-Nürnberg,
Krankenhausstrasse 12, D-8520 Erlangen, FRG

Martinet, N., Dr.
Service de Pneumologie, Hôpital Villemen, Rue de Nabecor, F-54000 Nancy,
FRANCE

Martinet, Y., Dr.
Service de Pneumologie, Hôpital Villemen, Rue de Nabecor, F-54000 Nancy,
FRANCE

McDonell, T., M.D.
Cardiovascular Pulmonary Laboratory, University of Colorado,
Health Sciences Center, Denver, Colorado 80262, USA

Mencia-Huerta, J.-M., M.D.
Institut Henri Beaufour, 1, avenue des Tropiques, F-91952 Les Ulis, FRANCE

Morris, A.H., M.D.
Division of Respiratory, Critical Care and Occupational Pulmonary Medicine, University of Utah Medical Center, 50 North Medical Drive, Salt Lake City, UT 84132, USA

Neuhof, H., Prof. Dr. med.
Zentrum Innere Medizin, Universität Gießen, Klinikstrasse 36, D-6300 Gießen, FRG

Obermaier, J., Dr. med.
Institut für Anästhesiologie und Operative Intensivmedizin, Zentralklinikum, Stenglinstrasse 2, D-8900 Augsburg, FRG

Pfeiffer, U.J., Priv.-Doz. Dr. med.
Institut für experimentelle Chirurgie, Technische Universität München, Ismaninger Strasse 22, D-8000 München 80, FRG

Pison, U., Dr. med.
Freie Universität Berlin, Universitätsklinikum Rudolf Virchow, Dept. Anesthesiology and Intensive Care Medicine, Augustenburger Platz 1, D-1000 Berlin, FRG

Pralat, U., Dr. med.
Zentrum Anästhesiologie, Abteilung IV, Medizinische Hochschule Hannover, D-3000 Hannover 51, FRG

Puter, G., Dr. med.
Univ.-Klinik für Anästhesiologie und Allgemeine Intensivmedizin, Anichstrasse 35, A-6020 Innsbruck, AUSTRIA

Putz, G., Dr. med.
Univ.-Klinik für Anästhesiologie und Allgemeine Intensivmedizin, Anichstrasse 35, A-6020 Innsbruck, AUSTRIA

Radermacher, P., Dr. med.
Institut für Anästhesiologie, Universität Düsseldorf, Moorenstrasse 5, D-4000 Düsseldorf, FRG

Rügheimer, E., Prof. Dr. med.
Institut für Anaesthesiologie, Universität Erlangen-Nürnberg Krankenhausstrasse 12, D-8520 Erlangen, FRG

Schoenberg, M.H., Dr. med.
Abteilung für Allgemeine Chirurgie, Klinikum der Universität Ulm, Steinhövelstrasse 9, D-7900 Ulm, FRG

Seeger, W., Priv.-Doz. Dr. med.
Zentrum Innere Medizin, Universität Gießen, Klinikstrasse 36,
D-6300 Gießen, FRG

Snatak, B., Dr. med.
Institut für Anästhesiologie, Universität Düsseldorf, Moorenstrasse 5,
D-4000 Düsseldorf, FRG

Stangl, K., Dr. med.
1. Medizinische Klinik, TU München, Ismaninger Strasse 22,
D-8000 München 8, FRG

Stuttmann, R., Dr. med.
Abteilung für Anästhesiologie, Städtische Krankenanstalten Köln-Merheim,
Ostmerheimer Strasse 200, D-5000 Köln 91, FRG

Sybrecht, G.W., Prof. Dr. med.
Abteilung für Pneumologie, Medizinische Universitätsklinik und Poliklinik,
D-6650 Homburg/Saar, FRG

Tschaikowsky, K., Dr. med.
Institut für Anaesthesiologie, Universität Erlangen-Nürnberg,
Krankenhausstrasse 12, D-8520 Erlangen, FRG

Voelkel, N.F., M.D.
Cardiovascular Pulmonary Laboratory, University of Colorado,
Health Sciences Center, Denver, Colorado 80262, USA

Wagner, W.W., Jr., Ph.D.
Indiana University, Medical Science 374, 635 Barnhill Drive, Indianapolis,
Indiana 46223, USA

Walmrath, D., Dr. med.
Zentrum Innere Medizin, Universität Gießen, Klinikstrasse 36,
D-6300 Gießen, FRG

Warner, A.E., M.D.
Department of Environmental Science and Physiology, Harvard University,
School of Public Health, 665 Huntington Ave, Boston, MA 02115, USA

Weber, P.C., Prof. Dr. med.
Institut für die Prophylaxe und Epidemiologie der Kreislaufkrankheiten,
Pettenkoferstrasse 9, D-8000 München 2, FRG

Weindler, J., Dr. med.
Klinik für Augenheilkunde, Universitätskliniken des Saarlandes, D-6650 Homburg/Saar, FRG

Weismann, D., Dr.
Drägerwerk AG, Moislinger Allee 53–55, D-2400 Lübeck, FRG

Wirtzfeld, A., Dr. med.
1. Medizinische Klinik, TU München, Ismaninger Strasse 22, D-8000 München 8, FRG

Wolff, G., Prof. Dr. med.
Klinik für Herz und Thoraxchirurgie, Universität Basel, Kantonsspital, CH-4031 Basel, SWITZERLAND

Zeravik, J., Dr. med.
Institut für Anästhesiologie und Operative Intensivmedizin, Zentralklinikum, Stenglinstrasse 2, D-8900 Augsburg, FRG

Contents

Part 6: Mechanics of Breathing and Surfactant

Part 7: The Respiratory Pump

Part 8: Artificial Ventilation

Part 1:

The Clinical Aspects of Respiratory Failure as a Result of Biochemical and Immunological Reactions: Endotoxin, Cytokines, and Receptors

E. Coli Sepsis-Induced Pulmonary Injury

P.A. Lee and B. Hinshaw

Sepsis-Induced Acute Lung Injury

Clinical Aspects

Sepsis-induced acute lung injury (ALI) is usually diagnosed in a setting of primary acute respiratory failure (ARF) in septic or bacteremic patients. ARF is present when arterial oxygen tension (PaO_2) is low, the alveolar to arterial oxygen gradient is greater than normal, and/or the arterial carbon dioxide tension ($PaCO_2$) is high in the absence of compensated metabolic alkalosis [1]. In the septic patient, ARF is considered synonymous with adult respiratory distress syndrome (ARDS). ARDS was first described by Ashbaugh et al. [2] and usually occurs within 3–7 days of the primary systemic insult [3]. Its occurrence is associated with numerous systemic illnesses (e.g., trauma, gastric content aspiration, immunosuppression); however, sepsis is the most common predisposition and has a higher mortality rate than other causes of ARDS [4, 5]. ARDS is characterized by hypoxemia, hyperventilation, ventilation-perfusion mismatch with 10%–20% A–V shunting, radiographic evidence of pulmonary edema (noncardiogenic pulmonary edema, NCPE) and normal capillary wedge pressures [6]. With uncomplicated ARDS, lung compliance decreases and severe hypoxemia ensues, requiring mechanical ventilation. In severe cases, this will progress to terminal hypoxia; however, few ARDS patients die from unresolved hypoxemia [7]. Nonpulmonary organ failure is most highly correlated with death in these patients. Mortality rates associated with ARDS alone are approximately 40%. In general, a 54% mortality rate is associated with failure of one organ in addition to the lungs and nearly 100% mortality with failure of four or more organ systems [7]. In patients who present with fulminant septic shock and subsequently develop ARDS, mortality rates are close to 90% [8]. Several concise reviews on the topic of sepsis-induced ALI in humans have been published recently [9, 10].

Experimental Animal Models

There are numerous different animal models of ARDS; however, most of these involve nonbacteremic insults. Many investigators employ gram-negative organism-derived endotoxins to produce "septic" ARDS [11]. While many of the pathophysiologic changes that occur with endotoxin infusion are similar to those induced by live bacteria, the full clinical spectrum of septic shock is not reproduced in models of endotoxic shock. There is a large difference between species with regard to quantity of endotoxin required to elicit a systemic response and qualitative pathophysiologic changes.

There are several well-developed models of live organism-induced septic ALI. Most notable are *Pseudomonas aeruginosa*-induced ARDS in sheep [12] and swine [13] and *E. coli*-induced ARDS in nonhuman primates [14, 15]. These models consistently reproduce the clinical course of septic ARDS. Quantitative pathophysiologic responses included: systemic hypotension, decreased cardiac output, hyperventilation, hypoxemia, NCPE, and pulmonary arterial hypertension. At necropsy, gross and histologic examination of the animals' lungs routinely reveals congestive atelectasis, intravascular congestion, interstitial edema, intra-alveolar cellular debris, and increased wet-to-dry lung ratios [16]. While the bacteremic model may be more difficult to evaluate and the extent (i.e., dose) of the insult difficult to quantify due to the combined actions of live bacteria and endotoxin released from dead organisms, it is a more clinically relevant model, qualitatively, in terms of elicited physiologic and pathologic changes. A more detailed description of the septic primate model developed in the authors' laboratory follows.

Sepsis and Septic ALI in the Nonhuman Primate

Details of the experimental model (animal preparation and protocol) have been described [14, 16] but will be briefly summarized below. Juvenile baboons (*Papio c. cynocephalus* or *Papio c. anubis*) were used in these studies. Animals were anesthetized (sodium pentobarbital) for the duration of the monitoring period (10 h). All animals received an LD_{100} of live *E. coli* (4×10^{10} organisms/kg) intravenously over 2 h. Measurements of physiologic parameters were taken hourly; blood samples for microbiologic, biochemical, hematologic, and blood gas analyses were drawn prior to the bacterial infusion and every 2 h thereafter. After completion of the experimental protocol (post-10 h), animals were monitored continuously for 36 h and then daily for a maximum of 7 days per animal. Gross post-mortem examinations were performed and tissue samples taken, fixed in buffered formalin, and submitted for histopathologic evaluation.

The progressive development of septic shock in this animal model can be divided on the basis of cardiopulmonary responses and pathologic findings and separated into two stages: early (hyperdynamic) and late (hypodynamic). Generally, the early stages encompass the first 6 h after initiation of the septic insult; the late stage refers to 10 or more h postinfusion of the *E. coli*.

Physiologic Changes

The physiologic, biochemical, and hematologic measurements routinely performed during these studies were: mean arterial blood pressure (MABP), heart and respiratory rates, cardiac output, pulmonary arterial and wedge pressures, core temperature, white blood cell (WBC) and platelet concentrations, hematocrit, fibrinogen level, serum glucose, blood urea nitrogen (BUN), creatinine and glutamate pyruvate transaminase (SGPT) concentrations, plasma lactate concentration, and arterial blood gases.

Early Stage. The early phase of septic shock is often referred to as the "hyperdynamic" phase. Cardiac output is either maintained or increased during this period in spite of a marked reduction in MABP. A reflex increase in heart rate occurs concomitant with the fall in MABP. The hyperdynamic state is also characterized by a slight increase in body temperature and an increase in respiratory drive. A slight increase in mean pulmonary arterial pressure may occur with no change in mean pulmonary wedge pressure. Normal or slightly decreased PaO_2 is evident with a significant fall in $PaCO_2$ and normal arterial pH (compensated metabolic acidosis). Notable changes in blood chemistries and hematology include: transient increase in serum glucose concentration (during infusion of bacteria) followed by a gradual decline below control values, significant decreases in WBC and platelet concentrations (differential WBC showing proliferation of immature cells, indicative of margination occurring), and a gradual decline in plasma fibrinogen levels. The latter is suggestive of early coagulopathic changes. No significant changes in BUN, creatinine, SGPT, or lactate occurred; early functional deficits in most organ systems (excluding the cardiopulmonary system) were not apparent.

The early compensatory hyperdynamic state may last several minutes to many hours depending on the severity of the septic insult. Animals maintaining adequate oxygenation and perfusion (prolonged hyperdynamic state) have a better chance for survival. In this lethal *E. coli* septic shock model the early phase is transient and animals progress into the hypodynamic (late) phase of shock.

Late Stage. The late hypodynamic phase of shock is characterized by: marked sustained hypotension with a decrease in cardiac output, tachycardia, hyperventilation, mild hyperthermia, hypoxemia, uncompensated metabolic acidosis, respiratory alkalosis, thrombocytopenia, leukopenia, decreased fibrinogen levels (to near 0% of control), and significant increases in biochemical markers of organ failure (BUN, creatinine, SGPT, lactate).

The primary physiologic abnormalities appear to be in the pulmonary and cardiovascular systems with secondary coagulopathic changes. Later in the development of septic shock multiple organ system failure is evident. The late changes in markers of renal and hepatic function are usually pre-terminal. The average survival time in this particular model is approximately 19 h.

Pathologic Findings

In order to obtain tissue samples for pathologic evaluation of early changes in this sepsis model, a subgroup of baboons, treated as described above, was killed at 6 h. A few of these animals were perfusion-fixed in situ with glutaraldehyde for electron-microscopic analysis.

Early Stage. Upon gross visual examination the lungs of animals killed within the first 6 h postinsult show few obvious lesions. There were some areas of focal petechial hemorrhage on the lung surface with notable gravitational atelectasis. Light-microscopic evaluation revealed: focal pulmonary edema, atelectasis, intravascular congestion with numerous red blood cells and polymorphonuclear leukocytes (PMN), and focal hemorrhage. Electron microscopy (EM) supported the above findings. Figure 1 is a transmission EM illustrating numerous PMNs and some red blood cells within the pulmonary capillary. Figure 2 is a scanning EM showing severe vascular congestion and mild extravasation routinely seen in the lungs of these animals. There was evidence of some alterations in the integrity of the pulmonary endothelium. Normally, the endothelial cell layer is in close apposition to the vascular lumen (Fig. 3A); within 2–4 h postbacterial infusion there was mild to moderate endothelial edema (Fig. 3B). There was also disruption of the continuity of the endothelial cell layer at sites of leukocyte adhesion. Other early alterations observed include: rounding of the alveolar spaces, edematous alveolar type I cells, and occasional intra-alveolar fluid accumulation.

Late Stage. Gross visual examination revealed heavy wet lungs, dark red to purple in color. Atelectasis was generalized and equally distributed throughout both lungs (no evidence of gravitational pooling). Occasional animals had

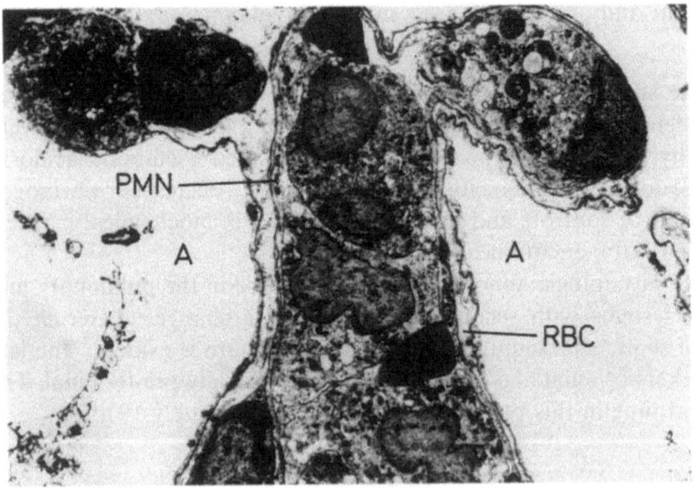

Fig. 1. Transmission electron micrograph of baboon pulmonary capillary and adjacent alveoli 30 min post-*E. coli* infusion. *A*, alveolar spaces; *RBC*, red blood cells; *PMN*, polymorphonuclear leukocytes

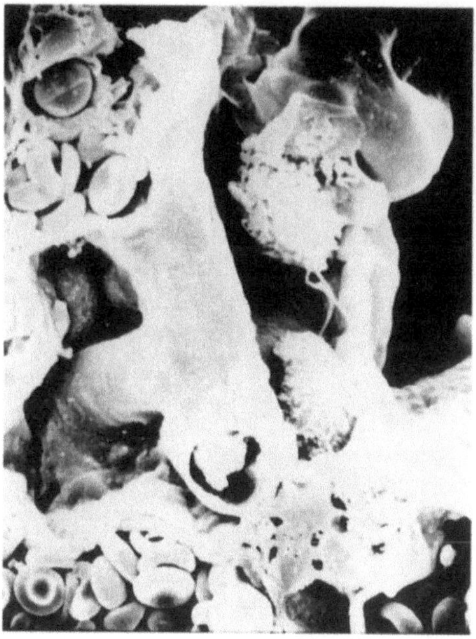

Fig. 2. Scanning electron micrograph of baboon lung showing capillary engorgement with RBC and neutrophils with platelet and fibrin strand adhesion

fulminant pulmonary edema with hemoptysis. Light-microscopic evaluation revealed marked diffuse pulmonary edema, intravascular congestion, interstitial edema, diffuse hemorrhage, and intravascular and intra-alveolar fibrin thrombi. All of these changes are consistent with the congestive atelectasis and diffuse alveolar damage (DAD) seen in humans. EM studies showed gross endothelial cell damage at sites of PMN adhesion and occasional vacuolization ("blebbing") of the endothelial cell layer (Fig. 4). There was significant alveolar type I cell damage and degenerative changes in type II cells (also consistent with DAD). Enhanced deposition of fibrin strands on the endothelial cell layer (Fig. 5A), compared with normal controls (Fig. 5B), was a frequent finding. This could favor the formation of platelet aggregates and exacerbate the existing coagulopathy.

Summary

Speculation

Putative mechanisms/mediators underlying the development of ARDS and subsequent development of multiple organ system failure are legion. There is little agreement on which mediators are primarily responsible for initiating the cascade of organ failure; however, there is a consensus that mediators released

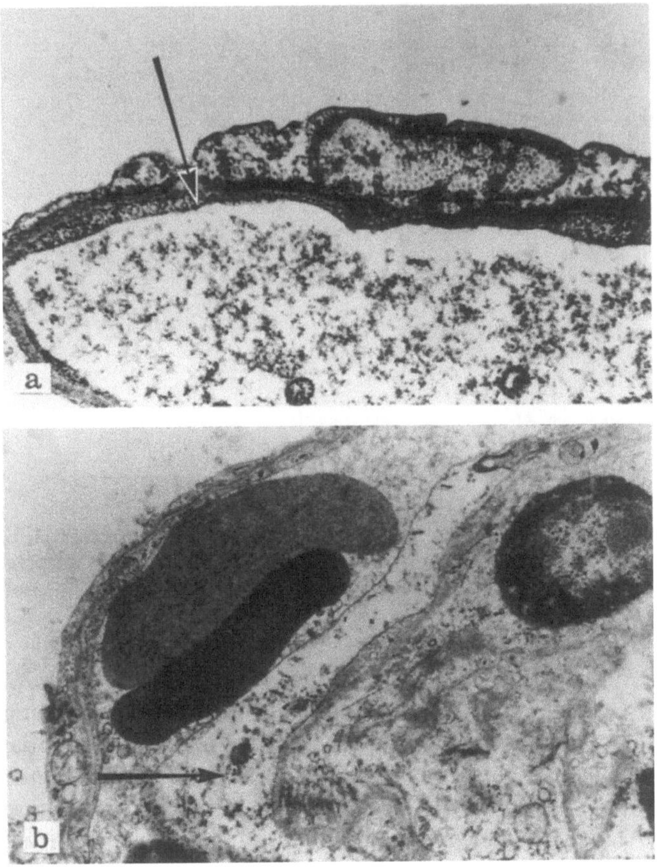

Fig. 3. A Normal baboon lung endothelium. **B** Pulmonary capillary endothelium showing moderately severe edema (*arrow*). Sample taken 4 h post-*E. coli* infusion

during sepsis act upon all physiologic systems, not just the pulmonary or cardiovascular systems. Although some organ systems may be more sensitive initially to these mediators (e.g., the lung), their mechanisms of action are not organ specific. Suggested mediators of sepsis-induced ALI/ARDS include: tumor necrosis factor (TNF), interleukins 1 and 2 (IL-1, IL-2), interferon-γ, bacterial toxins, complement, activated neutrophils and activated platelets, prostaglandins, lipoxygenase metabolites, fibrin-derived peptides, and oxygen free radicals.

Hinshaw et al. [17] have recently shown that administration of a monoclonal antibody to human TNF is beneficial in this lethal *E. coli* septic baboon model. TNF antibody administered during the course of the *E. coli* infusion improves both cardiovascular and pulmonary function and overall survival. All treated animals were permanent survivors (minimum 7 day survival). These

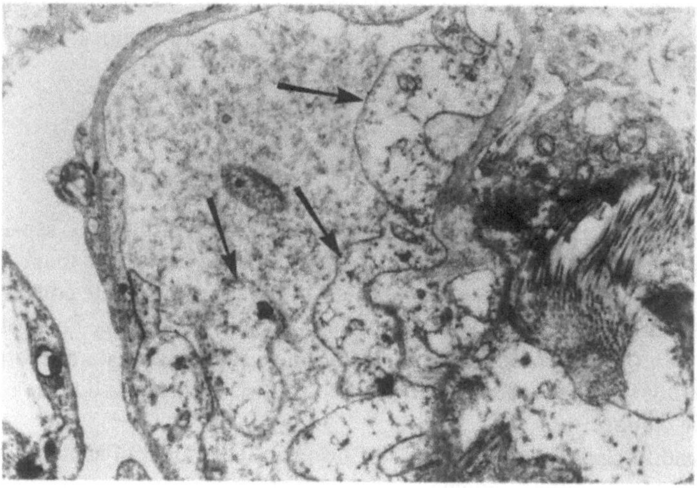

Fig. 4. Transmission electron micrograph of baboon lung taken 12 h post-*E. coli*. *Arrows* indicate areas of severe endothelial cell vacuolization; note that continuity of cell layer is not disrupted

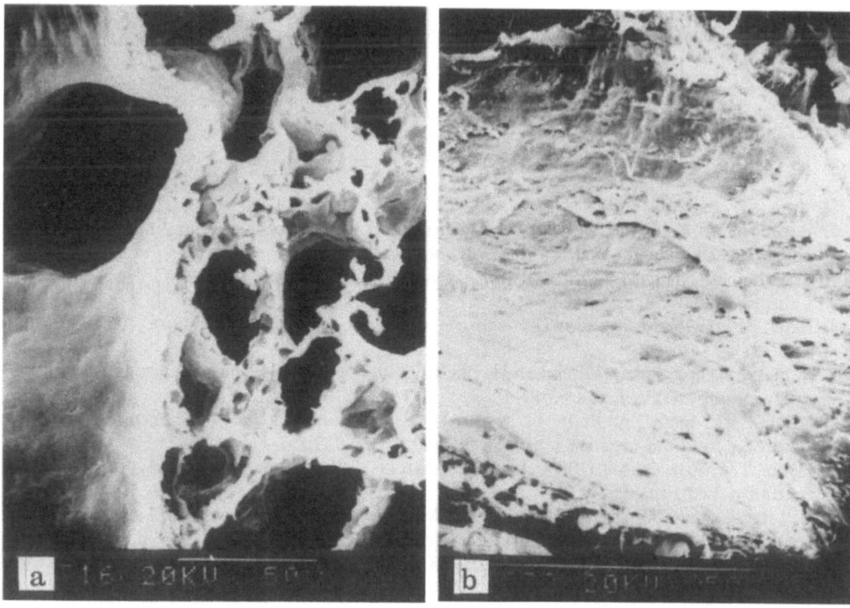

Fig. 5A, B. Transmission electron micrograph of normal pulmonary vascular endothelium (**A**) and post-*E. coli* infusion. (**B**) In the latter, some buckling of the endothelium is evident with marked fibrin strand deposition

studies suggest that TNF may be a mediator responsible for initiating the cascade of pathophysiologic changes that occur during septic shock, which ultimately leads to multiple organ system failure and death.

Conclusions

Ultrastructural changes in the lung occurring as a result of *E. coli*-induced sepsis are similar to those seen in human ARDS. Early changes reflect a marked inflammatory response with PMN accumulation in the lung, moderate congestion, and mild endothelial cell wall changes. Alterations in pulmonary function correlate well with these pathologic changes. Late structural changes are severe and are very similar to those seen in infants with hyaline membrane disease or diffuse alveolar damage.

Although endothelial disruption does not occur in this model of acute lung injury, the marked pulmonary edema and neutrophilic leukocyte infiltration suggest some defect in the pulmonary vascular permeability barrier. There are numerous humoral mediators which are capable of causing capillary leakage in the lung. The most popular candidates for causing septic ALI are the products of the macrophage/monocyte system: TNF and IL-1. Studies using a monoclonal antibody to human TNF in this *E. coli* septic baboon model suggest that interference with the actions of these cytokines early in the development of sepsis improves not only pulmonary function, but converts this model to one of a nonlethal bacteremia.

References

1. Pontoppidan H, Rie MA (1982) Pathogenesis and therapy of acute lung injury. In: Applied physiology in clinical respiratory care. Nijhoff, the Hague
2. Ashbaugh DG, Bigelow DB, Petty TL, Levine BE (1967) Acute respiratory disease in adults. Lancet 2:313
3. Baue AF (1975) Multiple progressive or sequential organ systems failure. Arch Surg 110: 779–781
4. Fein AM, Lippman M, Holtemann H (1983) The risk factors, incidence and prognosis of ARDS following septicemia. Chest 83:40–42
5. Kaplan RL, Sahn SA, Petty TL (1979) Incidence and outcome of the respiratory distress syndrome in Gram-negative sepsis. Arch Intern Med 139:867–869
6. Hyers TM, Fowler AA (1986) Adult respiratory distress syndrome: causes, morbidity and mortality. Fed Proc 45:25–29
7. Bell RC, Coalson JJ, Smith JD et al. (1983) Multiple organ system failure and infection in adult respiratory distress syndrome. Ann Intern Med 99(3):293–298
8. Jacobs ER, Bone RC (1983) Mediators of septic lung injury. Med Clin North Am 67(3): 701–715
9. Bersten A, Sibbald WJ (1989) Acute lung injury in septic shock. Crit Care Clin 5(1):49–79
10. Pepe PE (1986) The clinical entity of adult respiratory distress syndrome. Crit Care Clin 2:377–403
11. Brigham KL, Meyrick B (1986) Endotoxin and lung injury. Am Rev Respir Dis 133:913–927

12. Brigham KL, Woolverton WC, Blake LH, Staub NC (1974) Increased sheep lung vascular permeability caused by *Pseudomonas bacteremia.* J Clin Invest 54:792–804
13. Dehring DJ, Crocker SH, Wismar BL, Steinberg SM, Lowery BD, Cloutier CT (1983) Comparisons of live bacteria infusions in a porcine model of acute respiratory failure. J Surg Res 34:151–158
14. Hinshaw LB, Brackett DJ, Archer LT, Beller BK, Wilson MF (1983) Detection of the 'hyperdynamic state' of sepsis in the baboon during lethal *E. coli* infusion. J Trauma 23(5):361–365
15. Hangen DH, Bloom RJ, Stevens JH, O'Hanley P, Ranchod M, Collins J, Raffin TA (1987) Adult respiratory distress syndrome: a live *E. coli* septic primate model. Am J Pathol 126(2):396–400
16. Hinshaw LB, Coalson JJ, Benjamin BA, Archer LT, Beller BK, Kling OR, Hasser EM, Phillips RW (1978) *Escherichia coli* shock in the baboon and the response to adrenocorticosteroid treatment. Surg Gynecol Obstet 147:545–557
17. Hinshaw LB, Tekamp-Olson P, Chang ACK, Kuo G, Lee PA, Taylor FB, Murray CK, Peer GT, Emerson TE, Passey RB (1990) Survival of primates in LD_{100} septic shock following therapy with antibody to tumor necrosis factor. Circ Shock (in press)

Regulation of the Cellular Immune Response and Interaction with the Endothelium by Changes in Membrane Receptors

K. Tschaikowsky and M. Georgieff

Introduction

Combined with other organ failures, adult respiratory distress syndrome (ARDS) is still regarded as one of the most serious and most challenging problems of intensive care. Despite considerable therapeutical interventions, ARDS often proceeds to lung failure or contributes to the development of multiorgan failure. ARDS is characterized by an increased permeability of the lung endothelium and by changes in the lung vascular tonus, leading to impairments in gas exchange and in the microcirculation [6, 22, 24]. However, we still do not know the exact sequence of events eliciting this uniform response of the lung after a challenge by a variety of different primary diseases, e.g., sepsis, trauma, pancreatitis, or multiple transfusions.

Primarily mechanical impairments (i.e., trauma and hydrostatic edema) and dysfunctions in oxygen transport by erythrocytes (i.e., low blood flow, reduced oxygen saturation, and reduced hematocrit) leading to hypoxia were regarded as causes of acute organ failure. The role of leukocytes in the development of organ failure was, for a long time, of little concern.

Based on the results of immunological research, activated leukocytes are now regarded not only as functioning in specific and nonspecific immune defenses, but also as having a great potential for causing deleterious effects on the host organs.

Neutrophils [23] and macrophages are thought to play especially important key roles in the pathogenesis of acute lung failure after sepsis and trauma. By an excessive liberation of lysosomal enzymes, vasoactive eicosanoids, and toxic oxygen derived radicals they can cause increases in permeability, changes in vascular tonus, and damage to the endothelium of the lung vessels [10, 11, 14, 20, 29, 30].

As evidenced by many investigations, the sequestration of polymorphonuclear leukocytes (PMNs) in the lung is a crucial prerequisite for the full expression of the permeability lesion in ARDS. During lung failure one can regularly find an excess of adherent PMNs in the pulmonary microvasculature, lung lymph, and bronchoalveolar lavage. It has been demonstrated that, in the bronchoalveolar lavage of patients with ARDS, neutrophils constitute nearly 70% of the recovered cells in comparison to 1%–4% in normal volunteers and ventilated control patients [27]. The percentage of neutrophils correlated also with $AaDO_2$ and lung protein permeability.

Lysosomal enzymes such as elastase, glucoronidase, myeloperoxidase, and collagenase were often found in lung lymph and in the bronchoalveolar lavage [18, 27].

The most convincing evidence for the obligate role of neutrophils in the pathogenesis of ARDS is provided by lung injury models using neutropenic animals [2, 13, 15]. It could be shown that animals rendered neutropenic either did not develop or to a far lesser degree developed the lung permeability lesions usually demonstrable after microembolization, pancreatitis, or endotoxin infusion.

Further evidence for the pathogenetic relevance of PMNs was found by examining lung scintigraphs taken after injections of radioactively labeled autologous neutrophils.

In lung injury models [12] and in ARDS patients [26] a marked and prolonged increase in the sequestration of labeled PMNs in the lungs could be demonstrated by scintigraphy.

One may now ask which are the common mechanisms leading to this abnormal sequestration of neutrophils in the lung that can be seen in both sepsis- and trauma-induced ARDS. An enhanced chemotactic influx of neutrophil granulocytes to the lung has been suggested as one of the causes along with an increased adherence of neutrophils to the pulmonary endothelium.

During all inflammatory and traumatic processes chemotactic factors are produced. The most potent chemoattractants are the bacteria derived *N*-formyl peptides, the synthetic tripeptide *N*-formyl-methionyl-leucyl-phenylalanine (FMLP), and the endogenous mediators C5a and leukotriene (LT) B_4. In addition, a variety of factors from macrophages and endothelial cells or fibrin degradation products can form chemotactic gradients attracting granulocytes to the lung. Bound to their corresponding receptors in the granulocyte membrane, chemotactic factors not only induce chemotaxis, but also promote degranulation, aggregation, and release of oxygen derived radicals.

How can these important immune responses be modulated in sepsis and trauma to meet the requirements of an adequate immune defense? To answer this question researchers have investigated PMN FMLP receptors, which can bind bacterial chemoattractants, and have studied the influence of inflammatory mediators on their expression [8, 9, 17, 28]. It was demonstrated that: (a) FMLP receptors have two possible conformational states, binding ligands with high and low affinity, (b) mediators such as C5a, tumor necrosis factor (TNF), or granulocyte/macrophage colony-stimulating factor (GM-CSF) induce changes in the number or affinity of FMLP receptors in vitro, and (c) increased FMLP receptor expression is not based on a de novo synthesis but on a translocation of existing receptors from secondary granules to the granulocyte membrane.

Methods and Results

To assess the possible in vivo significance of this mediator-induced receptor increase, we studied FMLP receptors on granulocytes of septic patients.

Using isolated PMNs of healthy volunteers and septic patients, we measured both the number of high-affinity FMLP receptors and the total number of receptors by means of the binding of tritium-labeled FMLP at concentrations of 1 and 120 n*M*.

In addition, we assessed the stimulated (FMLP, phorbol myristate acetate) and nonstimulated production of oxygen superoxide per granulocyte by measuring the superoxide/dismutase inhibitable reduction of cytochrome c. During sepsis, there was a dramatic increase in both the expression of PMN high-affinity FMLP receptors (145%) and the total number of PMN FMLP receptors (91%). The PMNs of these patients also released significantly (60%) more oxygen superoxide after stimulation with FMLP (10^{-5} n*M*). These results indicate that septic processes induce a priming of neutrophils by increasing FMLP receptor expression, resulting in an enhanced immune response and increased toxic potency of these cells after subsequent stimulation.

After the influx of activated PMNs to the target tissue, the increased adherence of PMNs to the vascular endothelium is the second most important mechanism of nonspecific inflammatory reactions, including those that occur in ARDS. The enhanced adherence is mediated by quantitative and qualitative changes in the neutrophils and/or endothelial cells. Several studies have showed that mediators such as TNF and interleukin-1 (IL-1) are capable of inducing the expression of membrane glycoproteins of endothelial cells which promote an increased adherence of leukocytes [5, 19]. This effect has a lag time of several hours since these glycoproteins must first be synthesized by the endothelial cells. The rapid, initial sequestration of neutrophils in the lung demonstrated in ARDS after trauma and sepsis is therefore not likely to be caused by this protein synthesis dependent mechanism.

The following changes in granulocytes, which can take place within minutes after stimulation, seem to be responsible for their initial increased adherence to the endothelium:

1. *Changes in membrane potential*: Normally aggregation and adherence of granulocytes is inhibited by the negative resting potential on the surface of PMNs and endothelial cells. Following degranulation of neutrophils, this negative surface charge is decreased.

2. *Changes in blood flow*: Since Virchow, it has been assumed that the flow of blood cells has an impact on their adherence to the vessel wall. In a study on the adherence of PMNs to cultivated endothelial cells during quasilaminar flow conditions, Lawrence et al. found that adherence increased approximately four fold in response to a 50% reduction of the flow [16]. The reduced flow, however, seems rather to be a mechanical cofactor and is unlikely to produce stable adherence and activation of the PMNs per se. Nevertheless, it could provide a good explanation for why the most adherent PMNs are found in the postcapillary venules. Mediator-induced changes in neutrophils, which promote intimate

and prolonged contact between the activated granulocyte and the endothelial cell, are considered to have more pathogenetic relevance.

3. *Changes in intracellular cAMP*: Mediators that cause a decrease in intracellular cAMP induce a decrease in motility and an increased adherence of neutrophils. Factors such as prostaglandin (PG) E_1 and prostacyclin (PG) I_2, which increase intracellular cAMP, inhibit neutrophil adherence [7].

4. *Changes in the glycoprotein structure of the cell membrane*: In light of a series of in vitro and in vivo studies, the glycoprotein complex CD11/18 is believed to be one of the critical factors, presumably a sine qua non condition, promoting neutrophil adherence. By binding C3bi, a surface-bound fragment of the third component of complement, this glycoprotein complex facilitates phagocytosis and is therefore also considered to be a CR3 receptor.

Deficiency of this CR3 receptor (CD11b) is a rare autosomal recessive disorder affecting granulocyte adherence-related functions and is characterized clinically by depressed inflammatory responses and recurrent infections. Compelling evidence for the pathogenetic significance of this receptor was recently also found in two animal models: A monoclonal antibody against a subunit of the CR3 receptor (MoAb 60.3), given before a challenge prevented the inflammatory leukocyte infiltration of the skin usually observed after dermal injection of chemotactic factors [1] and increased significantly the survival rate after hemorrhagic shock [25].

In vitro studies were carried out to determine how CR3 receptor expression and the adherence of PMNs is modulated by inflammatory mediators and how this important immune response could be influenced by pharmacological and immunological means. In our studies, neutrophil granulocytes were isolated from venous blood of healthy volunteers by density gradient followed by hypotonic lysis of the remaining erythrocytes.

The percentage of neutrophil adherence to plasma-coated microtiter plates was measured radiometrically by labeling the cells with ^{51}Cr.

To assess CR3 receptor expression on the granulocyte membrane we developed a new enzyme immunoassay (EIA). The test principle is based on the binding of a monoclonal primary antibody to the CR3 receptor followed by the binding of an enzyme-labeled secondary antibody directed against the primary antibody. Nonspecific binding deducted, the assessed enzyme activity is a measure of the number of CR3 receptors.

To assess the influence of inflammatory mediators on CR3 receptor expression, we incubated isolated neutrophils for 35 min at 37 °C with ultrapure C5a, FMLP, recombinant TNF, and phorbol myristate acetate (PMA). All stimulated PMNs showed a 2- to 3.5-fold increase in CR3 receptor expression compared to the nonstimulated cells.

Similar results were also obtained by other investigators [3, 4, 21] and it was proposed that a change in the intracellular calcium level promotes this receptor increase. We therefore investigated to what extent the observed increase in receptor expression could be inhibited by calcium antagonists. For this purpose neutrophils were preincubated for 15 min with one of three different calcium antagonists: the calcium entry blocker verapamil, the intracellular effective agent TMB-8, and the calmodulin inhibitor trifluoperazine (TFP).

All applied calcium antagonists completely suppressed the increase in CR3 receptor expression induced by C5a, FMLP, and TNF. CR3 receptor expression in stimulated granulocytes treated with calcium antagonists was even somewhat below the baseline level of the nonstimulated cells, which were not preincubated with a calcium antagonist.

Surprisingly, the stimulatory effect of PMA, which is a calcium and receptor independent direct activator of protein kinase C, was also reduced by 10%–15%. This result suggests that the applied calcium antagonists may have additional, direct, inhibitory effects on this important enzyme.

Do calcium antagonists likewise influence the adherence of neutrophil granulocytes? To answer this question we first incubated isolated PMNs with C5a, FMLP, PMA, and TNF for 35 min at 37 °C. Similar to the results with CR3 receptor expression there was a significant 3- to 4.5-fold increase in neutrophil adherence. Prior to stimulation, the granulocytes were incubated again with one of the three different calcium antagonists. There was significant inhibition of neutrophil adherence with all administered antagonists, but of considerably different magnitudes. While verapamil and TMB-8 inhibited adherence by only 10%–35%, one could hardly find adherent neutrophils with the calmodulin inhibitor TFP.

Neutrophil adherence did not strictly parallel CR3 receptor expression; that is, an increase in CR3 receptor expression seems to not be necessary for increased neutrophil adherence. However, the existence of this receptor on the neutrophil membrane is an important requisite for PMN adherence, as could be seen in our experiments in which CR3 receptors were blocked with monoclonal anti-receptor antibodies (MAC 1). Preincubation of PMNs with this anti-CR3 receptor antibody resulted, in response to all stimuli, in an approximately 50% reduction in neutrophil adherence.

Conclusions

Our results provide evidence that the adherence of PMNs is essentially mediated by CR3 receptor bridging to the endothelial cell and that a calcium-calmodulin sensitive pathway and a reduced flow represent the intrinsic and extrinsic requirements of increased neutrophil adherence. Specific calcium antagonists and monoclonal antireceptor antibodies could therefore be useful tools to modulate cellular immune reactions participating in the development of ARDS and other organ failures. To what extent therapeutical advantages can be gained must be shown by future research.

References

1. Arfors KE, Lundberg C, Lindbom L, Lundberg K, Beatty PG, Harlan JM (1987) A monoclonal antibody to the membrane glycoprotein complex CD 18 inhibits polymorphonuclear leukocyte accumulation and plasma leakage in vivo. Blood 69:338–340
2. Barie PS, Tahamont M, Malik A (1982) Prevention of pulmonary vascular permeability in pancreatitis after granulocyte depletion in sheep. Am Rev Respir Dis 126:904–908
3. Berger M, O'Shea J, Cross AS, Folks TM, Chused TM, Brown EJ, Frank MM (1984) Human neutrophils increase expression of C3bi as well as C3b receptors upon activation. J Clin Invest 74:1566–1571
4. Berger M, Wetzler EM, Wallis RS (1988) Tumor necrosis factor is the major monocyte product that increases complement receptor expression on mature human neutrophils. Blood 71:151–158
5. Bevilacqua MP, Pober JS, Wheeler ME, Cotran RS, Gimbrone MA Jr. (1985) Interleukin 1 acts on cultured human vascular endothelium to increase the adhesion of polymorphonuclear leukocytes, monocytes, and related cell lines. J Clin Invest 76:2003–2011
6. Brigham KL (1982) Mechanisms of lung injury. Clin Chest Med 3:9–24
7. Chopra J, Webster RO (1988) PGE_1 inhibits neutrophil adherence and neutrophil-mediated injury to cultured endothelial cells. Am Rev Respir Dis 138:915–920
8. Fletcher MP, Gallin JI (1980) Degranulating stimuli increase the availability of receptors on human neutrophils for the chemoattractant fmet-leu-phe. J Immunol 124:1585
9. Fletcher MP, Gallin JI (1983) Human neutrophils contain an intracellular pool of putative receptors for the chemoattractant *N*-formyl-methionyl-leucyl-phenylalanine. Blood 62:792–799
10. Flick M, Hoeffel J, Staub N (1981) Superoxide dismutase prevents increased lung vascular permeability after air emboli in unanaesthetized sheep. Fed Proc 983:405
11. Harlan JM, Killen PD, Harker LA, Striker GE, Wright DG (1981) Neutrophil-mediated endothelial injury in vitro. J Clin Invest 68:1394–1403
12. Haslett C, Worthen GS, Giclas PC, Morrison DC, Henson JE, Henson PM (1987) The pulmonary vascular sequestration of neutrophils in endotoxemia is initiated by an effect of endotoxin on the neutrophil in the rabbit. Am Rev Respir Dis 136:9–18
13. Heflin AC Jr, Brigham K (1981) Prevention by granulocyte depletion of increased vascular permeability of sheep lung following endotoxemia. J Clin Invest 68:1253–1260
14. Henson P (1974) The immunologic release of constituents from neutrophilic leukocytes. J Immunol 107:1535–1546
15. Johnson A, Malik A (1982) Pulmonary edema after glass bead microembolization: protective effect of granulocytopenia. J Appl Physiol 52:155–162
16. Lawrence MB, McIntire LV, Eskin SG (1987) Effect of flow on polymorphonuclear leukocyte/endothelial cell adhesion. Blood 70:1284–1290
17. Mackin WM, Huang CK, Becker EL (1982) The formylpeptide chemotactic receptor on rabbit peritoneal neutrophils. J Immunol 129:1608–1611
18. McGuire WW, Spragg RG, Cohen AB, Cochrane (1982) Studies on the pathogenesis of the adult respiratory distress syndrome. J Clin Invest 69:543–553
19. Pohlman TH, Stannes KA, Beatty PG, Ochs HD, Harlan JM (1986) An endothelial cell surface factor(s) induced in vitro by lipopolysaccharide, interleukin 1, and tumor necrosis factor increases neutrophil adherence by a CDw18-dependent mechanism. J Immunol 136:4548–4553
20. Sacks T, Moldow CF, Craddock PR, Bowers TK, Jacobs HS (1978) Oxygen radicals mediate endothelial cell damage by complement-stimulated granulocytes. J Clin Invest 61:1161–1168
21. Socinski MA, Cannistra SA, Sullivan R, Elias A, Antman K, Schnipper L, Griffin JD (1988) Granulocyte-macrophage colony-stimulating factor induces the expression of the CD11b surface adhesion molecule on human granulocytes in vivo. Blood 72:691–697
22. Staub NC (1980) The pathogenesis of pulmonary edema. Prog Cardiovasc Dis 23:53–80
23. Tate RM, Repine JE (1983) Neutrophils and the respiratory distress syndrome. Am Rev Respir Dis 128:552–559
24. Tomashefski JF, Davies P, Boggis C, Greene R, Zapol W, Reid LM (1983) The pulmonary vascular lesions of the adult respiratory distress syndrome. Am J Pathol 112:112–126

25. Vedder NB, Winn RK, Rice CL, Chi EY, Arfors KE, Harlan JM (1988) A monoclonal antibody to the adherence-promoting leukocyte glycoprotein, CD 18, reduces organ injury and improves survival from hemorrhagic shock and resuscitation in rabbits. J Clin Invest 81:939–944
26. Warshawski FJ, Sibbald WJ, Driedger AA, Cheung H (1986) Abnormal neutrophil-pulmonary interaction in the adult respiratory distress syndrome. Am Rev Respir Dis 133:797–804
27. Weiland JE, Davis WB, Holter JF, Mohammed JR, Dorinsky PM, Gadek JE (1986) Lung neutrophils in the adult respiratory distress syndrome. Am Rev Respir Dis 133:218–225
28. Weisbart RH, Golde DW, Gasson JC (1986) Biosynthetic human GM–CSF modulates the number and affinity of neutrophil f-met-leu-phe receptors. J Immunol 137:3584–3587
29. Weissmann G, Smolen JE, Korchak HM (1980) Release of inflammatory mediators from stimulated neutrophils. N Engl J Med 303:27–34
30. Westaby S (1986) Mechanisms of membrane damage and surfactant depletion in acute lung injury. Intensive Care Med 12:2–5

Increased Expression of the Low-Affinity Receptor for IgE (FcεRII/CD23) on Rat Alveolar Macrophages

V. Lagente, B. Dugas, D. Hosford, J.M. Mencia-Huerta, and P. Braquet
Institut Henri Beafour, 1 av. des Tropiques, 91952 LESULIS (France)

Introduction

The demonstration that various cell types can express a receptor for the Fc fragment of immunoglobulin E (IgE) (FcεRII/CD23) distinct from that described on mast cells and basophils (FcεRI), was obtained from the use of IgE-coated erythrocytes, binding studies with radiolabelled IgE, and more recently by the use of monoclonal anti-Fcε receptor antibodies (Dessaint and Capron 1988). The expression of this receptor is regulated by various cytokines and, as described recently, by lipid mediators such as platelet-activating factor (PAF) and leukotriene B_4 (LTB_4) (Dugas et al. 1989, 1990). Both murine and human lymphocytes and monocytes/macrophages express FcεRII/CD23 and secrete a soluble IgE-binding factor structurally related to this receptor (sCD23), two phenomena now known to play a major role in the regulation of the IgE synthesis (Pène et al. 1988; Delespesse et al. 1989). In the present review the possible relationship between FcεRII/CD23 expression on rat alveolar macrophages and the immunological reaction involved during the late phase reaction of allergic asthma are briefly described.

The Late Phase Reaction of Allergic Asthma

Immediate and late falls in airway function are observed in asthmatic patients following inhalation of the allergen to which they are sensitive. The relevance of these early and late reactions to clinical asthma is unclear, and most of the asthmatic patients also presented an exaggerated response to a wide variety of inhaled stimuli. This phenomenon, referred to as bronchial hyperreactivity, may be linked to an exacerbated increase in airway resistance to airflow in the lung (Boushey et al. 1980). Surprisingly, despite the fact that various cell types and mediators, including cytokines, are recognized to play an important role in the regulation of IgE synthesis, the possibility that they could also contribute to the development of the late asthmatic response following antigen administration is presently undetermined. Moreover, experimental evidence suggests that some of the mast cell-derived mediators could contribute not only to the triggering of the immediate reaction but also to the initiation of the late response. Therefore, the possibility that immunological responses involving monocytes/macrophages and T and B lymphocytes and initiated by mast cell degranulation could occur following allergen stimulation of the lung and lead to an inflammatory reaction remains to be investigated.

In contrast to lymphocytes, alveolar macrophages have been extensively studied since they represent the vast majority of the cells present in bronchoalveolar lavages. Along with mast cells they probably represent the first cell type that is activated following allergen inhalation. Macrophages have multiple functions, including lysosomal enzyme release, free radical production, generation of PAF and other lipid mediators, and cell cytotoxicity. For example, IgE-dependent activation of rat alveolar macrophages induces the release of inflammatory mediators, such as LTC_4 (Rankin et al. 1982), and contributes to the pulmonary change during the late phase reaction. The recent demonstration that mast cells are capable of synthesizing and secreting various cytokines including IL-3, IL-4, IL-5, and IL-6 following IgE-dependent stimulation (Brown et al. 1987) strongly suggests that they play an important immunoregulatory role during allergic reactions. Finally, most of these cytokines have been suggested to be involved in the bronchopulmonary alterations observed during the late phase reaction of asthma. Therefore, despite the fact that allergic asthma has long been recognized as an immunological disease, it is now becoming evident that it involves processes initially thought to be restricted to the basic phenomenon of the immune response, i.e., monocyte/macrophage and T- and B-cell interactions.

The Role of PAF in Allergic Inflammation

Among the various mediators involved in allergic processes, PAF appears to play a central role, since it induces, directly or indirectly, a bronchoconstrictor response (reviewed in Braquet et al. 1987). In addition, this substance evokes a long-lasting alteration of the bronchopulmonary response to various agonists, including histamine or metacholine, and contributes to the recruitment of inflammatory cell types in the lung (Lellouch-Tubiana et al. 1988; reviewed in Mencia-Huerta et al. 1989). Besides these actions PAF may also play a role in lung pathology via the modulation of various immune processes. Indeed, PAF has a direct effect on lymphocyte proliferation, cytokine production, and cell-surface antigen expression (reviewed in Braquet and Rola-Pleszczynski, 1987). PAF has been also implicated in lymphocyte cytotoxicity (reviewed in Braquet and Rola-Pleszczynski 1987).

One way in which cytokines can contribute to allergic reactions is via the modulation of the release of various mediators, including PAF. Such a phenomenon, referred to as "priming," has been demonstrated to be operational in the case of cell responses induced by PAF (reviewed in Braquet et al. 1989a, b).

However, the secretion of PAF and cytokines are closely related since the phospholipid mediator has been shown to influence tumor necrosis factor (TNF), IL-1, and IL-6 production by rat and human macrophages (Mencia-Huerta et al. 1988; Bonavida et al. 1989) and IL-2 release by human peripheral mononuclear cells (Rola-Pleszczynski et al. 1987).

PAF is also involved in regulating the expression of FcεRII/CD23. Indeed, it has recently been demonstrated that incubation of monocytes and B lymphocytes, but not T lymphocytes, with PAF induced a dose-dependent increase in FcεRII/CD23 (Dugas et al. 1989; Paul-Eugène et al. 1990). Regarding B lymphocytes, the possibility that the PAF-dependent FcεRII/CD23 induction might be due to the endogenous production of secondary messengers from contaminating monocytes cannot be excluded. Indeed, PAF has been shown to induce leukotriene synthesis in phagocytes (reviewed in Braquet et al. 1987), and these autacoids, and especially LTB_4, potentiate FcεRII/CD23 expression, release of soluble FcεRII/CD23, and IgE secretion induced by IL-4 (Dugas et al. 1990; Paul-Eugène et al. 1991).

Expression of FcεRII/CD23 on Rat Alveolar Macrophages

The release of potent pro-inflammatory mediators by IgE-dependent mechanisms suggests that this immunoglobulin class could contribute to allergic reactions directly by activating FcεRII/CD23-bearing cells. Alveolar macrophages collected from allergic patients released lysosomal enzymes on addition of the specific allergen (reviewed in Dessaint and Capron 1988). Production of the sulfidopeptide leukotriene by alveolar macrophages stimulated with anti-IgE has also been reported (Rankin et al. 1982). The possibility that the cell surface FcεRII/CD23 on alveolar macrophages could be increased following antigen or PAF challenge is at present undetermined. We have therefore investigated the possible modulation of FcεRII/CD23 expression on alveolar macrophages from sensitized rats, challenged or not challenged with the antigen. In another set of experiments, the FcεRII/CD23 expression on rat alveolar macrophages stimulated by PAF in vivo was also evaluated.

Brown-Norway rats were placed twice, at an interval of 48 h, in a Plexiglas chamber (30 × 50 × 30 cm) and exposed to an aerosol of a saline solution containing ovalbumin (OA) 10 mg/ml for 30 min. A booster administration was performed under the same conditions after 14 days. When challenged with the antigen at day 21, sensitized rats developed a sustained bronchopulmonary response of about 30%, as calculated over the value obtained by clamping the trachea at the end of the experiment. By contrast, in the absence of the booster administration, rats developed a low bronchopulmonary response of about 10%–15%.

In these experiments alveolar macrophages from sensitized and antigen-challenged rats were obtained 24 h after the challenge by five successive

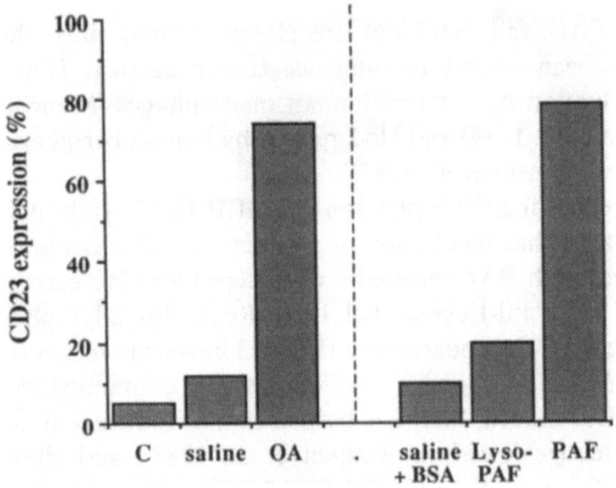

Fig. 1. Expression of FcεRII/CD23 on alveolar macrophages either from sensitized Brown-Norway rats challenged with ovalbumin (OA) aerosol of vehicule alone (saline) (*left panel*) or from Sprague-Dawley rats challenged by aerosol administration of PAF or lyso-PAF (500 μg/ml for 30 min) (*right panel*). *C*, Nonsensitized, unchallenged rats; *saline*, sensitized rats challenged with saline solution; *OA*, rats challenged with ovalbumin

bronchoalveolar lavages with a saline solution. The expression of FcεRII/CD23 was evaluated by flow cytometry using the BB10 monoclonal antibody (a generous gift from Dr. Monique Capron, Institut Pasteur, Lille). No expression of FcεRII/CD23 on alveolar macrophages from antigen-challenged, non-sensitized rats was observed. By contrast, 74% of the alveolar macrophages expressed FcεRII/CD23 after antigen stimulation by aerosol, compared to 11% following challenge with saline (Fig. 1).

In another set of experiments, aerosolized PAF (500 μg/ml for 30 min) induced after 24 h the expression of FcεRII/CD23 on 79% of the alveolar macrophages collected from non-sensitized rats. This is to be compared with the 20% expression of FcεRII/CD23 after administration by aerosol of the metabolite/precursor of PAF, lyso-PAF (500 μg/ml) (Fig. 1). These results obtained in an animal model strengthen the data obtained in vitro on human monocytes (Dugas et al. 1989; Paul-Eugène et al. 1990) and suggest a role for both FcεRII/CD23 and lipid mediators in the late phase of allergic reaction.

Concluding Remarks

The entry of allergen in lung tissue is followed by complex reactions whose consequence is the triggering and/or the perpetuation of pulmonary inflammation. Indeed, the antigen can stimulate several immunocompetent cell types present in the lung that are responsible for the initial steps of the allergic

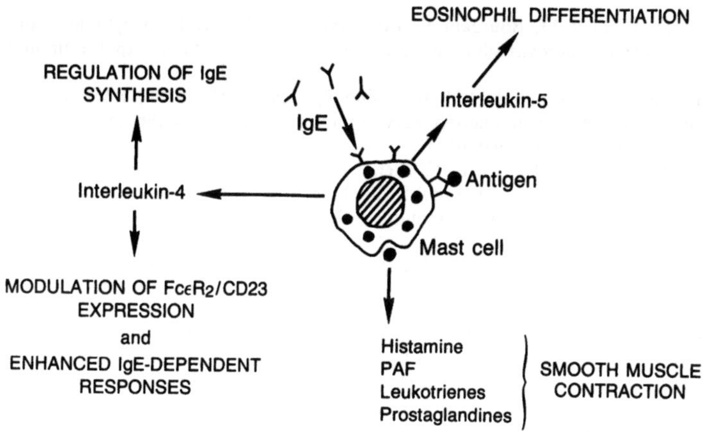

Fig. 2. Putative role of mast cells in the regulation of immune processes in the lung following antigen challenge

reaction such as IgE-producing cells and antigen-primed or activated T cells. In addition, antigen evokes the degranulation of mast cells and the release of various lipid mediators, the consequence being the initiation of the early phase reaction and alterations in the tissue response to further stimulation. This latter process is one of the major features of the late phase response of the allergic reaction. Furthermore, it is now evident that IgE-sensitized mast cells challenged with the specific antigen release PAF and various cytokines such as IL-4 and IL-5 in the microenvironment (Fig. 2). IL-4 induces the expression of FcεRII/CD23 on alveolar macrophages within a few hour in a process that is increased by PAF or LTB_4; these cells can then interact with IgE/antigen immune complexes and may result in an enhanced IgE-dependent response. In addition, challenge of alveolar macrophages expressing FcεRII/CD23 with the antigen may induce the generation of inflammatory mediators leading to the late phase reaction. Finally, the production of IL-5 by activated mast cells may play a role in the recruitment and local differentiation of eosinophil precursors. These possibilities indicate that mast cells could play a central role in the development of the allergic reaction, although in a quite different way from that initially suspected.

References

Bonavida B, Mencia-Huerta JM, Braquet P (1989) Effect of platelet-activating factor on monocyte activation and tumor necrosis factor production. Int Arch Allergy Appl Immunol 88:157–160

Boushey HA, Holtzmann MJ, Sheller JR, Nadel JA (1980) Bronchial hyperreactivity. Am Rev Respir Dis 121:389–413

Braquet P, Rola-Pleszczynski M (1987) The role of PAF in immunological responses. Immunol Today 8:345–352

Braquet P, Touqui L, Shen TY, Vargaftig BB (1987) Perspectives in platelet-activating factor research. Pharmacol Rev 39:97–145

Braquet P, Hosford D, Braquet M, Bourgain R, Bussolino F (1989a) Role of cytokines and platelet-activating factor in microvascular immune injury. Int Arch Allergy Appl Immunol 88:88–100

Braquet P, Paubert-Braquet M, Bourgain RH, Bussolino F, Hosford D (1989b) PAF/cytokine autogenerated feedback networks in microvascular immune injury: consequences in shock, ischemia and graft rejection. J Lipid Med 10:75–112

Delespesse G, Sarfati M, Hofstetter H, Frost H, Kilcher E, Suter U (1989) Human FcεRII and IgE binding factors. Int Arch Allergy Appl Immunol 88:18–22

Dessaint JP, Capron A (1988) Low-affinity immunoglobulin-E binding in asthma. Triangle 27:95–101

Dugas B, Paul-Eugène N, Mencia-Huerta JM, Braquet P (1989) Influence of platelet-activating factor on the expression of FcεRII/CD23 on normal mononuclear cells. Experta Medica Asia, Hong Kong pp 57–61

Dugas B, Paul-Eugène N, Gordon J, Spur BW, Braquet P, Mencia-Huerta JM (1990) Leukotriene B_4 potentiates the expression and the release of FcεRII/CD23 and proliferation and differentiation of human B lymphocytes induced by IL-4. J Immunol 145:3406–3411

Lellouch-Tubiana A, Lefort J, Simon MT, Pfister A, Vargaftig BB (1988) Eosinophil recruitment into guinea-pig lungs after PAF-acether and allergen administration: modulation by prostacyclin, platelet depletion and selective antagonists. Am Rev Respir Dis 137:948–952

Mencia-Huerta JM, Henane S, Sorlin B, Rola-Pleszczynski M, Pignol B, Braquet P (1988) Effect of platelet-activating factor on interleukin-1 release and synthesis by rat spleen adherent monocytes. In: Braquet P (ed) New trends in lipid mediator research, vol 1. Karger, Basel, pp 1–5

Mencia-Huerta JM, Hosford D, Braquet P (1989) Acute and long-term pulmonary effects of platelet-activating factor. Clin Exp Allergy 19:125–142

Paul-Eugène N, Dugas B, Picquot S, Lagente V, Mencia-Huerta JM, Braquet P (1990) Influence of interleukin-4 and of platelet-activating factor on the expression of the FcεRII/CD23 on human monocytes. J Lipid Med 2:95–101

Paul-Eugène N, Dugas B, Gordon J, Yamaoka K, Spur BW, Kolb JP, Mencia-Huerta JM, Braquet P (1991) Leukotriene B_4 potentiates the interleukin-4 dependent induction of Human IgE Synthesis. (submitted)

Pène J, Rousset F, Brière F, Chrétien I, Wideman J, Bonnefoy JY, de Vries JE (1988) Interleukin 5 enhances interleukin 4-induced IgE production by normal human B cells. The role of soluble CD23 antigen. Eur J Immunol 18:929–935

Rankin JA, Hitchcock M, Merill W, Bach MK, Brashler JR, Askenase PW (1982) IgE-dependent release of leukotriene C_4 from alveolar macrophages. Nature 297:329–331

Rola-Pleszcynski M, Pignol B, Pouliot C, Braquet P (1987) Inhibition of human lymphocyte proliferation and interleukin 2 production by platelet-activating factor (PAF-acether): reversal by a specific antagonist, BN 52021. Biochem Biophys Res Commun 142:754–760

Part 2:

Cellular Reactions and Interactions: Macrophages and Leukocytes

The Role of Alveolar and Intravascular Macrophages in Acute Lung Injury: New Methods and New Mechanisms

J.D. Brain and A.E. Warner

Introduction

Resident macrophages are central in defending the lungs against the assaults of particles and pathogens in inspired air. The phagocytic and microbicidal potential of macrophages is one of the major reasons why the lungs remain clean and sterile. Macrophages may also prevent allergy by ingesting and catabolizing inhaled foreign proteins. Alternatively, during some lung infections they may preserve and present antigens to lymphocytes and act cooperatively with other components of the immune system to enhance the immune response. At other times lung macrophages recognize and destroy neoplastic cells, thus preventing the development of cancer. Alveolar macrophages may also ingest effete type 1 and type 2 epithelial cells, red blood cells, and perhaps even some of the "worn out" surfactant (Brain 1985).

Regulatory Role of Macrophages

During the last several decades a mountain of evidence indicates that macrophages have roles that extend far beyond phagocytosis. They are secretory and regulatory cells; they can initiate and prolong inflammatory responses; they can stimulate the synthesis of extracellular matrix proteins. Thus, they both respond to their microenvironment and control the activities of other cells such as neutrophils, lymphocytes, and fibroblasts. Macrophages can secrete such diverse substances as lysosomal enzymes, interferon, components of complement, angiogenesis factor, plasminogen activator, cyclic nucleotides, leukotrienes, prostaglandins, inflammatory cytokines, and granulopoietins. Still other macrophage products may interact with complex systems such as those controlling clotting, fibrogenesis, fibrinolysis, as well as those regulating kinin and complement fragment generation.

Failure of Macrophage Function

Some of these activities reflect protective postures which help prevent lung disease, but at other times macrophages may be involved in processes leading to lung damage (Brain 1986). First, their defensive role can be compromised. Many investigators have shown that such diverse agents as viruses, silica, immunosuppressives, ethanol intoxication, cigarette smoke, air pollution, hypoxia, and hyperoxia can depress the ability of pulmonary macrophages to protect their host. Sometimes the agent or factor acts directly to kill or damage the macrophage. In other instances, particularly those situations involving pulmonary edema or altered acid-base balance, the macrophages themselves may be undamaged, but their activity may be indirectly depressed because of changes in their milieu, the pulmonary microenvironment.

Pathogenic Role of Macrophages

Secondly, there are situations in which pulmonary macrophages not only fail but directly contribute to the pathogenesis of pulmonary diseases. For example, the ingestion of particles (e.g., cigarette smoke), microbes, or endotoxin causes the release of lysosomal enzymes and oxygen radicals into the macrophage cytoplasm or the external environment. These substances may damage surrounding cells or the macrophage; dead or dying macrophages then release substances which can attract fibroblasts and elicit fibrogenic responses. This extracellular release of proteases and oxygen radicals can also alter the extracellular matrix or the activity of a variety of enzymes. When smoke or particles act to recruit more cells, to activate them, and to release proteolytic enzymes and oxygen radicals, then macrophages may be centrally involved in the development of lung disease. The same inhaled toxins may also elicit similar responses from other white blood cells such as polymorphonuclear leukocytes. Thus, even though macrophages defend the lungs, they can also injure the host while exercising their defensive role.

Types of Lung Macrophages

In the past, lung macrophages were usually exclusively equated with alveolar macrophages. However, macrophages exist not only in alveolar ducts and spaces, but also in other anatomic locations in the lungs (Brain 1988). They are present in airways (Brain et al. 1984b; Sorokin and Brain 1975) and connective tissue (Holt et al. 1985; Kobzik et al. 1987), in the pleural space (Zlotnik et al. 1982; Ackerman et al. 1980), and even in pulmonary capillaries.

Pulmonary Intravascular Macrophages

Since 1984, our laboratory has published a series of papers demonstrating that abundant resident macrophages within pulmonary capillaries of sheep, calves, goats, and cats avidly remove particles and pathogens from circulating blood (Warner and Brain 1984, 1986). Morphometry demonstrated that even normal sheep had more macrophages in pulmonary blood vessels than in their alveolar spaces (Warner et al. 1986). Pulmonary intravascular macrophages (PIMs) are large (20–80 μm diameter) mature macrophages that are bound to the endothelium of pulmonary capillaries. PIMs have morphologic features characteristic of differentiated macrophages including an indented nucleus, lysosomal granules, pseudopods, phagosomes and phagolysosomes, tubular micropinocytosis vermiformis structures, and a fuzzy glycocalyx (Fig. 1A). These ultrastructural features, especially the phagocytic vacuoles and micropinocytosis vermiformis, indicate the well-differentiated state of PIMs. They are not simply adherent monocytes. Phagosomes are a prominent feature in PIM cytoplasm, suggesting an active role for these cells in surveillance of the circulation. Thus, they are a member of that portion of the mononuclear phagocyte system (MPS) with access to the circulating blood. In a number of species, we have seen erythophagocytosis by PIMs.

PIMs form membrane adhesive complexes with underlying endothelial cells (Fig. 1A). These adhesions have an intercellular separation of 12–15 nm, and electron dense material is present both in the intercellular space and subjacent to the plasma membrane of both cells. A significant number of PIMs with easily demonstrated phagocytic function have been found in a number of species, including calves, sheep, pigs, goats, and cats (Warner and Brain 1984; Warner et al. 1986; Brain et al. 1988b). Figure 1B shows a macrophage in an alveolus of a sheep so that pulmonary intravascular and alveolar macrophages can be compared.

Physiologic and Pathophysiologic Role of PIMs

PIMs actively ingest particles such as iron oxide and gold colloid from the circulating blood (Warner and Brain 1986; Warner et al. 1986). Importantly, when such pathogenic agents as gram-negative bacteria and endotoxin are sequestered in the lungs, the subsequent inflammatory response is also localized there. We have found pulmonary inflammatory changes, including neutrophil recruitment, intravascular fibrin deposition and endothelial cell injury, as early as 1 h following localization of bacteria or endotoxin in the lungs (Warner et al. 1987, 1988). Figure 2A shows the appearance of sheep capillaries following intravenous injection of *Pseudomonas aeruginosa.* Figure 2B demonstrates that the cell responsible for pulmonary uptake of the circulating bacteria is the PIM.

We believe that rapid ingestion of pathogenic materials leads to secretion of inflammatory mediators from pulmonary intravascular macrophages. These mediators may include such cytokines as tumor necrosis factor, interleukin-1, platelet-activating factor, and a range of substances that may recruit and

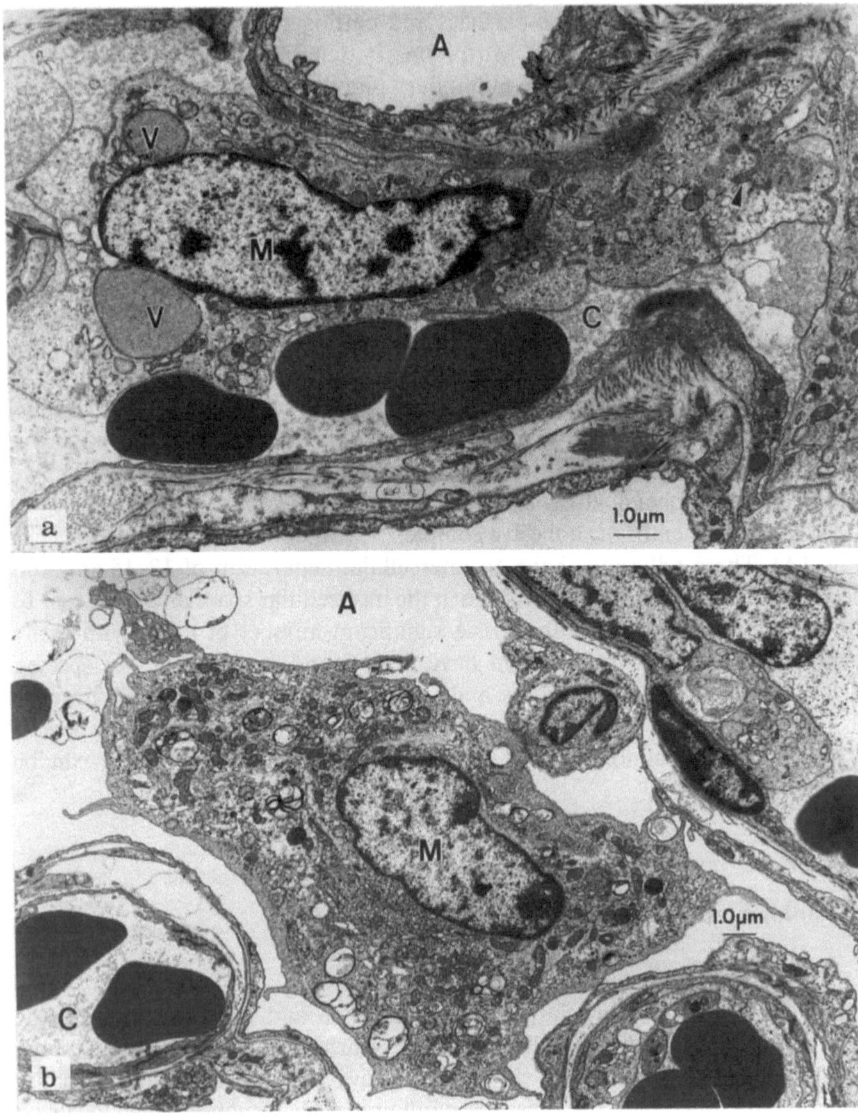

Fig. 1A, B. Comparison of sheep pulmonary intravascular and alveolar macrophages. **A** Pulmonary intravascular macrophage (*M*) within the capillary lumen (*C*) in sheep lung. The macrophage is closely apposed to the underlying capillary endothelium, has two prominent phagocytic vacuoles (*V*), and tubular membrane invaginations characteristic of micropinocytosis vermiformis (*arrow*); alveolar space (*A*) **B** Sheep alveolar macrophage within the alveolar space (*A*); capillary lumen (*C*). (Reprinted by permission from Warner et al. 1986. Copyright United States and Canadian Academy of Pathology)

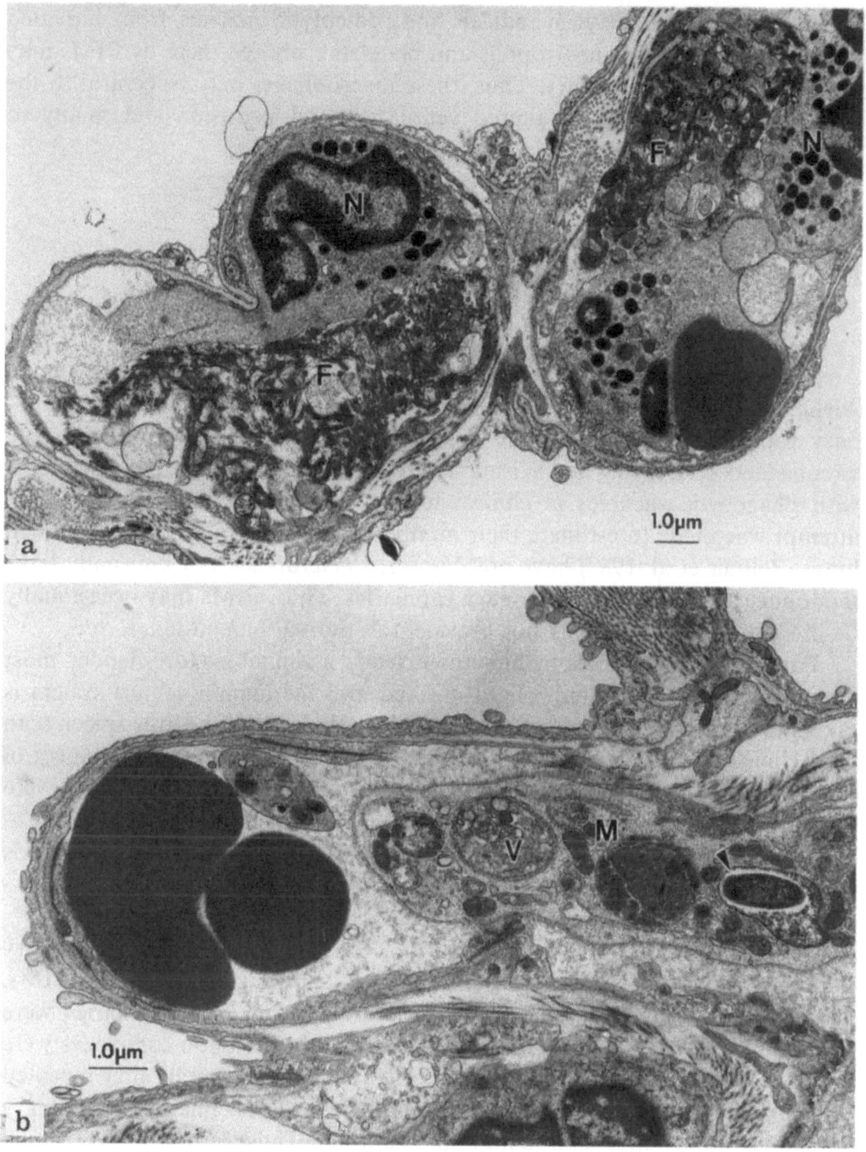

Fig. 2A, B. Pulmonary capillaries from sheep lungs after intravascular injection of *Pseudomonas aeruginosa*. **A** Ultrastructure of congested capillaries showing neutrophil (*N*) and fibrin (*F*) accumulation. **B** Pulmonary intravascular macrophage (*M*) showing phagocytic vacuole (*V*) and as ingested bacterial cell (*arrow*). (Reprinted by permission from Warner et al. 1987. Copyright American Lung Association)

activate neutrophils. Oxygen radicals and proteolytic enzymes from activated macrophages and from neutrophils and platelets recruited there by PIMs may then cause local tissue injury. Thus, these macrophages may be central to the chain of events leading to altered ventilation and perfusion and finally to respiratory distress.

Relevance of PIMs to Human Lung Injury

Are these experimental animal lung injury systems relevant as models of human ARDS? In other words, are there intravascular macrophages in human pulmonary capillaries? We believe the answer appears to be "few under normal circumstances". Dehring and Wismar (1989) have found large mononuclear cells with phagocytic vacuoles in clinical human lung biopsy specimens, but no attempt was made to estimate their number. Morphometric studies of human lungs (Zeltner et al. 1987) have not described macrophages or unusually large mononuclear cells in the pulmonary capillaries. Thus, PIMs may occasionally be present, but are probably not prevalent in normal human lungs.

Particle uptake studies in humans provide a similar picture. Under most circumstances, ^{99m}Tc-sulfur colloid injected into the human venous system is taken up by hepatic and splenic macrophages – the basis of the liver-spleen scan used clinically (George et al. 1980). There are, however, reported instances of lung uptake of colloidal radiopharmaceuticals, usually in humans with severe liver damage (Garty et al. 1984; Keyes et al. 1973). Lung uptake does appear to increase in some cases of pulmonary injury, however. For example, there is accumulation of radiolabeled fibrinogen or platelets in patients with ARDS (Quinn et al. 1987; Schneider et al. 1980).

We (Warner et al. 1989) found that prior endotoxemia enhances pulmonary uptake of injected particles in rats and rabbits – species lacking resident PIMs. Moreover, we found that mononuclear cells in pulmonary capillaries were responsible for the pulmonary uptake. Occasionally, adhesion complexes were found between mononuclear cells and capillary endothelial cells after repeated endotoxin administration. Cooper et al. (1988) also found enhanced pulmonary uptake in rabbits after endotoxin administration. Thus, certain kinds of lung injury may promote transient increases in phagocytically active mononuclear cells in pulmonary capillaries. This could be due to changes in adhesiveness at the level of the endothelial and/or circulating cells or it could reflect alterations in the deformability of the circulating monocytes. In turn these changes could lead to diminished transit time of circulating cells through the lungs and perhaps to adhesion and even PIM formation.

In addition to changes in the lungs or circulating white cells, enhanced pulmonary uptake may reflect reduced reticuloendothelial uptake in the liver and spleen. Molina et al. (1987) and Brain et al. (1987) studied the effects of blood substitutes on lung uptake. They showed that Kupffer cell function was compromised by the ingestion of perfluorochemical droplets. This led to increased lung uptake of *Pseudomonas aeruginosa* bacteria or cobalt oxide particles.

New Methods for Studying Lung Macrophages

This is an exciting time to be studying macrophages. New tools are becoming available to supplement classic approaches such as ultrastructure, biochemistry, and in vitro cell culture. Not only do we have an extensive repertoire of bioassays and immunologic assays for studying macrophage mediators, the tools of molecular biology such as the polymerase chain reaction now allow us to measure very small quantities of the RNA message responsible for the synthesis of these mediators. Moreover, in situ hybridization can be used to identify the cellular anatomic sites of mediator synthesis and to compare them to the distribution of disease within the lung. Flow cytometry is emerging as a valuable tool to study phagocytosis by macrophages and its associated oxidative burst (Kobzik et al. 1990).

Magnetometric Methods and Macrophages

Magnetic particles and sensitive magnetometers also serve as a new tool in cell biology (see reviews by Brain et al. 1988a, and Valberg and Brain 1988). Iron oxide particles are introduced into the lungs by inhalation or intratracheal instillation of magnetite or gamma hematite and are ingested by lung macrophages (Brain et al. 1984a). In species lacking PIMs, like the rat, these particles are ingested by hepatic and splenic macrophages following intravenous injection (Weinstock and Brain 1988). However, when species with abundant pulmonary intravascular macrophages are studied, these lung cells can be readily labelled by intravenous injection of magnetic dust.

These particles are easily recognized in living or fixed cells studied by light microscopy. They are also easily visualized by electron microscopy because of their electron density. Since the particles are magnetic, the motion of particle-containing organelles (primarily phagosomes and phagolysosomes) can be either measured or manipulated externally. Magnetic fields from particles ingested by mononuclear phagocytes in the lungs can be measured with fluxgate or with SQUID (superconducting quantum interference device) magnetometers. We have developed methods to use these magnetic particles to monitor the progression of phagocytosis, characterize organelle motion, and to measure cytoplasmic viscosity in normal and compromised cells.

Conclusion

Macrophages and other phagocytic cells occupy a central role in the pathogenesis of lung injury. These cells prevent infection, are involved in wound healing, but also contribute to lung disease when activated and/or damaged. Evidence suggests that phagocytic cells in lung capillaries have a key role in the response to bacteremia or septicemia. Continuing development of new methods will inevitably lead to additional insights into how macrophages are involved in lung injury and respiratory failure.

References

Ackerman N, Tomolonis A, Miran L, Kheifets J, Martinez S, Carter A (1980) Three day pleural inflammation: a new model to detect drug effects on macrophage accumulation. J Pharmacol Exp Ther 215:588–595

Brain JD (1985) Macrophages in the respiratory tract. In: Fishman AP, Fisher AB (eds) Circulation and nonrespiratory functions. American Physiological Society, Bethesda, pp 447–471 (Handbook of physiology, vol 1)

Brain JD (1986) Toxicological aspects of alterations of pulmonary macrophage function. Annu Rev Pharmacol Toxicol 26:547–565

Brain JD (1988) Lung macrophages – how many kinds are there? What do they do? Am Rev Respir Dis 137:507–509

Brain JD, Bloom SB, Valberg PA, Gehr P (1984a) Correlation between the behavior of magnetic iron oxide particles in the lungs of rabbits and phagocytosis. Exp Lung Res 6:115–131

Brain JD, Gehr P, Kavet R (1984b) Airway macrophages: the importance of the fixation method. Am Rev Respir Dis 129:823–826

Brain JD, Molina RM, Kreyling WG, Warner AE (1987) How do blood substitutes influence the fate of insoluble particles in the bloodstream and the extent of lung uptake? Am Rev Respir Dis 135:A211

Brain JD, Bloom SB, Valberg PA (1988a) Magnetometry – a tool for studying the cell biology of macrophages. In: Atsumi K, Kotani M, Ueno S, Katila T, Williamson SJ (eds) Biomagnetism '87. Tokyo Denki University Press, Tokyo, pp 10–17

Brain JD, Warner AE, Molina RM, DeCamp MM (1988b) Pulmonary intravascular macrophages are an important part of the mononuclear phagocyte system in ruminants and cats. Am Rev Respir Dis 137:A147

Cooper JA, McCandless BK, Ferro TJ, Malik AB (1988) Pulmonary intravascular phagocytic activity in rabbits and sheep. Am Rev Respir Dis 137:398A

Dehring DJ, Wismar BL (1989) Intravascular macrophages in pulmonary capillaries of humans. Am Rev Respir Dis 139:1027–1029

Garty I, Tal I, Daynan A (1984) Tc-99m colloid lung uptake in a rare case of Toxoplasmosis with liver involvement. Clin Nucl Med 9:310–313

George EA, Henderschott LR, Klos DJ, Donati RM (1980) Mechanism of hepatic extraction of gelatinized ^{99m}technetium sulfur colloid. Eur J Nucl Med 5:241–244

Holt PG, Degebrodt A, Venaille T, O'Leary C, Krska K, Flexman J, Farrell H, Shellam G, Young P, Penhale J, Robertson T, Papadimitriou JM (1985) Preparation of interstitial lung cells by enzymatic digestion of tissue slices: preliminary characterization by morphology and performance in functional assays. Immunology 54:139–147

Keyes JW Jr, Wilson GA, Quinonest JD (1973) An evaluation of lung uptake of colloid during liver imaging. J Nucl Med 14:687–691

Kobzik L, Godleski JJ, Barry BE, Brain JD (1987) Isolation and antigenic identification of hamster lung interstitial macrophages. Am Rev Respir Dis 138:908–914

Kobzik L, Godleski JJ, Brain JD (1990) Oxidative metabolism in the alveolar macrophage: analysis by flow cytometry. J Leukocyte Biol 47:295–303
Molina RM, Brain JD, Warner AE, DeCamp MM (1987) Blood substitutes alter the fate of bacteria in the blood and may place the lung at increased risk. Am Rev Respir Dis 135:A84
Quinn DA, Carvalhy AC, Geller E (1987) ^{99m}Tc fibrinogen scanning in adult respiratory distress syndrome. Am Rev Respir Dis 135:100–106
Schneider R, Zapol W, Carvalho A (1980) Platelet consumption and sequestration in severe acute respiratory failure. Am Rev Respir Dis 122:445–451
Sorokin SP, Brain JD (1975) Pathways of clearance in mouse lungs exposed to iron oxide aerosols. Anat Rec 181:581–626
Valberg PA, and Brain JD (1988) Lung particle retention and lung macrophage function evaluated using magnetic aerosols. J Aerosol Med 1:331–349
Warner AE, Brain JD (1984) Intravascular pulmonary macrophages in ruminants actively participate in reticuloendothelial clearance of particles. Fed Proc 43:1001
Warner AE, Brain JD (1986) Intravascular pulmonary macrophages: a novel cell removes particles from blood. Am J Physiol (Regulatory Integrative Comp Physiol) 19:R728–R732
Warner AE, Barry BE, Brain JD (1986) Pulmonary intravascular macrophages in sheep: morphology and function of a novel constituent of the mononuclear phagocyte system. Lab Invest 55:276–288
Warner AE, Molina RM, Brain JD (1987) Uptake of bloodborne bacteria by pulmonary intravascular macrophages and consequent inflammatory responses in sheep. Am Rev Respir Dis 136:683–690
Warner AE, DeCamp MM, Molina RM, Brain JD (1988) Pulmonary removal in circulatory endotoxin results in acute lung injury in sheep. Lab Invest 59:219–230
Warner AE, DeCamp MM, Bellows CF, Brain JD (1989) Endotoxemia enhances lung uptake of circulating particles in species lacking pulmonary intravascular macrophages. Am Rev Respir Dis 139:A158
Weinstock SB, Brain JD (1988) Comparison of particle clearance and macrophage phagosomal motion in liver and lungs of rats. J Appl Physiol 65:1811–1820
Zeltner TB, Caduff JH, Gehr P, Pfenninger J, Burri PH (1987) The postnatal development and growth of the human lung. I. Morphometry. Respir Physiol 67:247–267
Zlotnick A, Vatter A, Hayer RL, Blumenthal F, Crowle AJ (1982) Mouse pleural macrophages: characterization and comparison with mouse alveolar and peritoneal macrophages. J Reticuloendothel Soc 31:207–220

Pulmonary Fibrosis: Role of Inflammatory Cells in Local Injury and Fibrosis

Y. Martinet and N. Martinet

Diffuse interstitial fibrosis (DIF) of the lung is characterized by the abnormal deposition of extracellular matrix (collagens, elastin, proteoglycans) with a progressive loss of functional units [1, 2]. The sequence of events leading to lung fibrosis is thought to result from a stereotyped response of the lung to an initial injury. This response involves a local inflammatory reaction (alveolitis) and the accumulation of mesenchymal cells with extracellular matrix deposition (fibrosis) [3–5].

The inflammatory cells play an important role in fibrosis development by contributing to endothelial and epithelial cell injury and by directing mesenchymal cell accumulation. Regardless of its nature, the initiating process is responsible for a local injury with an inflammatory reaction which amplifies this injury and modulates the tissue repair with mesenchymal cells and extracellular matrix accumulation leading to fibrosis (Fig. 1). Altogether, the local injury, the inflammatory reaction, and the repair process with fibrosis result in the progressive loss of functional units [1–5].

Alveolitis

Alveolitis corresponds to the inflammatory reaction present in the lung [4, 5]. Alveolitis is evaluated by open lung biopsy, transbronchial biopsy, and, more importantly, by bronchoalveolar lavage (BAL). BAL allows the recovery from alveoli of inflammatory cells and gives an insight into the populations of inflammatory cells present in lung interstitium. BAL use has led to the description of different types of alveolitis depending upon the main inflammatory cell types and their associations: macrophages, lymphocytes, neutrophils, or eosinophils. For example, sarcoidosis is characterized by a macrophage-lymphocyte alveolitis while idiopathic pulmonary fibrosis is associated with a macrophage-neutrophil alveolitis.

Regarding lung fibrosis two diseases have been extensively studied: (1) the adult respiratory distress syndrome (ARDS), an acute disorder characterized by a rapid interstitial and intra-alveolar fibrosis with a poor prognosis [6–8]; and (2) idiopathic pulmonary fibrosis (IPF), a chronic disorder with progressive interstitial fibrosis, lung function deterioration, and a mean survival time of 5 years after onset of symptoms [9–11]. In both disorders, interstitial inflammation and progressive fibrosis lead to an “end stage lung.” The current

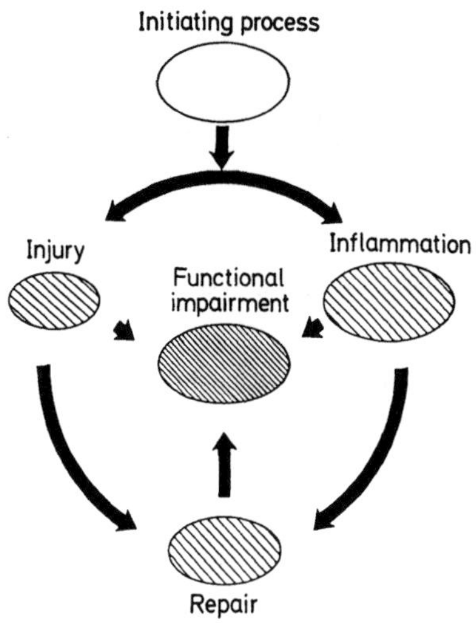

Fig. 1. Cellular events leading to functional impairment in diffuse interstitial lung fibrosis

understanding of these disorders implies that the nature of the mechanisms involved is identical, despite the multiplicity of the initiating processes.

Alveolitis in ARDS is at first defined by the presence of inflammatory cells, mostly polymorphonuclear neutrophil leukocytes (PMN), and platelets. After a few days, there is a progressive decrease in PMN concomitant with an increased number of macrophages.

IPF alveolitis is defined by the presence of PMN and macrophages. Therefore, in both disorders (ARDS and IPF), alveolitis is characterized by an increased cellularity with the abnormal presence of PMN.

PMN recruitment is thought to be related to the in situ presence of complement-derived factors and macrophage-derived chemotactic factors for neutrophils [4, 5]. The accumulation of macrophages may result from their limited ability to replicate, but more importantly from their recruitment from blood by the local presence of chemotactic factors such as monocyte chemotactic factor, platelet mediators, or extracellular matrix fragments [4, 5].

Lung Cell Injury

In the early stages (injury; Fig. 2) of ARDS (and of experimental ARDS) lung biopsies show the loss of capillary endothelial cells and of type I pneumocytes with evidence of local destruction of basement membranes creating gaps that allow the diffusion of serum proteins and the migration of mesenchymal cells into the alveoli [6–8].

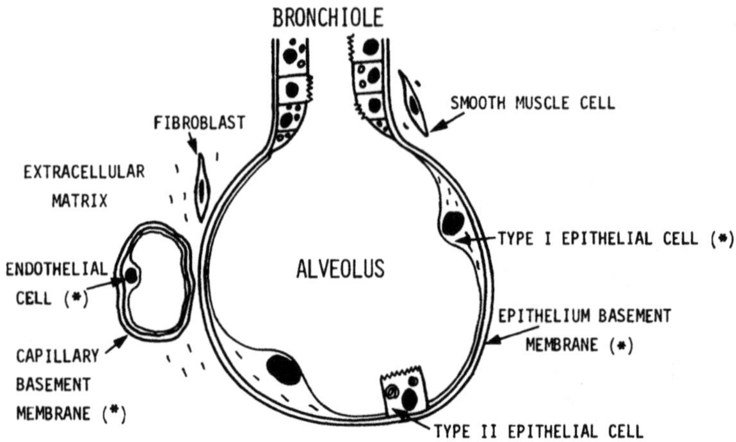

Fig. 2. Sites (*) of PMN mediated injury

Endothelial Cell Injury

Evidence of capillary endothelial cell injury is present in ARDS. This injury can induce cell necrosis as a result of the specific sensitivity of endothelial cells to several factors, such as oxidants. A progressive regeneration of endothelial cells is possible starting from intact areas. However, a chronic cycle of injury and endothelial cell regeneration (repair) initiates progressive vessel dysfunction [12].

Epithelial Cell Injury

Type I pneumocytes are very fragile cells that can be injured by the local presence of oxidants. Type II pneumocytes are more resistant and contribute to the repair process by dividing, expanding, and differentiating into type I pneumocytes. However, a chronic state of injury ends with cuboidal metaplasia with the abnormal presence in the alveoli of type II pneumocytes and/or epithelial cells migrating from the terminal bronchioles [12].

Role of PMN and Macrophages in Lung Cell Injury

The initiating process is responsible for the initial injury, but inflammatory cells contribute to its amplification (Fig. 1). PMN are likely to play a major role in lung cell injury, since activated neutrophils release several mediators cytotoxic for endothelial and epithelial cells [4, 5, 12]. Among them, oxidants ($O_2^{\bullet}$, H_2O_2, $\cdot OH$) are highly reactive metabolites with cytotoxic destructive potential. Hence,

PMN accumulation and activation in ARDS and in IPF implies an increased local burden of oxidants in these disorders. Furthermore, activated PMN release collagenases and a myeloperoxidase present, for example, in IPF patients' BAL fluid. These enzymes contribute to epithelial cell injury. Finally, extracellular matrixes (basal membranes for example) are other targets of PMN (e.g., one granulocyte collagenase is capable of a selective digestion of type I and type III collagens).

By releasing oxidants, activated macrophages may add to local cell injury [4, 5, 12], but this macrophage cytotoxic activity is limited. However, macrophages (and blood monocytes) may be involved, at least in septic ARDS, in lung cell injury by the release of tumor necrosis factor-α (TNF-α). TNF-alpha/cachectin is a macrophage mediator comprised of two to five identical 17 kDa chains [13, 14]. TNF-α is a mediator of cachexia and a cytotoxic factor for certain tumor cell lines. It induces shock by promoting PMN activation and adherence to endothelial cells with a local cytotoxicity ending in an increased capillary permeability and fluid leakage.

Fibrosis

Current Concepts of the Fibrotic Process

Fibrosis results from the local accumulation of mesenchymal cells (fibroblasts and smooth muscle cells) and the extracellular matrix produced by these cells [15]. This accumulation of mesenchymal cells is explained by: (1) the migration of these cells from surrounding areas to the site of inflammation and/or by (2) the local replication of these cells. Both mechanisms are present in ARDS and IPF. In ARDS, for example, mesenchymal cells migrate through the gaps created in the basement membrane. They eventually replicate in the alveoli and produce extracellular matrix leading to intra-alveolar fibrosis. Cell migration and replication depend upon the local presence, respectively, of chemotactic and growth factors.

In addition, an up-regulation of mesenchymal cell extracellular matrix production may contribute to the fibrotic process. Most observations suggest an increased collagen content in fibrotic lungs with a more selective deposition of type I vs type III collagen. This shift in collagen composition causes the fibrotic "rigidity" of the lung [4, 5, 12]. The mechanisms responsible for such an up-regulation are only partially understood. For example, transforming growth factor-β (TGF-β) increases collagen synthesis but inhibits its degradation by inducing the production of plasminogen activator inhibitor. TGF-β is a 25 kDa homodimer initially isolated from platelets and characterized by its ability to induce the phenotypic transformation of normal rat kidney (NRK) cells [16]. TGF-β is also a chemotactic factor for mesenchymal cells, stimulates fibroblast production of collagen and fibronectin, and inhibits fibroblast replication in the presence of optimal concentrations of growth factors.

Chemotactic factors released by inflammatory cells interact with mesenchymal cell membrane specific receptors [17]. They induce their migration along a concentration gradient of chemotactic factor. Macrophages are able to release several factors chemotactic for mesenchymal cells: platelet-derived growth factor (PDGF), fibronectin, and TGF-β.

The local replication of mesenchymal cells is related to the presence of different types of mediators acting on the fibroblast cell cycle [18, 19]. A resting fibroblast replicates only in the presence of two types of specific mediators: the first mediator gives a "competence" signal that allows the cell to leave its resting state (G_0) to enter its mitotic cycle. Then, the "competent" cell is able to respond to a second mediator, a "progression" factor, that signals the cell to complete its cycle and divide.

Activated macrophages release the "competence" factor PDGF and the "progression" factor insulin-like growth factor-1 (IGF-1).

PDGF, first purified from platelets, is a glycoprotein of 31 kDa composed of two different chains, A and B, bound by disulfide bonds. PDGF is a chemotactic and "competence" factor for mesenchymal cells [20].

IGF-1 is a monomer of 7.6 kDa initially isolated from serum. IGF-1 is a "progression" factor for fibroblasts. Recently, similar molecules showing the same biological activity, but with a 26 kDa molecular weight, have been isolated from several tissues and from alveolar macrophages [21].

Finally, inflammatory cells release other mediators that suppress the positive effects of growth factors on mesenchymal cell replication: TGF-β and prostaglandin E_2 (PGE_2) (Fig. 3). PGE_2 is a cyclooxygenase metabolite of arachidonic acid produced by several cell types. Beside modulating inflammation, PGE_2 inhibits mesenchymal cell replication in the presence of optimal concentrations of PDGF and IGF-1 [4, 5, 12].

Idiopathic Pulmonary Fibrosis

Most evidence suggests that macrophages play a central role in the modulation of mesenchymal cell accumulation in IPF. There is a local accumulation of

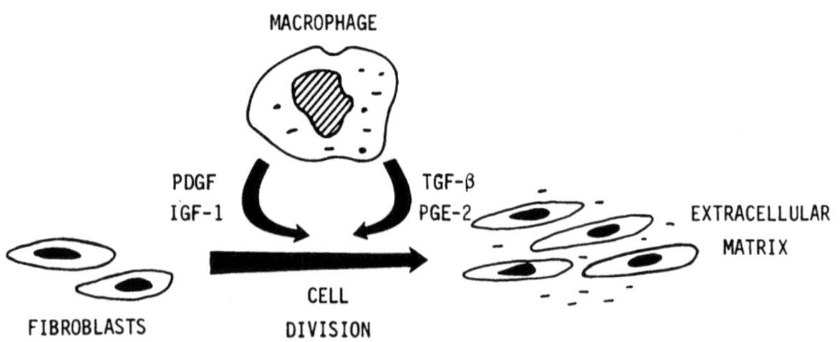

Fig. 3. Macrophage release of positive and negative mesenchymal growth signals

activated macrophages in IPF lung, and alveolar macrophages (AM) recovered by BAL release several mediators and express the genes coding for PDGF [22–25], fibronectin [26], TGF-β [27] and IGF-1 [21]. In addition, evaluation of IPF AM demonstrates that they spontaneously release increased amounts of PDGF [28], fibronectin [26, 29], and IGF-1 [21] in comparison to normal AM. In contrast, little data are available on TGF-β and PGE_2 spontaneous release by AM recovered from IPF patients.

Adult Respiratory Distress Syndrome

Evaluation of BAL fluid from patients with ARDS shows the presence of multiple mediators such as fibronectin [30–32] and PDGF [33].

During the early stage of ARDS the local edema suggests the presence of mediators leaked from plasma such as fibronectin and IGF-1. Platelets are also a potential source of other mediators like PDGF and TGF-β [34].

After a few days of disease progression, the accumulation of macrophages may contribute to ARDS fibrosis by releasing PDGF, IGF-1, and fibronectin. Finally, endothelial cells release PDGF after activation by addition of factor Xa and thrombin, two factors presumably involved in the pathogenesis of ARDS [35–37].

Conclusion

Regardless of the specific nature of the initiating event and of the acute or chronic evolution of each disorder, most evidence suggests a major role for inflammatory cells in lung cell injury and fibrosis.

References

1. Gabbiani G, Rungger-Brändle E (1981) The fibroblast. In: Glynn LE (ed) Tissue repair and regeneration. Elsevier/North-Holland, Amsterdam, pp 1–50
2. Leibovich SJ (1984) Mesenchymal cell proliferation in wound repair; the role of macrophages. In: Hunt TK, Heppenstall RB, Pines E, Rovee D (eds) Soft and hard tissue repair. Praegger, New York, pp 329–351
3. Rennard SI, Bitterman PB, Crystal RG (1984) Current concepts of the pathogenesis of fibrosis: lessons from pulmonary fibrosis. In: Berk P, Castro-Malaspina H, Wasserman LR (eds) Myelofibrosis and the biology of connective tissue. Liss, New York, pp 359–377
4. Crystal RG, Bitterman PB, Rennard SL, Hance AJ, Keogh BA (1984) Interstitial lung disease of unknown cause: disorders characterized by chronic inflammation of the lower respiratory tract. N Engl J Med 310:54–166
5. Crystal RG, Bitterman PB, Rennard SL, Hance AJ, Keogh BA (1984) Interstitial lung diseases of unknown cause: disorders characterized by chronic inflammation of the lower respiratory tract. N Engl Med 310:235–244

6. Petty TL (1982) Adult respiratory distress syndrome: definition and historical perspective. Clin Chest Med 3:3–7
7. Bachofen M, Weibel ER (1982) Structural alteration of lung parenchyma in the adult respiratory distress syndrome. Clin Chest Med 3:35–56
8. Lamy M, Fallat RJ, Koeniger E, Dietrich HP, Ratliff JL, Eberhart RC, Tucker HJ, Hill JD (1976) Pathologic features and mechanisms of hypoxemia in adult respiratory distress syndrome. Am Rev Respir Dis 114:267–284
9. Crystal RG, Fulmer JD, Roberts WC, Moss ML, Line BR, Reynolds HY (1976) Idiopathic pulmonary fibrosis: clinical, histologic, radiographic, physiologic, scintigraphic, cytologic and biochemical aspects. Ann Intern Med 85:769–788
10. Turner-Warwick M, Burrows B, Johnson A (1980) Cryptogenic fibrosing alveolitis: clinical features and their influence on survival. Thorax 35:171–180
11. Hance AJ, Crystal RG (1983) Idiopathic pulmonary fibrosis. In: Flenley DC, Petty TL (eds) Recent advances in respiratory medicine, vol 3. Churchill Livingstone, Edinburgh, pp 249–288
12. Phan SH (1989) Diffuse interstitial fibrosis. In: Massaro D (ed) Lung cell biology, Dekker, New York, pp 907–980
13. Tracey KJ, Lowry SF, Cerami A (1988) Cachectin/TNF-alpha in septic shock and septic adult respiratory distress syndrome. Am Rev Respir Dis 138:1377–1379
14. Martinet Y, Yamauchi K, Crystal RG (1988) Differential expression of the tumor necrosis factor/cachectin gene by blood and lung mononuclear phagocytes. Am Rev Respir Dis 138:659–665
15. Martinet Y (1988) Idiopathic pulmonary fibrosis, a model of the role of macrophage profibrotic mediators in fibrosis. In: Sorg C (ed) The alveolar macrophage. Regensberg and Biermann, Münster, pp 64–78
16. Sporn MB, Roberts AB, Wakefield LM, Assoian RK (1986) Transforming growth factor-beta: biological function and chemical structure. Science 233:532–534
17. Grotendorst GR, Paglia L, Mc Ivor C, Barsky S, Martinet Y, Pencev D (1985) Chemoattractants in fibrotic disorders. Ciba Found Symp 114:150–163
18. Pledger WJ, Stiles CD, Antoniades HN, Scher CD (1977) Induction of DNA synthesis in BALB/c3T3 cells by serum components: reevaluation of the commitment process. Proc Natl Acad Sci USA 74:4481–4485
19. Stiles CD, Capone GT, Scher CD, Atoniades HN, Van Wyk JJ, Pledger WJ (1979) Dual control of cell growth by somatomedins and platelet-derived growth factor. Proc Natl Acad Sci USA 76:1279–1283
20. Deuel TF, Huang JS (1984) Platelet-derived growth factor: structure, function and roles in normal and transformed cells. J Clin Invest 74:669–676
21. Rom WN, Basset P, Fells GA, Nukiwa T, Trapnell BC, Crystal RG (1988) Alveolar macrophages release an insulin-like growth factor I-type molecule. J Clin Invest 82:1685–1693
22. Shimokado K, Raines EW, Madtes DK, Barrett TB, Benditt EP, Ross R (1985) A significant part of macrophage-derived growth factor consists of at least two forms of PDGF. Cell 43:277–286
23. Martinet Y, Bitterman PB, Mornex JF, Grotendorst GR, Martin GR, Crystal RG (1986) Activated human monocytes express the c-*sis* proto-oncogene and release a mediator showing PDGF-like activity. Nature 319:158–160
24. Mornex JF, Martinet Y, Yamauchi K, Bitterman PB, Grotendorst GR, Chytil-Weir A, Martin GR, Crystal RG (1986) Spontaneous expression of the c-*sis* gene and release of a platelet-derived growth factor-like molecule by human alveolar macrophages. J Clin Invest 78:61–66
25. Martinet Y, Jaffe HA, Yamauchi K, Betsholtz C, Westermark B, Heldin CH, Crystal RG (1987) Platelet-derived growth factor (PDGF) B-chain gene expression by activated blood monocytes precedes the expression of the PDGF A-chain gene. Fed Proc 46:1996 A
26. Yamauchi K, Martinet Y, Crystal RG (1987) Modulation of fibronectin gene expression in human mononuclear phagocytes. J Clin Invest 80:1720–1727
27. Yamauchi K, Basset P, Martinet Y, Crystal RG (1987) Normal human alveolar macrophages express the gene coding for transforming growth factor-beta, a protein with a capacity to suppress fibroblast growth. Am Rev Respir Dis 135:66 A
28. Martinet Y, Rom WN, Grotendorst GR, Martin GR, Crystal RG (1987) Exaggerated spontaneous release of platelet-derived growth factor by alveolar macrophages from patients with idiopathic pulmonary fibrosis. N Engl J Med 317:202–209

29. Rennard SI, Hunninghake GW, Bitterman PB, Crystal RG (1981) Production of fibronectin by the human alveolar macrophage: mechanism for the recruitment of fibroblast to sites of tissue injury in interstitial lung diseases. Proc Natl Acad Sci USA 78:147–151
30. Schoenberger CI, Rennard SI, Bitterman PB, Fukuda Y, Ferrans VJ, Crystal RG (1984) Paraquat-induced pulmonary fibrosis. Role of the alveolitis in modulating the development of fibrosis. Am Rev Respir Dis 129:168–173
31. Dubaybo BA, Thet LA (1986) Changes in lung tissue and lavage fibronectin after paraquat injury in rats. Res Comm Chem Pathol Pharmacol 51:211–220
32. Peters JH, Ginsberg MH, Bohl BP, Sklar LA, Cochrane CG (1986) Intravascular release of intact cellular fibronectin during oxidant-induced injury of the in vitro perfused rabbit lung. J Clin Invest 78:1596–1603
33. Snyder LS, Harmon KR, Hertz MI, Henke CA, Bitterman PB (1988) ARDS: role of platelet-derived growth factor in acute alveolar fibrosis. Am Rev Respir Dis 137:415
34. Sporn MB, Roberts AB (1986) Peptide growth factors in inflammation, tissue repair, and cancer. J Clin Invest 78:329–332
35. Dicorleto PE, Bowen-Pope DF (1983) Cultured endothelial cells produce a platelet-derived growth factor-like protein. Proc Natl Acad Sci USA 80:1919–1923
36. Harlan JM, Thompson PJ, Ross R, Bowen-Pope DF (1986) Alpha-thrombin induces the release of platelet-derived growth factor-like molecule (s) by cultured human endothelial cells. J Cell Biol 103:1129–1133
37. Gajdusek C, Carbon S, Ross R, Nawroth P, Stern D (1986) Activation of coagulation releases endothelial cell mitogens. J Cell Biol 103:419–428

Part 3:

Mediators and Nonspecific Effectors: Eicosanoids, Proteases and Oxygen Radicals

Eicosanoids and Acute Respiratory Failure – Pathophysiologic and Therapeutic Aspects

W. Seeger, D. Walmrath, and F. Grimminger

Bacterial sepsis is the most consistent factor associated with acute respiratory distress syndrome (ARDS) in adults [1–3]. Moreover, acute diffuse lung injury of different etiologies is often complicated by nosiocomial pneumonia [4–5]. In experimental models septic lung failure is mimicked by the application of lipolysaccharide compounds of gram-negative bacteria (endotoxins) and plenty of detailed information is available on the mechanisms of lung injury by these agents. There is evidence for a critical role of circulating inflammatory cells and activation of several humoral mediator systems, e.g., complement, arachidonic acid (AA) metabolites, reactive oxygen species, and proteases, has been documented; this field has recently been reviewed by Brigham and Meyrick [6, 7].

Only very little information is available on abnormalities inflicted by "non-endotoxin toxins" in the pulmonary circulation. The present contribution will focus on the effects of bacterial exotoxins, particularly *Escherichia coli* hemolysin, on hemodynamics, fluid balance, and gas exchange of isolated rabbit lungs. The role of lung eicosanoid generation, which mediates a variety of the toxin effects in this organ, will be particularly addressed. The second part will then focus on the presently available evidence of eicosanoid involvement in the pathogenesis of ARDS under clinical conditions and on possible therapeutic approaches merging from the role of eicosanoids. In the experiments with isolated rabbit lungs three bacterial exotoxins were used: *Staphylococcus aureus* alpha-toxin, *Escherichia coli* hemolysin, and *Pseudomonas aeruginosa* cytotoxin. The basic mechanisms of membrane attack by these exotoxins have been discussed [8–10]. All toxins attack outer membranes of different target cells, including inflammatory competent cells. Discrete hydrophilic transmembranous pores are formed, the effective diameter of which has been characterized. In a variety of cells this pore formation is followed by marked extra-intracellular calcium flux and subsequent marked stimulation of lung eicosanoid metabolism [11–14]. The experimental data given in the present contribution will particularly focus on the hemolysin of *Escherichia coli*. This hemolysin is the only secretory protein of *E. coli*; it has a molecular weight of 107–111 kDa; it creates hydrophilic transmembranous pores with an effective diameter of about 2 nm in a variety of target membranes; and these pores exhibit some cation selectivity [8, 9]. An enhanced pathogenicity of hemolysin-forming *E. coli* compared to non-hemolysin-forming *E. coli* has been documented in a variety of experimental models. Whereas hemolysin producing strains are infrequently encountered in the normal fecal flora, approximately 50% of *E. coli* strains causing pyelonephritis and septicemia in humans are toxin producers, thus supporting the role of this bacterial agent as an important virulence factor.

Experiments were performed in a model of isolated perfused and ventilated rabbit lung, the details of which have previously been described. This model allows the parallel measurement of a variety of physiologic variables including pulmonary artery pressure, pulmonary vascular resistance, capillary filtration coefficient (water permeability of the pulmonary microcirculation), lung weight gain, and inflation pressure. Metabolites of arachidonic acid including prostanoids, thromboxane, leukotrienes and hydroxyeicosatetraenoic acids (HETEs) can be extracted from the recirculating blood-free perfusion fluid and from the bronchoalveolar lavage fluid and are identified by a variety of chromatographic techniques as previously described [17–19].

When hemolysin-forming *E. coli* bacteria, taken in their log growth phase, are added to the blood-free perfusate of an isolated rabbit lung, a dose- and time-dependent increase in pulmonary artery pressure is noted (Fig. 1). There is steep pressure rise within 20–30 min after use of 10^6 *E. coli*/ml, whereas 10^3 *E. coli*/ml provoke a moderate and late increase in pulmonary vascular resistance after 3–4 h [20]. In contrast, isogenic non-hemolysin-forming *E. coli* bacteria provoke only a very moderate and late increase in pulmonary artery pressure even at a high concentration of 10^6 *E. coli*/ml. Moreover, the application of hemolysin-forming *E. coli* in isolated rabbit lungs causes a dose- and time-dependent increase in the capillary filtration coefficient. This is measured

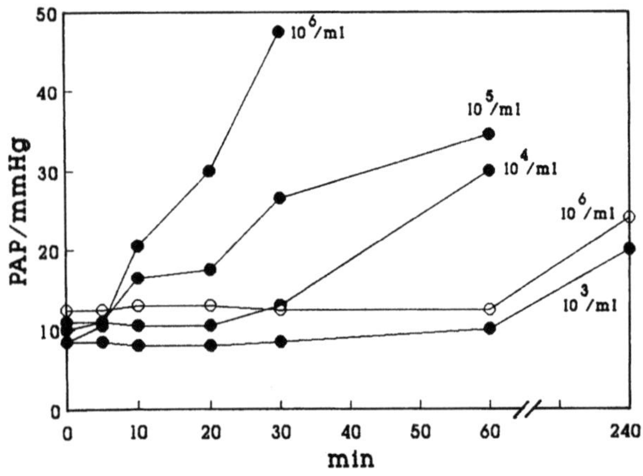

Fig. 1. Increase in pulmonary artery pressure (*PAP*) induced by hemolysin-forming *E. coli*. Different concentrations of hemolysin-forming *E. coli* were added to the recirculating Krebs-Henseleit albumin buffer of isolated rabbit lungs (*closed circles*). This procedure resulted in a dose- and time-dependent increase in pulmonary artery pressure. Controls with a high concentration of isogenic non-hemolysin-forming *E. coli*, in contrast, caused only a moderate pressor response after a delay of 4 h (*open circles*). All points reflect a mean of two independent experiments

at constant microvascular pressure in order to suppress vascular pressure-induced alterations of lung weight gain. At a concentration of 10^6 *E. coli* bacteria/ml, a more than ten times increase in the capillary filtration coefficient within 30–60 min was observed; at 10^5 *E. coli*/ml a similar severe increase in the microvascular permeability is noted within 120 min, and 10^4 *E. coli*/ml provoke virtually a doubling of the capillary filtration coefficient within 4 h [20]. Again, isogenic non-hemolysin-forming *E. coli* bacteria are virtually ineffective even at a concentration of 10^6/ml in this model. These marked biophysical increases in pulmonary vascular resistance and in pulmonary microvascular permeability are paralleled by a time- and dose-dependent release of the hemolysin into the recirculating perfusate. Moreover, these alterations can be completely mimicked by application of the isolated bacterial toxin to fresh isolated rabbit lungs in the absence of bacteria. In the concentration range between 0.05 and 5 hemolytic units/ml, corresponding to approximately 5–500 ng toxin/ml, a pulmonary artery pressure response corresponding to that upon application of hemolysin-forming *E. coli* is noted [21]. These pressure responses are accompanied by a dose-dependent release of thromboxane A_2 and prostacyclin into the recirculating perfusion fluid, as shown in Fig. 2.

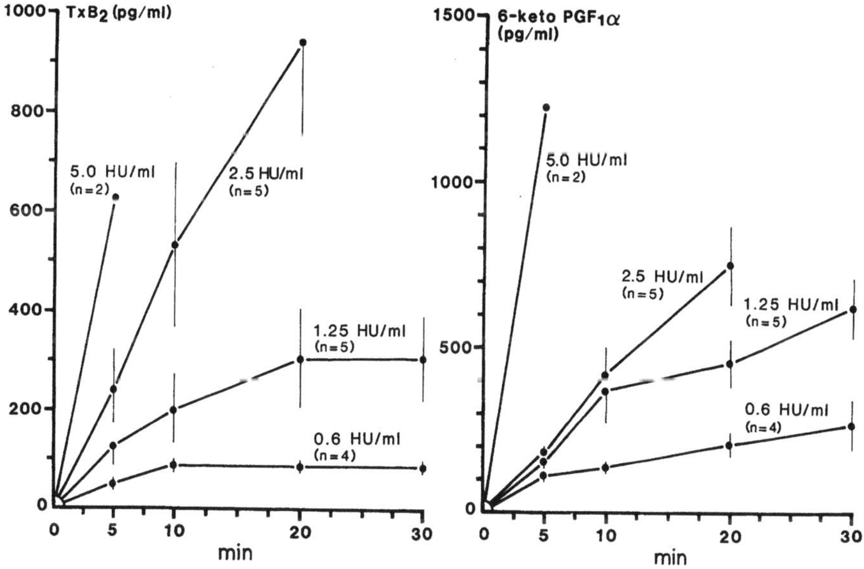

Fig. 2. Dose-dependence and time course of *E. coli* hemolysin-induced prostanoid release into the Krebs–Henseleit albumin buffer of isolated rabbit lungs. Isolated *E. coli* hemolysin was admixed to the buffer fluid in the absence of live bacteria at the given final concentrations before recirculation; 1 hemolytic unit, *HU* per ml corresponds to 100 ng/ml of this bacterial agent; The concentrations of thromboxane A_2 (*TXB_2*) and prostacyclin (measured as *6-keto-$PGF_{1\alpha}$*) in the recirculating buffer fluid at different times after administration of the various doses of hemolysin are given. All concentrations of the bacterial agent caused significant pressure responses, and in the studies with application of 2, 5, and 5 units hemolysin/ml the perfusion had to be stopped before termination of the 30 min period because of a total weight gain surpassing 20 gram. From [21]

Studies with various pharmacological agents including cyclooxygenase inhibitors, thromboxane synthetase inhibitors, and thromboxane antagonists clearly show that the hemolysin evoked thromboxane is primarily responsible for the pressure response noted upon application of this bacterial agent. Thromboxane surpasses the vasodilatory effect of the simultaneously generated prostacyclin. In addition to its effect on lung hemodynamics hemolysin causes a marked alteration of gas exchange as depicted in Fig. 3 [22]. There is a severe mismatch of ventilation and perfusion characterized by a bimodal distribution of the ventilation-perfusion ratio. Preliminary experimental evidence suggests that this ventilation-perfusion mismatch is again primarily caused by pulmonary thromboxane generation, causing "irregular" vasoconstriction throughout the rabbit lung. Moreover, a marked increase in true shunt flow due to alveolar edema formation or atelectasis is noted. Preliminary data presently suggest that this feature of gas exchange disturbance is caused by the hemolysin-induced permeability increase with subsequent leakage of protein-rich edema into the alveolar space. Thus, hemolysin-induced pulmonary thromboxane generation appears to be responsible for pulmonary artery pressure response and bimodality of ventilation-perfusion distribution in the isolated rabbit lung. The hemolysin-induced increase in lung vascular permeability, however, as well as the subsequent alveolar edema formation, accompanied by severe shunt flow, are also observed in the presence of cyclooxygenase and thus thromboxane inhibition and thus must be ascribed to different mechanisms.

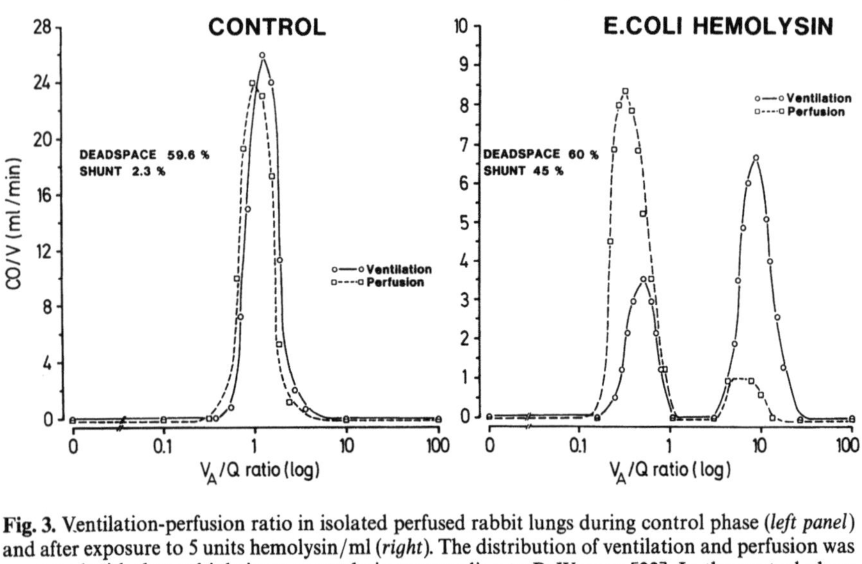

Fig. 3. Ventilation-perfusion ratio in isolated perfused rabbit lungs during control phase (*left panel*) and after exposure to 5 units hemolysin/ml (*right*). The distribution of ventilation and perfusion was measured with the multiple inert gas technique according to P. Wagner [22]. In the control phase a unimodal VQ distribution centered at a ratio of 1 with only minimal shunt flow was noted. After application of hemolysin a bimodal distribution of ventilation and perfusion occurred, accompanied by a marked shunt flow in this isolated lung; *CO*, cardiac output; *V*, ventilation; *Q*, perfusion

Are arachidonic acid lipoxygenase products responsible for these alterations? Presently, this question cannot completely be resolved but several lines of evidence suggest a contribution of lung lipoxygenase metabolism of arachidonic acid to the bacterial toxin-induced lung permeability increase. The hemolysin attack in the rabbit lung is accompanied by the dose- and time-dependent release of leukotrienes (LT) including LTC_4, LTD_4, LTE_4, and LTB_4, 5-HETE, and 12-hydroxyheptadecatrionic acid (12-HHT) into the recirculating perfusate (unpublished data). This profile of lipoxygenase product release corresponds to that obtained in the presence of another bacterial exotoxin, *Pseudomonas aeruginosa* cytotoxin, in the present model (Fig. 4). Similar to *E. coli* hemolysin, *Pseudomonas* cytotoxin causes a delayed but severe increase in lung vascular permeability, accompanied by the release of LTs (and HETEs) into the recirculating perfusate and into the bronchoalveolar space (Fig. 4). In the presence of the lipoxygenase inhibitor AA 861 the cytotoxin-induced generation of LTs and HETEs is substantially suppressed [24]. Moreover, in the presence of this lipoxygenase inhibitor the cytotoxin-induced increase in lung vascular permeability is markedly reduced and delayed, however, not completely inhibited. Thus, lipoxygenase products of arachidonic acid, separated upon exposure of the lung microvasculature to the *Pseudomonas* cytotoxin, appear to be involved in the toxin-induced increase in lung vascular permeability. Nonetheless, additional mechanisms, possibly including tumor necrosis factor generation in the lung and direct effects of the toxin on endothelial cells, must be assumed.

Presently it is not clear which lipoxygenase products of arachidonic acid are responsible for the lung permeability increase. Direct application of cysteinyl-LTs (LTC_4, LTD_4, or LTE_4) or LTB_4 into the intravascular space of blood-free perfused lungs does not reproduce an increase in vascular permeability [16, 25, 26]. Thus, HETEs may be of importance in this context, as suggested by experiments with lipoxygenase inhibitors, which affected the arachidonic acid-induced lung permeability increase [16], and as recently suggested for 5-HETE and 15-HETE in isolated guinea pig lungs [27]. It may, however, be a major difference whether these lipoxygenase products are offered to the lung vascular endothelium from the luminal side (as reproduced by bolus application of these agents), are generated within pulmonary cells and possibly endothelial cells (see below), or are like albumin to these cells. Moreover, lung lipoxygenase metabolism of arachidonic acid is even more complicated in the presence of granulocytes adhering to the endothelial surface. Under these circumstances intercellular cooperation in eicosanoid generation ensues as depicted in Fig. 5 [18, 19, 28]. Upon adherence to the endothelial surface the profile of neutrophil arachidonic acid metabolism is altered: there is a reduction of 5-HETE generation with predominance of LTA_4 generation (precursor of LTs) within the 5-lipoxygenase pathway. The unstable LT precursor LTA_4 is, however, not released into the extravascular space, as observed in experiments in vitro with rapid hydrolysis to nonenzymatic products, but is transferred to different acceptor cells including lung endothelial cells. By this mechanism the

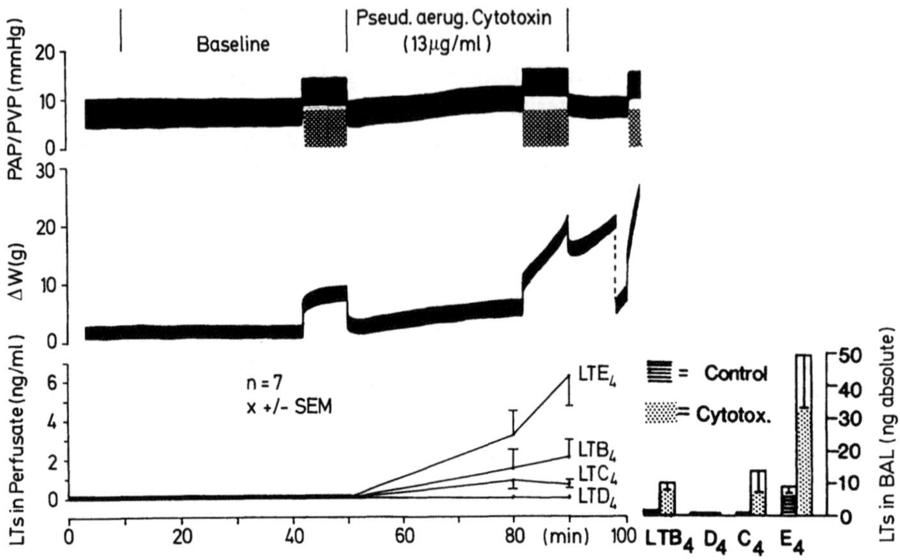

Fig. 4. Increase in pulmonary vascular permeability and leukotriene generation in isolated rabbit lungs exposed to *Pseudomonas aeruginosa* cytotoxin. Pulmonary artery pressure, *PAP*; pulmonary venous pressure, *PVP*, indicated by *shaded area* if different from O; and lung weight gain, *W*; the *vertical lines* indicate changes of perfusion fluid. The lung was perfused with Krebs-Henseleit buffer. A sequence of three pulmonary venous pressure challenges were induced (*shaded areas*). Each of these maneuvers caused an instantaneous rise in PAP, an immediate rise in lung weight (assumed to represent mainly filling of the vascular compartment), and a slower phase of weight gain (assumed to represent mainly fluid filtration), from which the capillary filtration coefficient is calculated. Under baseline conditions this venous pressure challenge evokes a flat curve of fluid filtration corresponding to a low capillary filtration coefficient with only very small net weight gain after discontinuation of the pressure elevation. After exposure to the *Pseudomonas* cytotoxin, the venous pressure elevation causes a steep slope of fluid filtration, indicative of a several-fold increase in the capillary filtration coefficient accompanied by marked net weight gain (the *dotted line* between the 2nd and 3rd venous challenge indicates baseline readjustment due to already marked weight gain at this time). During baseline conditions no considerable amounts of leukotriene (*LTs*) C_4, D_4, E_4, or B_4 are measured in the recirculating perfusate. However, marked amounts of these lipoxygenase products of arachidonic acid are released in the presence of the bacterial agent. Moreover, analysis of the bronchoalveolar lavage fluid (BAL) of cytotoxin exposed lungs, but not of control lungs, reveals an accumulation of these lipid mediators in the bronchoalveolar space

enzymatic equipment of lung endothelial cells is evidently used to form large amounts of cysteinyl-LTs from the granulocyte-derived LTA_4. Lung endothelial acceptor cells, e.g., interstitial or intra-alveolar macrophages, must be assumed to take up neutrophil-derived LTA_4 with rapid subsequent conversion to the chemotactic agent LTB_4. This way a chemotactic gradient into the intra-alveolar space might be created by the granulocyte itself. Moreover, there is evidence that granulocytes are "fed" by endothelial cells with arachidonic acid, thus perpetuating the generation of LTA_4 and LTA_4-derived products. In summary, this intercellular cooperation in lung lipoxygenase metabolism results in a potentiation of eicosanoid generation, particularly in the generation of LTs,

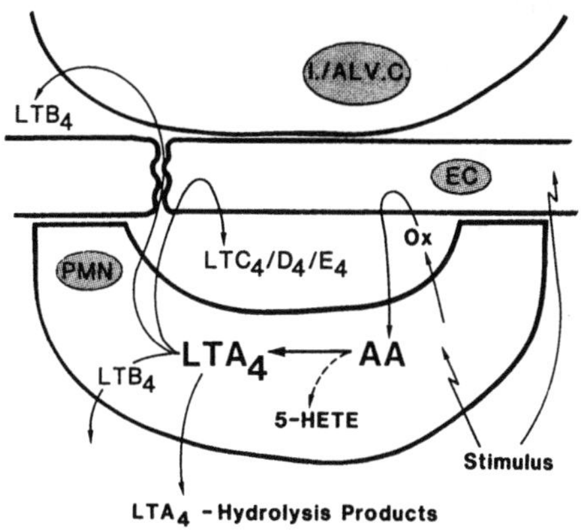

Fig. 5. Cooperative leukotriene generation upon granulocytes sticking in the pulmonary microcirculation. An adhering granulocyte (*PMN*), endothelial cells (*EC*), and an interstitial or an alveolar cell (1., ALV. C.), which is not further characterized, are indicated. Under these circumstances, the granulocyte-derived leukotriene precursor LTA_4 is transferred into endothelial and non-endothelial acceptor cells with subsequent formation of leukotriene C_4, D_4, E_4, and B_4. Secretion of LTA_4 into the free intravascular space with subsequent generation of nonenzymatic hydrolysis products of this leukotriene precursor is reduced under these circumstances. Moreover, stimulation of endothelial cells, possibly by neutrophil-derived oxidants, must be assumed to "feed" the adhering granulocyte with arachidonic acid, thus potentiating the overall sum of leukotrienes formed in this model of cooperative eicosanoid synthesis

and in an alteration of mediator profile compared to stimulation of granulocytes in vitro. Presently it is, however, not yet known how these complex mechanisms of transcellular eicosanoid generation in the lung microvasculature are related to biophysical alterations encountered under conditions of marked stimulation of lung eicosanoid generation.

The main results of the presented experimental data are summarized in Fig. 6. Based on the effects of bacterial exotoxins in isolated lungs as a model of septic ARDS it was shown that stimulation of lung cyclooxygenase metabolism of arachidonic acid with predominance of thromboxane generation is primarily responsible for the increase in pulmonary artery pressure, for a bimodality in perfusion-ventilation distribution (mismatch), and, most probably due to postcapillary vasoconstriction, for an increase in lung microvascular pressure. Stimulation of lung lipoxygenase metabolism causes a large variety of products including LTs and HETEs, which are not of major importance for lung pressure rise and microvascular pressure rise in the isolated rabbit lung. Concerning this vasoactivity of LTs and HETEs, however, there may be major species differences. In the rabbit lung the lipoxygenase metabolism of arachidonic acid is related to an increase in the capillary filtration coefficient with subsequent formation of protein-rich interstitial and alveolar edema, followed by marked shunt flow. Lung-derived LTB_4 and 5-HETE are relevant for the induction of granulocyte adherence and diapedesis. Corresponding effects related to stimulation of lung eicosanoid metabolism as evoked by bacterial toxins have been observed upon induction of the terminal complement complex and in the presence of fibrin monomer and granulocyte-derived hydrogen peroxide in this model [29–31].

What is in the evidence for a contribution of eicosanoids to the pathogenesis or the perpetuation of inflammatory events in ARDS under clinical conditions?

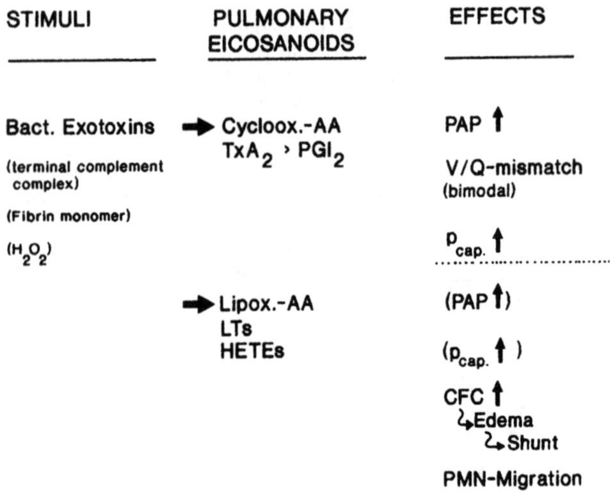

Fig. 6. Summary of pulmonary effects evoked by bacterial exotoxins and related to cyclooxygenase products and lipoxygenase products of arachidonic acid; *AA*, arachidonic acid; *TX*, thromboxane; *PG*, prostaglandin; *LT*, leukotriene; *HETE*, hydroxyeicosatetraenoic acid; *PAP*, pulmonary artery pressure; *V/Q*, ventilation/perfusion ratio; p_{cap}, capillary pressure; *CFC*, capillary filtration coefficient; *PMN*, polymorphonuclear granulocyte. For details see text

Studies with bronchoalveolar lavage showed increased levels of thromboxane and lipoxygenase products of arachidonic acid in the lavage fluid. In 15 out of 17 lavage samples from patients with ARDS, LTB_4 or its metabolites 20-hydroxy-LTB_4 and 20-COOH-LTB_4 were detected, and the end product of omega-oxidation 20-COOH-LTB_4 was the quantitatively predominant compound, detected in the range of 0.3–2.7 ng/ml perfusate [32]. In contrast, in none of eight lavage samples from patients with cardiogenic edema and none of ten lavage samples from healthy volunteers these LTs were detected. Stephenson et al. recently showed evidence for the presence of cysteinyl-LTs (LTC_4 and LTD_4) in the lavage fluid of patients at risk of ARDS and at even higher levels of patients with established ARDS by using immunological methods, though direct chromatographic evidence for these lipoxygenase products of arachidonic acid was not given. Thus, there is evidence for increased concentrations of eicosanoids, at least in the bronchoalveolar space, in the lungs of patients with ARDS, and future studies with improved analytical techniques will most probably support these findings.

Is there also evidence for a pathogenetic role of these lipid mediators in the development of respiratory failure under clinical circumstances? The main obstacle to answering this question at the present time is the lack of availability of specific inhibitors and/or antagonists, which can be used under clinical circumstances. Substances that are presently used in clinical trials are the vasodilatory prostanoids prostaglandin E_1 and prostacyclin. Continuous central venous infusion of these short-lived vasodilatory agents causes a decrease of the augmented pulmonary vascular resistance in patients with ARDS, accompanied by an increase of cardiac output, as shown in a variety of studies [34–39]. In a subgroup of ARDS patients with a predominance of pulmonary hypertension an acute and far-reaching alteration of pulmonary hemodynamics can be achieved by these agents, as demonstrated in an example in Fig. 7. However, two recent publications with measurements of ventilation-perfusion distribution using multiple inert gas analysis showed that the decrease in pulmonary vascular resistance was accompanied by an increase in the perfusion of non-ventilated

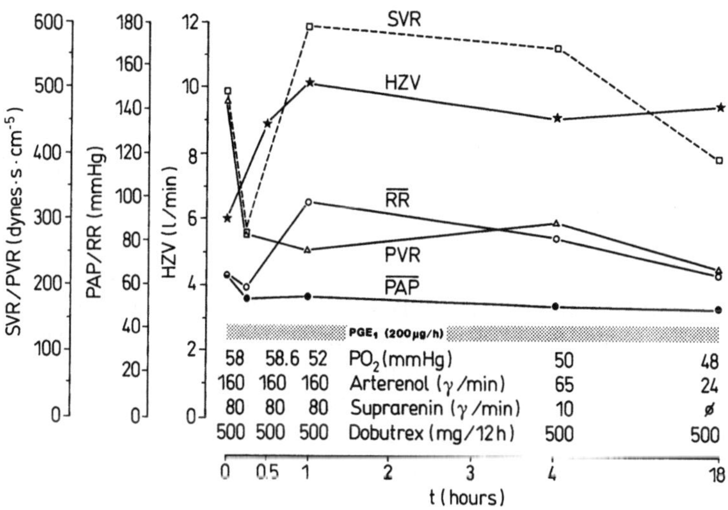

Fig. 7. Clinical example of an acute effect of high dose prostaglandin (*PG*) E_1 on pulmonary hemodynamics. The example gives data from a 41 year old female patient, who suffered from chronic allergic alveolitis with accompanying interstitial fibrosis and who acquired a severe superinfection with bacteria and *Candida albicans*. An extremely severe deterioration of gas exchange developed: in spite of mechanical ventilation with 100% oxygen an arterial PO_2 of only 55–60 mmHg was achieved. Moreover, the patient developed critical hemodynamic conditions. Due to an overall septic state she had a low systemic vascular resistance (*SVR*), which could not be increased even by high doses of norepinephrine (*Arterenol*). Due to a several-fold increase in pulmonary vascular resistance *PVR*), right heart failure with low cardiac output occurred. In spite of high doses of dobutamine (*Dobutrex*) and epinephrine (*Suprarenin*) a cardiac output (*HZV*) sufficient for the septic state could not be achieved. The patient had a low systemic arterial pressure (*RR*) and a high pulmonary artery pressure (*PAP*), and a hemodynamic shock state with increasing generation of lactate developed. Assuming massive pulmonary vasoconstriction superimposed on anatomically fixed increased resistance in the lung of this patient, PGE_1 as vasodilator was given to counteract suspected effects of vasoconstrictive prostanoids. At the high dose of 200 µg PGE_1/h, the pulmonary vascular resistance could nearly be halved, whereas the systemic vascular resistance, after a short initial drop, remained more or less constant. This resulted in a markedly reduced afterload of the right ventricle with subsequent increases in cardiac output and systemic arterial pressure. During this therapeutic approach only a slight decrease of arterial PO_2 was noted, and oxygen delivery markedly increased in parallel with the increase in cardiac output. This marked effect of PGE_1 application could be maintained, even upon reduction of norepinephrine and epinephrine application, for more than 18 h. This instantaneous effect of a high dose application of a vasodilative agent demonstrates a marked contribution of vasospasm to the increase in pulmonary vascular resistance due to diffuse distribution of inflammatory events in the lung of this patient

areas, i.e., an increase in shunt flow, in the majority of ARDS patients [38, 39]. This increase in true shunt flow is partially outweighed by an increase in venous oxygenation due to the rising cardiac output, which reduces the contribution of the shunted blood to the drop in arterial oxygenation. Nevertheless, there is a decrease in arterial oxygenation in most ARDS patients treated by infusion of prostaglandin E_2.

At the present time it is not clear whether a similar negative influence on ventilation-perfusion distribution is also achieved by application of prostacyclin in ARDS patients. In spite of a possible decrease in arterial oxygen content, oxygen delivery rises in virtually all patients treated with prostaglandin E_1 or prostacyclin [40] due to the increase in cardiac output. It is presently not clear whether this increase in oxygen delivery is accompanied by an increase of whole body oxygen uptake, which surpasses the increasing oxygen uptake attributable to a rise in heart work. A marked increase in oxygen uptake during administration of 5 ng prostacyclin/kg body weight in 27 critically ill ARDS patients has been documented by Bihari et al. [40]. These authors speculate that this increased oxygen uptake might reduce the tendency to develop multiple organ failure in these patients. It is, however, presently not proven whether the incidence of additional organ failure in ARDS patients can be reduced by prostacyclin application and whether this vasodilatory prostanoid causes an improvement of outcome. Such an improvement in overall survival in ARDS patients was noted in a prospective trial using a 7-day infusion of prostaglandin E_2 in surgical patients with acute respiratory failure [37]. This finding could, however, not be confirmed by multicenter studies. Thus, the present conclusion concerning vasodilatory prostanoids is that they can be used to decrease pulmonary vasoconstriction and therefore to increase cardiac output in individual patients; however, one must be aware of possible adverse effects on ventilation-perfusion distribution (increase in shunt flow). There also is no clear evidence for a decrease in the development of additional organ failures or an improvement of overall survival at the present time.

Neither prostanoid possesses "pulmonary specificity" nor "intrapulmonary specificity." The former means that both prostaglandin E_1 and prostacyclin cause vasodilation not only in the pulmonary vasculature but also in the peripheral circulation with resulting decrease of systemic vascular resistance. Theoretically, this effect should be much less upon use of prostaglandin E_1, as this prostanoid is metabolized during one passage in the pulmonary circulation by more than 75%. Measurements under experimental and clinical conditions of respiratory failure have, however, shown that the rate of lung PGE_1 metabolism (pulmonary extraction of this agent) is markedly depressed under these circumstances. This finding may explain why in the majority of ARDS patients the decrease in pulmonary vascular resistance is accompanied by a corresponding decrease in systemic vascular resistance. The lack of "intrapulmonary specificity" is illustrated by the example of hemolysin-induced perfusion-ventilation mismatch demonstrated in Fig. 8. Following this example of septic ARDS, it might be very useful to antagonize the hemolysin triggered unphysiologic

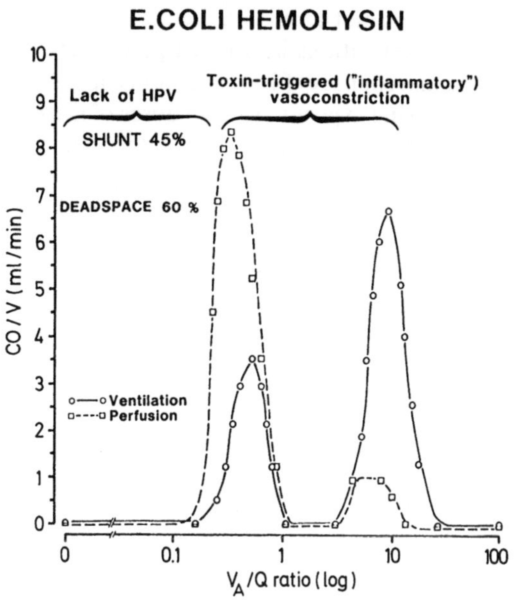

Fig. 8. Deterioration of gas exchange induced by *E. coli* hemolysin in isolated rabbit lungs, assumed to be caused by toxin triggered (thromboxane-mediated) vasoconstriction and by a lack of hypoxic pulmonary vasoconstriction (*HPV*). For details see legend of Fig. 3

("inflammatory") vasoconstriction, which appears to be responsible for the noted bimodal distribution of ventilation and perfusion. At the same time, however, the marked perfusion of nonventilated lung areas, i.e., the shunt flow, should not be further increased. This means that a suitable antagonist should inhibit vasoconstriction induced by inflammatory mechanisms but should not reduce the hypoxic vasoconstriction (Euler–Lilljestrand mechanism). It might even be desirable to strengthen the hypoxic vasoconstriction under these circumstances, which appears to be principally possible, as documented in a recent investigation on the effects of almitrine in gas exchange in ARDS patients [43].

An additional pharmacological approach to influence lung eicosanoid metabolism which can be used under clinical conditions is the application of high doses of corticosteroids. These agents have been shown to reduce phospholipase activity via induction of lipocortin in a variety of cell systems. A reduction of the generation of cyclooxygenase products and lipoxygenase products of arachidonic acid can thus be expected. Controlled clinical studies using high dose corticosteroids in patients with ARDS have, however, not shown any beneficial effects of this treatment on the development of the disease and the outcome of patients, but rather an increased rate of secondary infections was noted [44–48]. How can these results be reconciled with a possible role of eicosanoids in ARDS? First, corticosteroids have a large number of different effects on various cell and mediator systems, i.e., they are nonspecific in terms of arachidonic acid metabolism, and their overall effect can hardly be predicted from their various biological efficacies. Second, corticosteroids were given quite late in the course of ARDS in some of the above mentioned clinical studies.

Third, even high doses of corticosteroids do not at all completely inhibit lung eicosanoid metabolism. Experimental investigations in isolated pulmonary endothelial cells [49] and in isolated lung macrophages [50] have shown a marked reduction of eicosanoid metabolism following exposure to high doses of methylprednisolone. Pulmonary mast cells, however, do not respond to high dose corticosteroids in terms of arachidonic acid metabolism, and experimental studies using the model of isolated rabbit lungs showed only a very moderate influence of rabbit or lung pretreatment with high dose corticosteroids on bacterial exotoxin evoked arachidonic acid metabolism (unpublished results). Summing up, lack of evidence for a beneficial effect of corticosteroids in ARDS does not rule out a possible significance of eicosanoids in the pathogenesis of this syndrome. For a definitive evaluation of a role of these lipid mediators in the initiation or perpetuation of ARDS clinical studies with specific antagonists and/or inhibitors will be necessary. Among those, inhibitors or antagonists of thromboxane or a combination of both (the latter may be particularly profitable for pharmacological reasons), inhibitors or antagonists of LTs or a combination of both, and inhibitors of HETE generation or antagonists of these agents may be of particular interest.

Several variables should be influenced by these agents. First, they should inhibit excessive vasoconstriction triggered by inflammatory events without simultaneous inhibition of hypoxic vasoconstriction. If possible, hypoxic vasoconstriction, i.e., deviation of blood flow from nonventilated areas to ventilated areas, should even be reinforced. An inhibition of post-capillary venoconstriction triggered by inflammatory events would contribute to a reduction in microvascular pressure and thus to a reduction in lung edema formation. Second, a reduction in permeability increase in the pulmonary microvasculature may be expected from these agents. Capillary endothelial as well as alveoloepithelial permeability with the consequences of protein-rich interstitial and intra-alveolar edema should be addressed in this regard. Third, a reduction of pulmonary generation of chemotactic eicosanoids should result in a reduced lung vascular adherence and migration of granulocytes and thus in reduced perpetuation of inflammatory events centered around these cells. Fourth, oxygen delivery and possibly whole body oxygen uptake may be increased by the use of inhibitors and/or antagonists of vasoconstrictor eicosanoids, which might have considerable impact on the development of multi organ failure. Inhibitors and/or antagonists of eicosanoid metabolism may thus have a possible future role in prevention or treatment of acute respiratory failure; however, definitive answers await clinical studies.

References

1. Fowler AA, Hamman RF, Zerbe GO, Benson KN, Hyers TM (1985) Adult respiratory distress syndrome. Prognosis after onset. Am Rev Respir Dis 132:472–478

2. Montgomery AB, Stager MA, Carrico CJ, Hudson LD (1985) Causes of mortality in patients with the adult respiratory distress syndrome. Am Rev Respir Dis 132:485–489
3. Petty TL (1985) Indicators of risk, course, and prognosis in adult respiratory distress syndrome (ARDS). Am Rev Respir Dis 132:471–472
4. Andrews CP, Coalson JJ, Smith JD, Johanson WG (1981) Diagnosis of nosocomial pneumonia in acute, diffuse lung injury. Chest 80:254–258
5. Bodey GP, Jadeja L, Elting L (1985) *Pseudomonas* bacteremia. Arch Intern Med 145: 1621–1629
6. Brigham KL, Meyrick B (1984) Interactions of granulocytes with the lung. Circ Res 54: 623–635
7. Brigham KL, Meyrick B (1986) Endotoxin and lung injury. Am Rev Respir Dis 133: 913–927
8. Bhakdi S, Tranum-Jensen J (1987) Damage to mammalian cells by proteins that form transmembrane pores. Rev Physiol Biochem Pharmacol 107:148–223
9. Bhakdi S, Tranum-Jensen J (1988) Damage to cell membranes by pore-forming bacterial cytolysins. Prog Allergy 40:1–43
10. Lutz F (1986) Interactions of *Pseudomonas aeruginosa* cytotoxin with plasma membranes from Ehrlich ascites tumor cells. Naunyn Schmiedebergs Arch Pharmacol 332:103–110
11. Seeger W, Suttorp N, Hellwig A, Bhakdi S (1986) Non-cytolytic terminal complement complexes may serve as calcium gates to elicit leukotriene generation in human polymorphonuclear leukocytes. J Immunol 137:1286–1293
12. Suttorp N, Seeger W, Dewein E, Bhakdi S, Roka L (1985) Staphylococcal alpha-toxin induced PGI_2 production in endothelial cells: role of calcium. Am J Physiol 248:C127–C134
13. Suttorp N, Seeger W, Uhl J, Lutz F, Roka L (1985) *Pseudomonas aeruginosa* cytotoxin stimulates prostacyclin production in cultured pulmonary artery endothelial cells: Membrane attack and calcium influx. J Cell Physiol 123:64–72
14. Suttorp N, Seeger W, Zucker-Reimann J, Roka L, Bhakdi S (1987) Mechanism of leukotriene generation in polymorphonuclear leukocytes by staphylococcal alpha-toxin. Infect Immun 55:104–110
15. Seeger W, Walmrath D, Menger M, Neuhof H (1986) Increased lung vascular permeability after arachidonic acid and hydrostatic challenge. J Appl Physiol 61:1781–1788
16. Seeger W, Menger M, Walmrath D, Becker G, Grimminger F, Neuhof H (1987) Arachidonic acid lipoxygenase pathways and increased vascular permeability in isolated rabbit lungs. Am Rev Respir Dis 136:964–972
17. Schulz R, Seeger W (1986) Release of leukotrienes into the perfusate of calcium-ionophore stimulated rabbit lungs: influence of 5-lipoxygenase inhibitors. Biochem Pharmacol 35: 183–193
18. Grimminger F, Becker G, Seeger W (1988) High yield enzymatic conversion of intravascular leukotriene A_4 in blood-free perfused lungs. J Immunol 141:2431–2436
19. Grimminger F, Menger M, Becker G, Seeger W (1988) Potentiation of leukotriene generation following sequestration of neutrophils in isolated lungs. Blood 72:1687–1692
20. Seeger W, Obernitz R, Thomas M, Walmrath D, Bhakdi S (1991) Effect of hemolysin-forming *Escherichia coli* in isolated rabbit lungs 143:797–805
21. Seeger W, Walter H, Suttorp N, Bhakdi S (1989) Thromboxane-mediated hypertension and vascular leakage by low doses of *Escherichia coli* hemolysin in rabbit lungs. J Clin Invest 84: 220–227, 1989
22. Walmrath D, König R, Grimminger F, Neuhof H, Seeger W (1990) Effect of bacterial exotoxins on ventilation-perfusion-mismatch in isolated lungs (to be published)
23. Seeger W, Walmrath D, Neuhof H, Lutz F (1986) Pulmonary microvascular injury induced by *Pseudomonas aeruginosa* cytotoxin in isolated rabbit lungs. Infect Immun 52:846–852
24. Grimminger F, Birkemeyer R, Seeger W (1991) *Pseudomonas aeruginosa* cytotoxin provokes leukotriene generation in isolated rabbit lungs 163:362–370
25. Albert RK, Lamm WJE, Henderson WR, Bolin RW (1989) Effect of leukotrienes B_4, C_4, and D_4 on segmental pulmonary vascular pressures. J Appl Physiol 66:458–464
26. Noonan TC, Selig WM, Burhop KE, Burgess CA, Malik AB (1988) Pulmonary microvascular response to LTB_4: effects of perfusate composition. J Appl Physiol 64:1989–1996
27. Burhop KE, Selig WM, Malik AB (1988) Monohydroxyeicosatetraenoic acids (5-HETE and 15-HETE) induce pulmonary vasoconstriction and edema. Circ Res 62:687–698
28. Grimminger F, Kreusler B, Schneider U, Becker G, Seeger W (1990) Influence of microvascular

adherence on neutrophil leukotriene generation – evidence for cooperative eicosanoid synthesis. J Immunol 144:1866–1872
29. Seeger W, Hartmann R, Neuhof H, Bhakdi S (1989) Local complement activation, thromboxane-mediated vasoconstriction and vascular leakage in isolated lungs – role of the terminal complement sequence. Am Rev Respir Dis 139:88–99
30. Seeger W, Neuhof H, Hall J, Roka L (1988) Pulmonary vasoconstrictor response to soluble fibrin in isolated lungs: possible role of thromboxane generation. Circ Res 62:651–659
31. Seeger W, Suttorp N, Schmidt F, Neuhof H (1986) The glutathione redox cycle as a defense system against H_2O_2-induced prostanoid formation and vasoconstriction in rabbit lungs. Am Rev Respir Dis 133:1029–1036
32. Seeger W, Grimminger F, Barden M, Becker G, Lohmeyer J, Heinrich D, Lasch HG (1991) Leukotrienes detected in the bronchoalveolar lavage fluid of patients with non-cardiogenic pulmonary edema, but not in those with cardiogenic edema Intensive Care Med. 17:1–6
33. Stephenson AH, Lonigro AJ, Hyers TM, Webster RO, Fowler AA (1988) Increased concentrations of leukotrienes in bronchoalveolar lavage fluid of patients with ARDS or at risk for ARDS. Am Rev Respir Dis 138:714–719
34. Appel PL, Shoemaker WC (1984) Hemodynamic and oxygen transport effects of prostaglandin E_1 in patients with adult respiratory distress syndrome. Crit Care Med 12:528
35. Tokioka H, Kobayashi O, Otha Y, Wakabayashi T, Kosaka F (1985) The acute effects of prostaglandin E_1 on the pulmonary circulation and oxygen delivery in patients with the adult respiratory distress syndrome. Intensive Care Med 11:61–64
36. Shoemaker WC, Appel PL (1986) Effects of prostaglandin E_1 in adult respiratory distress syndrome. Surgery 99:275–282
37. Holcroft JW, Vassar MJ, Weber CJ (1986) Prostaglandin E_1 and survival in patients with the adult respiratory distress syndrome. Ann Surg 203:371–378
38. Melot C, Lejeune P, Leeman M, Moraine JJ, Naeije R (1989) Prostaglandin E_1 in the adult respiratory distress syndrome. Am Rev Respir Dis 139:106–110
39. Radermacher P, Santak B, Becker H, Falke KJ (1989) Prostaglandin E_1 and nitroglycerin reduce pulmonary capillary pressure but worsen ventilation-perfusion distributions in patients with adult respiratory distress syndrome. Anesthesiology 70:601–606
40. Bihari D, Smithies M, Gimson A, Tinker J (1987) The effects of vasodilation with prostacyclin on oxygen delivery and uptake in critically ill patients. N Engl J Med 317:397–403
41. Gillis CN, Pitt BR, Wiedemann HP, Hammond GL (1986) Depressed prostaglandin E_1 and 5-hydroxytryptamine removal in patients with adult respiratory distress syndrome. Am Rev Respir Dis 134:739–744
42. Cox JW, Andreadis NA, Bone RC, Maunder RJ, Pullen RH, Ursprung JJ, Vassar MJ (1988) Pulmonary extraction and pharmacokinetics of prostaglandin E_1 during continuous intravenous infusion in patients with adult respiratory distress syndrome. Am Rev Respir Dis 137:5–12
43. Reyes A, Roca J, Rodriguez-Roisin R, Torres A, Ussetti P, Wagner PD (1988) Effect of almitrine on ventilation-perfusion distribution in adult respiratory distress syndrome. Am Rev Respir Dis 137:1062–1067
44. Bernard GR, Luce JM, Sprung CL, Rinaldo JE, Tate RM, Sibbald WJ, Kariman K, Higgins S, Bradley R, Metz CA, Harris TR, Brigham KL (1987) High-dose corticosteroids in patients with the adult respiratory distress syndrome. N Engl J Med 317:1565–1570
45. Luce JM, Montgomery AB, Marks JD, Turner J, Metz CA, Murray JF (1988) Ineffectiveness of high-dose methylprednisolone in preventing parenchymal lung injury and improving mortality in patients with septic shock. Am Rev Respir Dis 138:62–68
46. Bone RC, Fisher CJ, Clemmer TP, Slotman GJ, Metz CA, Balk RA, The Methylprednisolone Severe Sepsis Study Group (1987) A controlled clinical trial of high-dose methylprednisolone in the treatment of severe sepsis and septic shock. N Engl J Med 317:653–658
47. The Veterans Administration Systemic Sepsis Cooperative Study Group (1987) Effect of high-dose glucocorticoid therapy on mortality in patients with clinical signs of systemic sepsis. N Engl J Med 317:659–665
48. Bone RC, Fisher CJ, Clemmer TP, Slotman GJ, Metz CA, The Methylprednisolone Severe Sepsis Study Group (1987) Early methylprednisolone treatment for septic syndrome and the adult respiratory distress syndrome. Chest 92:1032–1036
49. Suttorp N, Galanos C, Neuhof H (1987) Endotoxin alters arachidonate metabolism in pulmonary endothelial cells. Am J Physiol 253:C384–C390

50. Balter MS, Eschenbacher WL, Peters-Golden M (1988) Arachidonic acid metabolism in cultured alveolar macrophages from normal, atopic and asthmatic subjects. Am Rev Respir Dis 138:1134–1142
51. Schleimer RP, Schulman ES, MacGlashan DW (1983) Effects of dexamethasone on mediator release from human lung fragments and purified human lung mast cells. J Clin Invest 71:1830–1835

Dietary Modification of the Arachidonic Acid Cascade

P.C. Weber

Introduction

Eicosanoids, the oxygenation products of arachidonic acid (AA; C20:4n − 6) or related 20-carbon polyunsaturated fatty acids, are involved in the pathophysiology of the acute phase response and in allergic, atherothrombotic, and chronic inflammatory disorders. Interference with eicosanoid formation is characteristic of steroidal and nonsteroidal antiinflammatory agents, antiplatelet and other cardiovascular drugs, and – in conjunction with the eicosanoid receptor blockers – a target of refined pharmacological intervention strategies. A change in the arachidonic acid cascade and eicosanoid-dependent cellular functions may also be achieved by a nutritional modification of the eicosanoid precursor fatty acid pool.

During the last few years the biochemistry of marine long-chain n − 3 fatty acids, their eicosanoids and their influence on the arachidonic acid cascade has attracted much attention. Eicosanoids and related lipid mediators, such as 1,2 diacylglycerol (DAG) or platelet activating factor (PAF), function as a modulatory device in stimulus-response coupling and cell to cell communication. The scheme in Fig. 1 shows that some eicosanoids, like thromboxane A_2 (TXA_2) and leukotriene (LT) B_4, might amplify an initial (Ca^{2+}-related) signal for cell activation by stimulating specific membrane receptors coupled to phospholipases, (PLS) (e.g., PLC, PLA_2), thereby further increasing intracellular Ca^{2+} concentrations. Other eicosanoids, such as prostaglandin (PG)I_2 or PGD_2 – via an increase in cAMP – might, on the contrary, blunt an initial signal for cell activation by decreasing intracellular Ca^{2+}-release. Pharmacological modification of phospholipases, cyclooxygenase and lipoxygenase activities, or eicosanoid receptors and/or nutritional modification of membrane fatty acid composition, and thus the eicosanoid precursor pool, lead to a qualitative change in the spectrum of eicosanoids formed, which, in turn, might alter these regulators of cell function.

Nutrition and the Eicosanoid System

Under our "western" dietary conditions, arachidonic acid is by far the dominant precursor fatty acid for eicosanoid formation. This is at variance with the

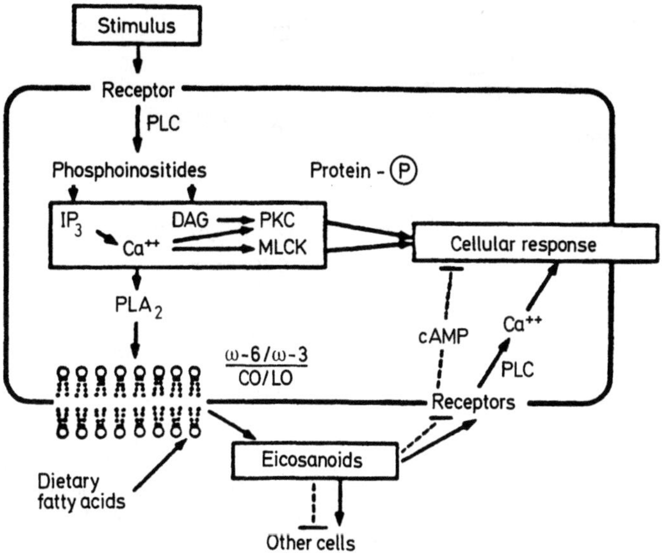

Fig. 1. The putative role of n − 6 and n − 3 eicosanoid precursor fatty acids in membrane phospholipids, as determined by dietary intake, and their eicosanoids in the modulation of stimulus-response coupling and cell to cell communication. *PLC*, phospholipase C; IP_3, inositol triphosphate; *DAG*, 1,2 diacylglycerol; *PKC*, protein kinase C; *MLCK*, myosin light chain kinase; PLA_2 phospholipase A_2; *CO*, cyclo-oxygenase; *LO*, lipoxygenase; *Protein-P*, phosphorylated proteins

putative diet of our ancestors which had always been much lower in total fat but relatively rich in n − 3 fatty acids. In the mammalian organism fatty acids belonging to different families, such as n − 3 and n − 6 fatty acids, cannot be interconverted (Fig. 2). Nutritional intake, therefore, determines the fatty acid composition of phospholipids in plasma and in cell membranes. Short- and long-chain n − 6 and n − 3 fatty acids in the diet are rapidly absorbed and incorporated into plasma lipids over a period of hours. Most incorporation of these fatty acids into cellular membrane phospholipids takes longer and appears to occur during cell formation, at least under in vivo conditions in the unstimulated cell. In vivo in the adult organism the formation of the eicosanoid precursor fatty acids from their respective short-chain parent fatty acids, C18: 2n − 6 or C18:3n − 3, is a slow process. This implies that the long-chain eicosanoid precursor fatty acids in the diet might have a more direct and immediate effect on the eicosanoid precursor pool.

The desaturation step from n − 6 fatty acids to n − 3 fatty acids is carried out exclusively in the green leaves of plants, algae, and phytoplankton to form linolenic acid (LA; C18:3n − 3) from linoleic acid (LA; C18:2n − 6). Higher in the marine food chain there is accumulation of the long-chain n − 3 derivatives of C18, 3n − 3, i.e., eicosapentaenoic (EPA; C20:5n − 3) and docosahexaenoic (DCHA; C22:6n − 3) acids, in the lipids of zooplankton and fish. Several independent lines of evidence suggest that an increased intake of long-chain

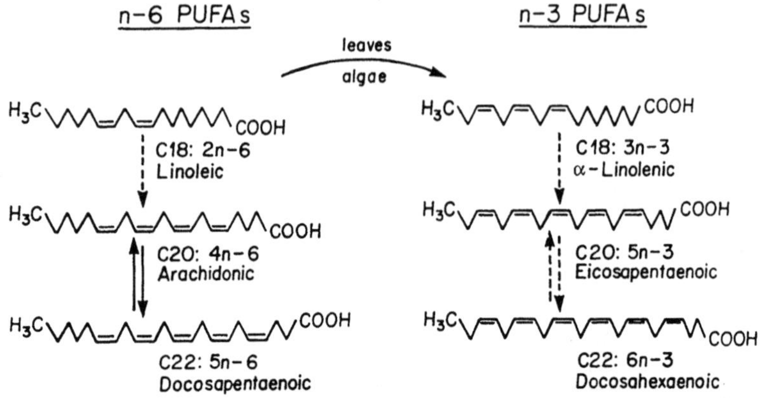

Fig. 2. Relation of important polyunsaturated fatty acids (*PUFAs*) of the n − 6 and n − 3 classes. The transformations depicted by the *arrows* incorporate two or more reaction steps. The chemical and spatial formulas of the fatty acids are shown. For example, in *C18 : 2n − 6*, the chemical formula for linoleic acid, *C18* indicates the number of carbon atoms and *2 t*he number of unsaturated carbon–carbon double bonds, the position of which is shown in the adjacent spatial formula. *n − 6* denotes both the number of carbon atoms from the methyl end of the molecule to the first double bond and the class of fatty acid. The *arching arrow* indicates that only in leaves and algae is n − 6 linoleic acid desaturated to form n − 3 α-linolenic acid, the progenitor of the n − 3 class of fatty acids

n − 3 fatty acids leads to a reduction of atherothrombotic, allergic, chronic inflammatory, and proliferative disorders.

Functional Effects of Dietary n − 3 Fatty Acids

Diets enriched in n − 3 fatty acids induce a series of functional alterations that may underlie their beneficial effects, i.e., reduced vascular reactivity and platelet aggregatability, reduced chemotaxis of white blood cells and cellular proliferation, and reduced formation of cytokines and growth factors. These changes probably contribute to the experimentally induced reduction of cell proliferation, reduced thrombus and atheroma formation, blunted inflammatory and immune reactions, and retarded tumor growth seen after administration of dietary n − 3 fatty acids in animal experiments and in human studies.

Biochemical Effects of n − 3 Fatty Acids

Dietary EPA and DCHA, which partially replace AA and LA in a specific time- and dose-dependent manner in plasma and in certain cellular phospholipid subclasses, induce a series of biochemical events (Fig. 3). Once incorporated into

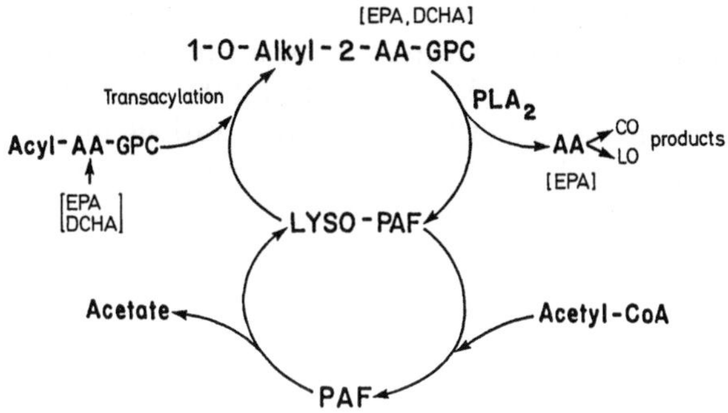

Fig. 3. The role of EPA and DCHA in the modification of the PAF precursor pool

cellular membranes, EPA and DCHA are less readily released upon cell stimulation, thus reducing substrate availability for eicosanoid generation and decreasing potent amplification mechanisms to which AA metabolites contribute, e.g., as a cellular response to injury. In addition to reducing the level of AA and most often its eicosanoid derivatives, the $n-3$ fatty acids EPA and DCHA, which can be retroconverted to EPA, serve as precursors to a class of eicosanoids with an attenuated spectrum of biological activity: TXA_3, formed in small quantities in $n-3$ fatty acid enriched platelets, in addition to significantly reduced TXA_2 formation, is almost inactive as a platelet aggregator and vasoconstrictor. LTB_5, formed from EPA in neutrophils and monocytes/macrophages, is one order of magnitude less active as a chemotactic agent compared to LTB_4, which is also reduced after prolonged dietary intake of $n-3$ fatty acids. In contrast PGI_3, which is formed from dietary $n-3$ fatty acids in amounts of up to 50% of an unchanged synthesis of PGI_2, is biologically as active as PGI_2 in inhibiting platelet aggregation and reducing vascular tone.

The formation of PAF is also reduced by $n-3$ fatty acids through interference with the turnover of the PAF precursor pool. Altogether, the data indicate that it is possible in humans – by nutritional means – to change plasma and cell membrane phospholipid fatty acid composition, the arachidonic acid cascade, the spectrum of biologically highly active eicosanoids and other lipid mediators, and the production of potent peptide mediators such as interleukin-1 (IL-1), tumor necrosis factor (TNF), and platelet-derived growth factor (PDGF), thereby inducing an antithrombotic, antiinflammatory, and antiproliferative state.

Future Studies

Further evaluation of the relationship of $n-6$ vs $n-3$ fatty acids and their oxygenated metabolites to membrane receptor function, modulation of transmembranous signaling mechanisms, formation of 1,2 DAG or PAF, and CA^{2+}-

release should contribute to a better understanding of the role of these mediators and their precursor fatty acids in cell function. Some interesting areas for future research can already be identified. These include: (a) the study of the effects of dietary precursors on eicosanoid formation from various long- vs short-chain n − 6 and n − 3 fatty acids; (b) the reabsorption, organ distribution, cellular and phospholipid subclass incorporation of eicosanoid precursor fatty acids; and (c) the potential role of n − 6 and n − 3 fatty acids in the modification of the prothrombotic and inflammatory response as it relates, for example, to the function of monocytes/macrophages and regulation of T-lymphocytes.

Bibliography

1. Dyerberg, J, Bang, HO, Stoffersen E, Moncada S, Vane JR (1978) Eicosapentaenoic acid and prevention of thrombosis and atherosclerosis? Lancet 1:117–119
2. Fischer S, Weber PC (1984) Prostaglandin I_3 is formed in vivo in man after dietary eicosapentaenoic acid. Nature 307:165–168
3. Lee TH, Hoover RL, Williams JD, Sperling RI, Ravalese J, Spur BW, Robinson D, Corey EJ, Lewis RA, Austen KF (1985) Effect of dietary enrichment with eicosapentaenoic and docosahexaenoic acids on in vitro neutrophil and monocyte leukotriene generation and neutrophil function. N Engl J Med 312:1217–1224
4. v Schacky C, Weber PC (1985) Metabolism and effects on platelet function of the purified eicosapentaenoic and docosahexaenoic acids in humans. J Clin Invest 76:2446–2450
5. Siess W, Weber PC, Lapetina EG (1985) Different functions of phosphoinositide turnover and arachidonate metabolism for platelet activation. In: Bailey JM (ed) Prostaglandins, leukotrienes and lipoxins. Plenum, New York
6. Strasser T, Fischer S, Weber PC (1985) Leukotrine B_5 is formed in human neutrophils after dietary eicosapentaenoic acid. Proc Natl Acad Sci USA 82:1540–1543
7. Weber PC, Fischer S, v. Schacky C, Lorenz R, Strasser T (1986) The conversion of dietary eicosapentaenoic acid to prostanoids and leukotrienes in man. Prog Lipid Res 25:273–276
8. Weber PC (1989) Epidemiologische und biochemische Studien über n − 3 Fettsäuren in der Prävention der Atherosklerose. Internist (Berlin) 30:283–390
9. Leaf A, Weber PC (1988) Cardiovascular effects of n − 3 fatty acids. N Engl J Med 318:549–557
10. Weber PC (1989) Clinical studies on the effects of n − 3 fatty acids on cells and eicosanoids in the cardiovascular system. J Int Med 225:61–68

Proteinases as Mediators of the Disturbance of Pulmonary Vascular Permeability in Sepsis, Polytrauma, and ARDS

H. Neuhof and H. Fritz

Introduction

A series of humoral alterations are a characteristic finding in sepsis, polytrauma, and other affections, which are often followed by an acute lung failure (ARDS, adult respiratory distress syndrome) or multiple organ failure (MOF). Based on experimental and clinical findings, the cooperation of a variety of mediators and mediator systems are responsible for causing the disturbance of vascular tone and permeability and inducing the morphological transformation which finally may result in the failure of vital organs. Beside the classical mediators, such as catecholamines, histamine, serotonin, and bradykinin, increasing attention has recently focused on metabolites of arachidonic acid, cytokines, and products from circulating or resident inflammatory cells. Of all these humoral and cellular alterations the activation and liberation of proteinases seems to play an essential role with regard to loss of capillary barrier function and interstitial edema formation.

Vascular Effects Directly or Indirectly Induced by Nonspecific and Selective Proteolysis

Proteinases influence vascular permeability in two ways (Fig. 1). First of all they are able to destroy the vessel wall by nonspecific proteolysis. Besides this direct action, however, proteinases are components of the three classical cascade systems which are activated and controlled by selective proteolysis. Upon activation all these, the complement system, the kallikrein-kinin system, and the coagulation and fibrinolytic system generate factors which directly influence vascular tone and permeability (Belew et al. 1978; Yamamoto and Cochrane 1981; Neuhof and Lasch 1984). Moreover, each of these systems can activate a number of target cells and stimulate pulmonary arachidonic acid metabolism resulting in the release or production of mediators with potent vascular effects (Neuhof et al. 1987). Thus, aggregation and degranulation of neutrophils is caused by the complement factors C_{3a} and C_{5a} (Becker et al. 1974; Craddock et al. 1977), by plasma kallikrein (Wachtfogel et al. 1983) and Hageman factor XIIa (Wachtfogel et al. 1986), and the fibrinogen split product D (Manwaring and

Selective Proteolysis	Nonspecific Proteolysis
by:	by:
specific serine - proteinases	**nonspecific cysteine-, serine-, aspartatic-, and metalloproteinases**
XIIa, kallikrein, thrombin, C_1-esterase, etc.	elastase, cathepsins, collagenases, plasmin, etc.
from:	from:
Kallikrein - Kinin and complement systems	**granulocytes, macrophages, mast cells,**
Coagulation and fibrinolytic systems	**injured tissue, etc.**
Activation of the classical cascade systems	**Destruction of basement membranes and other structural elements**

Fig. 1. Systemic and local effects following the activation and liberation of proteinases

Curreri 1982). Besides granulocytes, a series of other mediator producing cells, such as macrophages, platelets, and mast cells, are activated by products of these cascade systems. Thus, the prophylactic and therapeutic concept of proteinase inhibition does not aim to prevent or block the destructive proteolysis of tissue only. Instead, it should be possible to prevent or reduce the generation and release of mediators by influencing the activities of the humoral cascade systems with specific proteinase inhibitors.

Granulocytes and Macrophages as Mediator Sources

Polymorphonuclear granulocytes (PMN) are considered to be the main sources of mediators which affect the endothelial and epithelial barriers of the lung capillaries and alveoli, respectively, in ARDS (Tate and Repine 1983; Brigham and Meyrick 1984) (Fig. 2). Granulocytes are activated by a great variety of stimuli, such as complement factors, kallikrein, products of coagulation and fibrinolysis, bacterial toxins, stimuli for phagocytosis, and many others. Activated PMN stick to the endothelium of the plumonary circulation (Schlag et al. 1980), where in close contact with the vessel wall they release their lysosomal proteinases, liberate lactoferrin and myeloperoxidase, generate toxic oxygen products, and synthesize leukotrienes and other arachidonic acid metabolites. This release reaction is reflected by increasing plasma levels of PMN-elastase-α_1-proteinase inhibitor complexes and of lactoferrin and myeloperoxidase (Dittmer et al. 1986). The released proteinases, such as elastase, cathepsins, and others, are able to lyse fibronectin, the glue of the endothelial cells, and to split

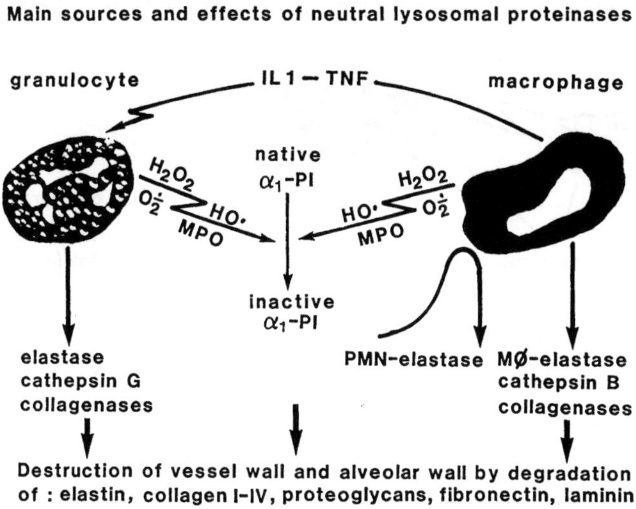

Fig. 2. Action and interaction of granulocytes and macrophages following activation

structural elements of the basement membrane and vessel wall (Fritz and Jochum 1984).

Oxygen radicals which are generated during the burst reaction of PMN have a direct cytotoxic and permeability enhancing effect on cultured endothelial cells and on isolated perfused rat and rabbit lungs (Varani et al. 1985; Shasby et al. 1982; Tate et al. 1982). In addition, toxic oxygen products generated by PMN or produced outside the cells from released myeloperoxidase and lactoferrin inactivate endogenous α_1-proteinase inhibitor (Zaslow et al. 1983) and thus create the conditions for an unlimited proteolytic attack on the vessel wall.

Alveolar macrophages and resident and intravascular macrophages are further potent sources of proteinases, reactive oxygen products, and other mediators influencing vascular permeability (Nathan 1987). In contrast to PMN, which are only able to release their stored proteinases once upon stimulation, macrophages are able to resynthesize their enzymes and thus sustain a prolonged release.

Different Pathomechanisms in Pulmonary Edema Formation

To understand the role of proteinases in the pathogenesis of pulmonary edema, the different pathomechanisms in edema formation have to be considered with regard to their therapeutic consequences (Fig. 3). In contrast to cardiogenic pulmonary edema induced by elevated capillary pressure due to congestive

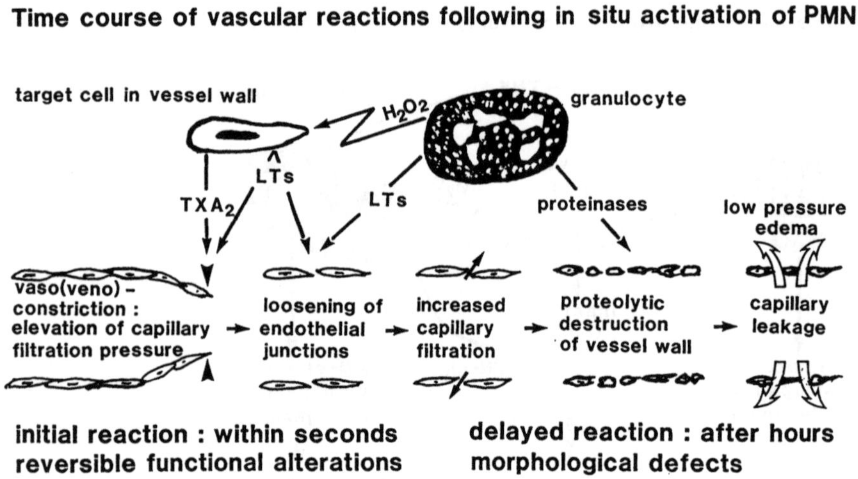

Fig. 3. Pathomechanisms involved in interstitial edema formation

heart failure, the edema in sepsis and ARDS occurs because of alterations in the microcirculation and microvessels. In principle, two different pathomechanisms have to be considered: The formation of interstitial edema in the early stage in animal models and in the early stages of sepsis, polytrauma, and ARDS in patients seems to be caused above all by functional alterations which are reversible, by changing microvascular tone and increasing capillary filtration pressure, and by altering the endothelial cell shape, thus loosening inter-endothelial junctions. By this mode of action, the classical mediators histamine and bradykinin (Joris et al. 1972) and the more recently described lipoxygenase products of arachidonic acid are known to cause interstitial edema. We have studied the effect of lipoxygenase products of arachidonic acid on pulmonary vascular permeability in the model of isolated perfused and ventilated rabbit lungs. The induction of interstitial edema by these eicosanoids requires simultaneous elevation of the capillary filtration pressure and can be blocked by an inhibitor of 5-lipoxygenase (Seeger et al. 1987).

In contrast to the almost reversible increasing vascular permeability in the early phases, the delayed vascular leakage, which occurs in the later phases of sepsis and ARDS, even with low filtration pressures, seems to be caused by a different pathomechanism.

Recent observations give much reason to believe that the disturbance of pulmonary vascular permeability in the later phase of ARDS is due to structural injury to the vessels and alveoli caused by lysosomal proteinases from granulocytes and macrophages. Thus, free activity of PMN elastase in the presence of inactivated α_1-proteinase inhibitor (α_1-PI) was found in bronchoalveolar lavage fluid from patients in later stages of ARDS by Cochrane et al. (1983). Zaslow et al. (1983) have shown that α_1-PI is inactivated by oxidation caused by hydrogen peroxide and myeloperoxidase from activated granulocytes. Further indication of the causal role of elastase in the process of endothelial cell injury by granulocytes was supplied by Smedly et al. (1986) by means of an endothelial monolayer assay.

Experimental Studies in Isolated Rabbit Lungs

To investigate the action of PMN proteinases within the pulmonary microcirculation, we performed studies in isolated perfused and ventilated rabbit lungs.

In this model lungs are perfused with Krebs-Henseleit starch buffer solution in a closed circuit and are ventilated by means of a Starling pump. The lungs are suspended on an electronic balance whereby changes in lung weight, indicating edema formation, are monitored continuously. The pressure in the pulmonary artery and in the left atrium are recorded simultaneously to reveal changes in pulmonary vascular resistance.

When PMN elastase was added to the perfusion fluid, lung weight increased continuously after a latent period of about 15 min, reflecting the formation of interstitial edema. However, pulmonary artery pressure remained unchanged, indicating that the edema was a true permeability edema and not caused by hemodynamic changes in filtration pressure.

To study the reaction of stimulated granulocytes within the pulmonary circulation, human PMN were isolated by centrifugation through a Percoll gradient. Following the injection of an average of 150 ml of these isolated PMN, the cells remained in the pulmonary circulation but did not induce changes in vascular resistance or permeability during a control period of 4–6 h, as long as they were not additionally stimulated. However, upon stimulation of the PMN with antigen-antibody complexes or heat-denaturated immunoglobulins, which were added to the perfusion fluid, pulmonary artery pressure and lung weight increased. The rise in pulmonary vascular resistance was caused by thromboxane, whose generation was induced by the burst reaction of the granulocytes. The pressure increase could be blocked by a thromboxane receptor antagonist, whereas the edema formation continued. When PMN were stimulated in vitro and injected into the pulmonary circulation after finishing their burst reaction, there was no occurrence of either thromboxane generation or a pressure reaction.

Using prestimulated PMN or PMN stimulated within the pulmonary circulation, vascular leakage developed, as reflected by an increase in lung weight. In both situations the latent period was more than 1 h. Edema formation was paralleled by an increasing level of PMN elastase in the perfusion fluid. Electron microscopy of such lungs showed vacuolated granulocytes which stuck to the endothelium of alveolar capillaries. The endothelial cells were injured and partially loosened from the vessel wall below the contact area and interstitial edema had developed. The edema formation could be largely suppressed by the addition of the proteinase inhibitor Eglin c to the perfusion fluid (Fig. 4). Similarly Eglin c prevented the increase in fluid passage through monolayers of cultured endothelial cells, following their exposure to supernatants of activated granulocytes (Suttorp et al. 1989) (Fig. 5).

Eglin c is a potent elastase-cathepsin G inhibitor from the leech *Hirudo medicinalis* (Seemüller et al. 1986). In comparison to the protective effect of Eglin c, which is resistant to inactivation by oxidation, α1-PI failed to inhibit edema formation when PMN were stimulated in situ. Catalase has proven to be ineffective under these experimental conditions in preventing inactivation of α1-PI by oxygen radicals from granulocytes.

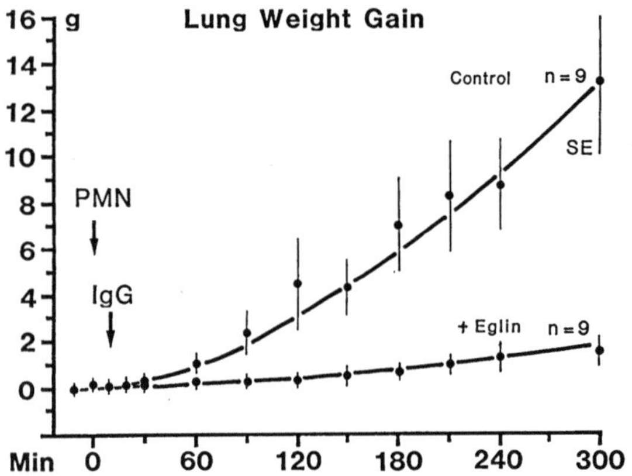

Fig. 4. Interstitial edema formation in an isolated perfused rabbit lung following the injection of human granulocytes into the pulmonary circulation and subsequently stimulated in situ by addition of heat-denaturated IgG to the perfusion fluid. The vascular leakage can be prevented by prior addition of Eglin c to the perfusate.

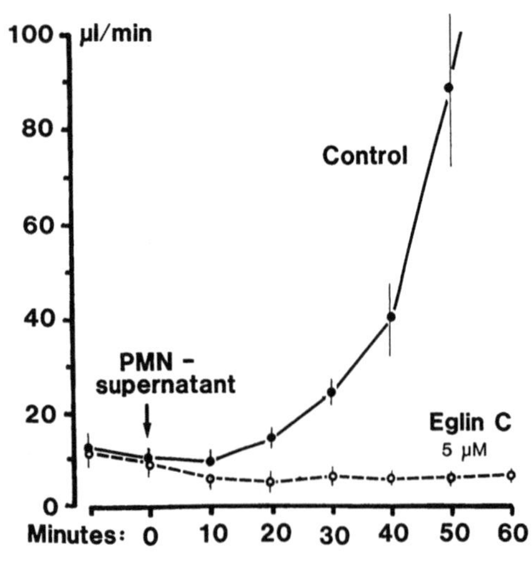

Fig. 5. Enhancement of fluid passage through a confluent monolayer of endothelial cells, cultured on polycarbonate filter membranes, following the addition of supernatants from PMA-stimulated granulocytes. The increase in permeability can completely be prevented by prior application of Eglin c. (modified graph according to Suttorp et al. 1989)

Conclusion

The disturbance of pulmonary vascular permeability in sepsis and ARDS is caused by a complex pathomechanism in which a variety of mediators are involved. Of these arachidonic acid metabolites, toxic oxygen species, and proteinases can be considered as important end products which directly affect the endothelial and epithelial barriers.

Of these key end products, proteinases from granulocytes and probably also from macrophages seem to be mainly responsible for the pulmonary vascular leakage that occurs in the later stages of sepsis and ARDS. Based on this pathophysiological aspect, future concepts for prophylaxis and therapy should include blockers and antagonists of arachidonic acid metabolism, antioxidants, and, last but not least, proteinase inhibitors which are resistant to inactivation by oxidation.

References

Becker EL, Showell HJ, Henson PM, Hsu LS (1974) The ability of chemotactic factors to induce lysosomal enzyme release. J Immunol 112:2047–2054

Belew M, Gerdin B, Porath J, Saldeen T (1978) Isolation of vasoactive peptides from human fibrin and fibrinogen degraded by plasmin. Thromb Res 13:983–994

Brigham KL, Meyrick B (1984) Interactions of granulocytes with the lungs. Circ Res 54:623–635

Cochrane CG, Spragg R, Revak SD (1983) Pathogenesis of the adult respiratory distress syndrome – evidence of oxidant activity in bronchoalveolar lavage fluid. J Clin Invest 71: 754–761

Craddock PR, Hammerschmidt D, White JG, Dalmasso AP, Jacob HS (1977) Complement (C5a)-induced granulocyte aggregation in vitro. J Clin Invest 60:260–264

Dittmer H, Jochum M, Fritz H (1986) Freisetzung von granulozytärer Elastase und Plasmaprotein-veränderungen nach traumatisch-hämorrhagischem Schock. Unfallchirurg 89:160–169

Fritz H, Jochum M (1984) Granulocyte proteinases as mediators of unspecific proteolysis in inflammation: a review. In: Selected topics in clinical enzymology 2. De Gruyter, Berlin, pp 305–327

Joris I, Manjo G, Ryan GB (1972) Endothelial contraction in vivo: a study of the rat mesentery. Virchows Arch [B] 12:73–83

Manwaring D, Curreri PW (1982) Platelet and neutrophil sequestration after fragment D-induced respiratory distress. Circ Shock 9:75–80

Nathan CF (1987) Secretory products of macrophages. J Clin Invest 79:319–326

Neuhof H, Lasch H-G (1984) Interactions between intravascular coagulation and tissue perfusion. Clin Hemorheol 4:5–13

Neuhof H, Seeger W, Suttorp N (1987) Activation of the pulmonary arachidonic acid system and its consequences for hemodynamics and fluid balance. In: Schlag G, Redl H (eds) First Vienna shock forum: pathophysiological role of mediators and mediator inhibitors in shock. Liss, New York, pp 289–300

Schlag G, Voigt WH, Redl H, Glatzl A (1980) Vergleichende Morphologie des posttraumatischen Lungenversagens. Anasth Intensivther Notfallmed 15:315–339

Seeger W, Menger M, Walmrath D, Becker G, Grimminger F, Neuhof H (1987) Arachidonic acid lipoxygenase pathways and increased vascular permeability in isolated rabbit lungs. Am Rev Respir Dis 136:964–972

Seemüller U, Dodt J, Fink E, Fritz H (1986) Proteinase inhibitors of the leech *Hirudo medicinalis* (hirudins, bdellins, eglins). In: Barrett, Salvesen (eds) Proteinase inhibitors. Elsevier, Amsterdam pp 337–359

Shasby DM, Vanbenthuysen KM, Tate RM, Shasby SS, McMurtry I, Repine JE (1982) Granulocytes mediate acute edematous lung injury in rabbits and in isolated rabbit lungs perfused with phorbol myristate acetate: role of oxygen radicals. Am Rev Respir Dis 125:443–447

Smedly LA, Tonnesen MG, Sandhaus RA, Haslett C, Guthrie LA, Johnston RB (1986) Neutrophil-mediated injury to endothelial cells – enhancement by endotoxin and essential role of neutrophil elastase. J Clin Invest 77:1233–1243

Suttorp N, Nolte A, Neuhof H (1989) Bedeutung der granulozytären Elastase für die endotheliale Permeabilität. In: Suttorp N (ed) Zellbiologische Untersuchungen zur Pathogenese des akuten Atemnotsyndroms des Erwachsenen. Habilitationsschrift, University of Giessen

Tate RM, Vanbenthuysen KM, Shasby DM, McMurtry IF, Repine J (1982) Oxygen-radical-mediated permeability edema and vasoconstriction in isolated perfused rabbit lungs. Am Rev Respir Dis 126:802–806

Tate RM, Repine JE (1983) State of the art – neutrophils and the adult respiratory distress syndrome. Am Rev Respir Dis 128:552–559

Varani J, Fligiel SEG, Till GO, Kunkel RG, Ryan US, Ward PA (1985) Pulmonary endothelial cell killing by human neutrophils. Lab Invest 53:656–663

Yamamoto T, Cochrane CG (1981) Guinea pig hageman factor as a vascular permeability enhancement factor. Am J Pathol 105:164–175

Zaslow MC, Clark RA, Stone PJ, Calore JD, Snider GL, Franzblau C (1983) Human neutrophil elastase does not bind to alpha$_1$-protease inhibitor that has been exposed to activated human neutrophils. Am Rev Respir Dis 128:434–439

The Involvement of Oxygen Radicals and Their Derivatives in ARDS

M.H. Schoenberg and H.G. Beger

Introduction

A remarkable array of clinical settings is associated with noncardiogenic pulmonary edema and respiratory failure, described as ARDS. The pathophysiology and pathology are similar; thus, it is tempting to infer that the pathogenesis is similar as well. This has led investigators to search for common pathogenetic events with the hope that a single intervention might be effective, regardless of the etiology of ARDS.

One of the most common clinical settings in which ARDS occurs is gram-negative sepsis. Early descriptions of the pathology of noncardiogenic pulmonary edema (now commonly referred to as ARDS) cited pulmonary sequestration of leukocytes in the capillaries and neutrophil migration into the interstitial and alveolar space (Bachhofen and Weibel 1977). This accumulation of polymorphonuclear neutrophil leukocytes (PMN) in the lungs is followed by ultrastructural evidence of pulmonary endothelial damage (Riede et al. 1978). Physiological responses include marked pulmonary hypertension, and, later, increased permeability of the exchange vessels (Brigham et al. 1983). The temporal relationship between the accumulation and migration of neutrophils and the structural and physiological changes in the lung have led to the hypothesis that PMN leukocytes are involved in the pathogenesis of ARDS. Various inciting events, perhaps including activation of the complement system (especially C5a), may cause the sequestration of neutrophils in the lung. Subsequent neutrophil stimulation induces the release of toxic neutrophil products, contributing to acute edematous lung injury.

This hypothesis is supported by the observation that, experimentally, the increase in pulmonary permeability is significantly diminished by neutrophil depletion (Heflin and Brigham 1981).

Moreover, in the bronchoalveolar lavage of patients with ARDS dramatic increases of neutrophils and their products were reported, re-emphasizing the potential involvement of these inflammatory cells in the syndrome (McGuire et al. 1982).

Despite these observations, it seems unlikely that complement activation and subsequent granulocyte accumulation alone are sufficient to explain the severe and prolonged lung injury seen in patients suffering from ARDS.

The endothelial alterations observed after accumulation of granulocytes in the lung and the activation of granulocytes per se inevitably lead to microthrombosis in the capillaries and venules. In turn, intravascular coagulation facilitates the accumulation of inflammatory cells; both interactions therefore constitute a positive feedback cycle and stimulate each other (Gerdin et al. 1982).

It was shown experimentally that cyclooxygenase and lipoxygenase metabolites of arachidonic acid are increased in lung lymph during sepsis. Prostaglandin metabolites and thromboxane thus appear to mediate both changes in lung mechanics and pulmonary vasoconstriction. Concomitantly, lipoxygenase products may play a role in both the inflammatory response and the increase in vascular permeability (Brigham and Duke 1985; Ogletree et al. 1982).

In regard to the early morphological and functional alterations in ARDS it seems likely, that accumulation and activation of PMN microemboli lead to a disturbed microcirculation, subsequent tissue hypoxia, and enhanced prostaglandin and leukotriene metabolism. These are essential for the development of acute respiratory failure. In spite of their completely different pathophysiological effects, these pathomechanisms have one thing in common: They all induce an enhanced generation of oxygen radicals.

The Generation of Oxygen Radicals by Granulocytes

The main source of oxygen radicals in ARDS seems to be activated PMNs leukocytes. Under normal conditions PMN leukocytes flow along the endothelium of the capillaries and venules. Due to inciting events, i.e., stimulation of the complement system, especially C5a, during septic shock, these leukocytes adhere, sometimes firmly, to the endothelium of the vessels. In some instances neutrophils obstruct the capillaries, adding to the microcirculatory disturbances. Later granulocytes migrate, most likely through interendothelial junctions, to the extravascular space (Hammerschmidt et al. 1980; Marchesi and Florey 1960). In addition to secreting enzymes, such as proteases, synthesizing and releasing mediators (i.e., prostaglandins), PMN leukocytes produce upon stimulation and/or phagocytosis oxygen radicals. The generation of oxygen radicals during phagocytosis is called "respiratory burst" (Babior 1978).

It thereby seems likely that the released mediators, proteases, and O_2 radicals react with each other, potentiating their adverse effects. It was recently shown that proteases enhance the generation of oxygen radicals in macrophages. O_2 radicals, in turn, oxidize α_1-protease inhibitor, which potentiates the effects of proteases released from granulocytes.

In vitro studies showed that endotoxin, normally found in patients suffering from gram-negative sepsis, primes neutrophils. When subsequently activated, these neutrophils produce more superoxide radicals and release more lysosomal enzymes than cells not triggered by endotoxin (Haslett et al. 1985).

It should be noted that there are three other sources of oxygen radicals unrelated to the respiratory burst of neutrophils. Small amounts of O_2 radicals can be generated by: (1) mitochondrial damage, (2) by the xanthine oxidase pathway during tissue ischemia, and (3) by enhanced arachidonic acid metabolism.

The Generation of Free Radicals After Tissue Hypoxia and Reoxygenation

Impaired microcirculation, due to intravascular coagulation and the release of vasoactive substances, can induce severe pulmonary tissue ischemia. After a certain period of incomplete ischemia the mitochondria are damaged. Consequently, the electron transport chain does not function adequately. Normally oxygen is reduced to H_2O via the cytochrome oxidase system by adding four electrons to an oxygen molecule in one step. The damaged mitochondria add only one electron after the other to the oxygen molecule, producing the intermediate metabolites superoxide, H_2O_2, and $OH^{\dot{-}}$ (Boveris 1977). These metabolites are released intracellularly and lead to irreversible damage (Fig. 1).

The major source of oxygen free radicals in ischemic and reperfused tissue, however, appears to be due to the enzyme xanthine oxidase. The nascent enzyme exists as xanthine dehydrogenase and accounts for about 90% of the total activity in healthy tissue. The dehydrogenase form of this enzyme degrades hypoxanthine and xanthine, metabolites of purine metabolism, into uric acid, thus reducing oxidized nicotinamide adenine dinucleotide (NAD) (Stirpe and Della Corte 1969).

Tissue ischemia initiates a chain of adverse events. The lack of oxygen stops the production of ATP, although the use of ATP continues. ATP is degraded into ADP, AMP, and finally to hypoxanthine. Further metabolism to uric acid is not possible, due to hypoxia; hence, hypoxanthine accumulates in the tissue (Deuticke et al. 1966). At the same time, as the energy charge of the cells decreases, the normal calcium gradient across cell membranes cannot be maintained. This leads to a net influx of calcium into the cytosol. Increased intracellular calcium concentrations activate proteases, which in turn convert xanthine dehydrogenase into xanthine oxidase (Roy and McCord 1983) (Fig. 2).

After local reperfusion or after primary therapy, that is, after reoxygenation of the ischemic tissue, xanthine oxidase metabolizes the accumulated hypoxanthine to uric acid. This reaction produces large quantities of superoxide and its derivatives, which are detrimental to cell membranes (Schoenberg et al. 1985) (Fig. 3).

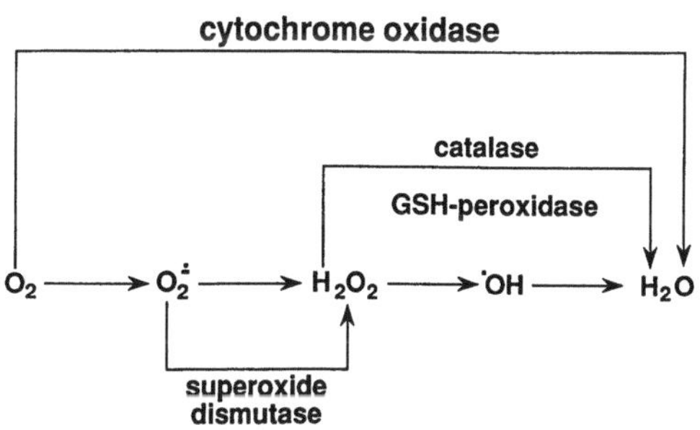

Fig. 1. The normal and univalent pathway for reduction of molecular oxygen and the enzymatic defense mechanisms detoxifying the radical intermediates

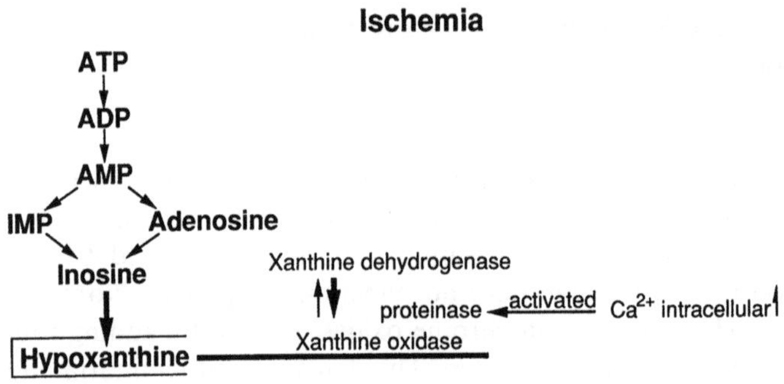

Fig. 2. Mechanisms converting xanthine dehydrogenase into xanthine oxidase during tissue ischemia

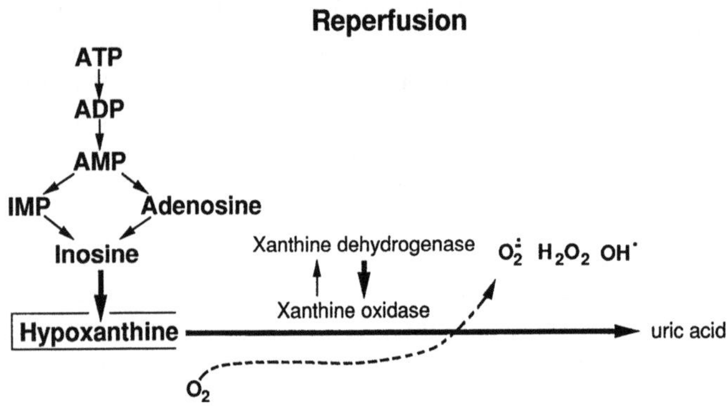

Fig. 3. Generation of oxygen free radicals after re-oxygenation of the former ischemic tissue

Oxygen Free Radicals and Arachidonic Acid Metabolism

High concentrations of arachidonic acid derivatives in sepsis, one of the main causes of ARDS, are not only due to an inhibited inactivation, but also to an increased de novo synthesis stimulated by endotoxin (Oettinger et al. 1983).

Increased formation of the prostaglandin (PG) endoperoxide PGG_2 and its subsequent conversion to PGH_2, PGE_2, PGF_2, and PGD_2 result, at the same time, in an enhanced production of oxygen radicals and their derivatives (Moncade and Vane 1979). In addition, also increased lipoxygenase-mediated metabolism generates oxygen radicals (Schrör 1984).

Effects of Oxygen Free Radicals

All biological substances, such as proteins, polysaccharides etc., react with oxygen free radicals. Most susceptible, however, are polyunsaturated fatty acids

(PUFA), which are present in high concentrations in cellular membranes. Reaction of free radicals with these constituents of the membrane leads to lipid peroxidation within the membranes with subsequent disruption of both liposomal and cellular membranes. Peroxidation of PUFA is a chain reaction resulting in the generation of lipid hydroperoxides, lipid peroxide radicals, and fragmentation products such as malondialdehyde. Once started, this radical chain reaction only terminates if lipid radicals react with each other or with radical scavengers (Buege and Aust 1978).

In vitro experiments by Mead and co-workers showed that the structural and steric composition of the biological membrane constitutes the optimal prerequisite for the propagation of radical chain reactions (Mead 1976). Moreover, lipid hydroperoxides leave the intracellular space and are able to "export", by the formation of alcoxy radicals, radical reactions in tissues other than the primary damaged ones (Safar 1984). Extensive peroxidative alterations ultimately lead to cell death (Slater 1984).

Damage to this extent, occurring in the endothelial layer of the capillaries and venules, results in an increased permeability with extravasation of plasma and even erythrocytes (Del Maestro et al. 1984).

Besides their direct damaging effects on the tissue free radicals seem to produce in the plasma a chemotactic factor which triggers the accumulation of granulocytes in the tissue involved. Furthermore, free radical-stimulated granulocytes adhere to the capillary wall (leukocyte sticking) and in some instances even plug the entire vessel (Björk and Arfors 1982). As mentioned above, stimulation, especially phagocytosis, of these inflammatory cells induces a respiratory burst, which generates oxygen free radicals, thus enabling the granulocyte to kill bacteria (Babior 1978).

Oxygen free radicals indirectly stimulate, due to the generation of lipid peroxides, arachidonic acid metabolism and lead to increased concentrations of PGs, thromboxanes, and leukotrienes, which add to the permeability changes and micro- and macrocirculatory derangements observed (Marshall et al. 1984) (Fig. 4). Apparently, oxygen radicals stimulate, in turn, those pathophysiological mechanisms which previously led to the generation of these radicals. This feedback system initiates several vicious circles, ultimately resulting in irreversible tissue damage.

Due to their high reactivity, the presence of oxygen free radicals cannot be determined directly. The concept of free radical involvement in the pathophysiology of acute respiratory failure is therefore based on circumstantial evidence and in vitro studies. The early morphological alterations, compared to the functional changes in ARDS, as outlined above, support the notion that oxygen radicals are responsible for at least some of the lung injury observed. They cannot be regarded as direct proof.

Chemical generators of oxygen radicals, used in an experimental setting, induce similar morphological and functional alterations as seen in the early phase of ARDS. Tate et al. (1982, 1984) could show in an isolated perfused lung model, that oxygen radicals added to or artificially produced in the perfusate

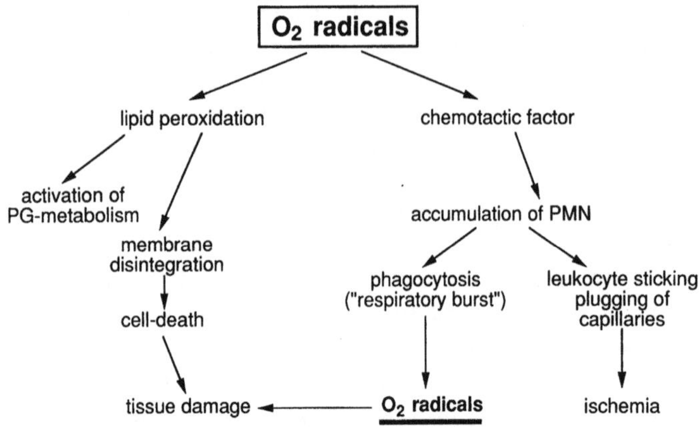

Fig. 4. The effects of oxygen free radicals on the tissue, PMN leukocytes, and prostaglandin metabolism

caused lung edema due to enhanced permeability, increased thromboxane generation, and vasoconstriction in the pulmonary circulation. Similarly, Johnson and Ward demonstrated that the intratracheal instillation of chemical generators of oxygen radicals in rats caused acute lung injury, as determined by histological damage and accumulation of labeled albumin in the lung tissue (Johnson et al. 1981).

Concerning the direct effects of oxygen radicals, it was shown recently that there is a quantitative correlation between the intensity of lung injury induced by endotoxemia and the appearance of lipid peroxidation products, i.e., conjugated dienes, malodialdehyde, and Schiff bases, in the plasma and lung tissue (Ward et al. 1985; Demling et al. 1986). Cochrane and co-workers measured increased levels of lipid hydroperoxides and a reduced activity of α_1 protease inhibitor in the bronchoalveolar lavage of patients suffering from early stage ARDS (Cochrane et al. 1983).

There is, however, another possible way to assess the importance of oxygen free radicals in sepsis. The effects of oxygen-derived free radicals can be blocked either by the substitution of protective enzymes, such as superoxide dismutase (SOD) and catalase, which are normally present in high concentrations in cells, or by treatment with free radical scavengers. These enzymes and scavengers are highly specific substances detoxifying oxygen free radicals. Their beneficial effects after treatment can therefore serve as indirect proof for the postulated involvement of free radicals in the pathomechanism of septic shock. Concomitantly, they also point out a new option for treatment (Fig. 5). In a growing number of studies this inductive and indirect way to obtain evidence has been employed.

Various experimental models were used to produce lesions comparable to the alterations seen in ARDS. Johnson et al. induced an increase in lung vascular permeability and pulmonary vascular resistance by the infusion of

Enzymatic agents	superoxide dismutase catalase glutathione peroxidase
Scavengers	dimethyl sulfoxide dimethyl thiourea benzoate salicylate mannitol N-acetyl cysteine vitamine E
Iron chelators	deferoxamine apolactoferrin 2, 3-dihydroxybenzoic acid
Inhibitors	allopurinol

Fig. 5. Different substances protecting against or inhibiting the generation of oxygen radicals

80 U/kg thrombin into sheep (Johnson et al. 1986). The authors could demonstrate that treatment with SOD attenuated the increases in permeability and vascular resistance. Ward et al. activated the complement system by i.v. injection of cobra venom factor into rats and induced an acute lung injury, as reflected by increased vascular permeability and morphological damage to the lung vascular endothelial cells. They demonstrated a quantitative correlation between lung injury and the concentration of lipid peroxidation products (conjugated dienes). Moreover, pretreatment with radical scavengers (SOD, catalase, DMSO, dimethylthiourea, and desferoxamine) prevented the morphological alterations and lipid peroxidation in the lung tissue without interfering with the accumulation of neutrophils in the lung interstitial capillaries (Ward et al. 1985). Similarly, Gee and co-workers activated the complement system by i.v. administration of zymosan-activated plasma, thus exposing the pulmonary endothelial cells to activated blood leukocytes. SOD prevented the formation of lung edema and the increase in thromboxane, supporting the hypothesis that free radicals enhance arachidonate metabolism (Gee et al. 1987). Taylor et al. produced a fulminant edema by intrapulmonary infusion of α-naphthylthiourea (ANTU) in dogs (Taylor et al. 1985). Pretreatment with SOD, DMSO, and hydroxyurea prevented ANTU damage in at least 50% of all animals. In addition, inhibition of the arachidonate system by ibuprofen attenuated the lesions; allopurinol-treated and neutropenic animals were not protected. The authors concluded that HO· is responsible for the damage seen and is generated by enhanced arachidonic acid metabolism (Martin et al. 1987). Recently, Grosso et al. studied the effects of pulmonary hypoperfusion in an isolated rat lung model. The authors showed that ischemia and reperfusion of lung tissue leads to a nonhydrostatic pulmonary edema due to endothelial damage. The damage is mediated by oxygen radicals generated by xanthine oxidase metabolism (Grosso et al. 1989). The various experimental models and effects of different treatments, however, leave many questions, concerning the mechanisms responsible for tissue damage, unanswered.

Most research work focused on the participation of free radicals and their derivatives in the development of ARDS lung injury induced by infusion of *E. coli* endotoxin into unanesthetized sheep. The animals were treated with SOD, catalase, and the scavenger *N*-acetylcysteine in order to prevent the development of ARDS. (Till et al. 1982; Bernard et al. 1984; Traber et al. 1985). The results, however, are inconsistent, although the experimental models were comparable. *N*-acetylcysteine and catalase attenuated the pathophysiological and histological changes in the lung after endotoxin infusion, whereas SOD treatment failed to have any beneficial effect. Not only free radicals, but also cyclooxygenase metabolites and proteases are probably responsible for the endotoxin-induced injury of the lung (Brigham and Meyrick 1986). Nevertheless, *N*-acetylcysteine is a free radical scavenger which is already clinically available and can be given in large amounts without adverse effects.

Summary and Conclusion

Lung cell injury, as seen in the early phase of ARDS, is at least partly mediated by the generation of oxygen radicals. Inflammatory cells, especially granulocytes, are one if not the major source of these toxic oxygen species, but intracellular generation of free radicals probably also adds to the lesions observed. Likewise, granulocyte-derived proteases and enhanced PG and leukotriene metabolism may also be responsible for some of the early alterations in the development of ARDS. Moreover, the balance between proteases and antiproteases could be important. The fact that oxygen radicals can inactivate antiproteases and, in turn, that antiproteases can act as free radical scavengers suggests a complex relationship among several mediators of ARDS.

Experimentally, various other scavengers have proven to effectively attenuate morphological and functional changes observed in the early phase of ARDS. Some of them (*N*-acetylcysteine) are already being used clinically and can be given in large amounts without adverse effects. Therefore, there is hope that this new pathophysiological and therapeutical concept will soon also prove to be relevant for patients suffering from ARDS.

References

Babior BM (1978) Oxygen-dependent microbial killing by phagocytes. N Engl J Med 298:659–668

Bachhofen M, Weibel ER (1977) Alterations of the gas exchange apparatus in adult respiratory insufficiency associated with septicemia. Am Rev Respir Dis 116:589–615

Bernard GR, Lucht WD, Niedermeyer ME (1984) Effect of *N*-acetylcysteine on the pulmonary response to endotoxin in the awake sheep and upon in vitro granulocyte function. J Clin Invest 73:1772–1784

Björk J, Arfors KE (1982) Oxygen radicals and leucotriene B_4 induced increase in vascular leakage is mediated by PMN-leucocytes. Agents Actions [Suppl] 11:63–73

Boveris A (1977) Mitochondrial production of superoxide radical and H_2O_2. In: Jöbsis FF (ed) Oxygen and physiological function. Professional Information Library, pp 67–82

Brigham K, Duke S (1985) Prostaglandins and lung disease: adult respiratory distress syndrome. Semin Respir Med 7:11–16

Brigham KL, Meyrick B (1986) Endotoxin and lung injury. Am Rev Respir Dis 133:913–927

Brigham KL, Begley CJ, Bernard GR, Loyd JE, Lucht WD et al. (1983) Septicemia and lung injury. Clin Lab Med 3:719–744

Buege JA, Aust SD (1978) Microsomal lipid peroxidation. Methods Enzymol 52:941–948

Cochrane CG, Spragg R, Revak SD (1983) Pathogenesis of the adult respiratory distress syndrome. Evidence of oxidant activity in bronchoalveolar lavage fluid. J Clin Invest 71:754–761

Del Maestro RF, Björk J, Arfors KE (1984) Increased permeability induced by enzymatically generated free radicals. Microvasc Res 22:239–254

Demling RH, Lalonde C, Jin L, Ryan P, Fox R (1986) Endotoxemia causes increased lung tissue lipid peroxidation in unanesthetized sheep. J Appl Physiol 60(6):2094–2100

Deruticke B, Gerlach E, Dickermann R (1966) Abbau freier Nucleotide im Herzen, Skelettmuskel, Gehirn und Leber der Ratte bei Sauerstoffmangel. Pflugers Arch 192:239–245

Gee MH, Margiotta M, Tahamont MV, Flynn JT (1987) Free-radical generation in complement-induced pulmonary dysfunction. In: Taylor AE, Matalon S, Ward PA (eds) Physiology of oxygen radicals. Williams and Wilkins, Baltimore, pp 187–199

Gerdin B, Sandler H, Saldeen T (1982) Pulmonary insufficiency in the rat intravascular coagulation and inhibition of fibrinolysis. II. Investigations on edema formation and morphology, Eur Surg Res 14:252–261

Grosso MA, Brown JM, Viders DE, Mulvin DW et al. (1989) Xanthine oxidase derived oxygen radicals induce pulmonary edema via direct endothelial injury. J Surg Res 46:355–360

Hammerschmidt DE, Weaver LJ, Hudson LD et al. (1980) Association of complement activation and elevated plasma C5a with adult respiratory distress syndrome: pathophysiological relevance and possible prognostic value. Lancet 1:947–949

Haslett C, Henson PM, Guthrie CLA (1985) Modulation of multiple neutrophil functions by preparative methods or trace concentrations of bacterial lipopolysaccharide. Am J Pathol 119:101–110

Heflin AC, Brigham KL (1981) Prevention by granulocyte depletion of increased vascular permeability of sheep lung following endotoxinemia. J Clin Invest 68:1253–1260

Johnson A, Perlman MB, Blumenstock FA, Malik AB (1986) Superoxide dismutase prevents the thrombin-induced increase in lung vascular permeability: role of superoxide in mediating the alterations in lung fluid balance. Circ Res 59:405–415

Johnson KJ, Fantone JC, Kaplan J, Ward PA (1981) In vivo damage of rat lungs by oxygen metabolites. J Clin Invest 67:983–993

Marchesi VT, Florey HW (1960) Electron micrographic observations on the emigration of leucocytes. J Exp Physiol 45:343–348

Marshall PJ, Kulmacz RJ, Lands WEM (1984) Hydroperoxides, free radicals and prostaglandin synthesis. In: Bors W, Saran M, Tait D (eds) Oxy-radicals in chemistry and biology. De Gruyter, Berlin, pp 299–308

Martin D, Allison RC, Taylor AE (1987) Hydroxyl radical damage produced by ANTU In: Taylor AE, Matalon S, Ward PA (eds) Physiology of oxygen radicals. Williams and Wilkins, Baltimore, pp 131–143

McGuire WW, Spragg RG, Cohen AM, Cochrane CG (1982) Studies on the pathogenesis of ARDS. J Clin Invest 69:543–553

Mead JF (1976) Free radical mechanisms of lipid damage and consequences for cellular membranes. In: Pryor WA (ed) Free radical in biology. Academic, New York, pp 51–68

Moncade S, Vane JR (1979) Pharmacology and endogenous role of prostaglandin endoperoxides, thromboxane A2, and prostacyclin. Pharmacol Rev 30 (3):293–331

Oettinger W, Walter G, Jensen U et al. (1983) Endogenous prostaglandin F2 in the hyperdynamic state of severe sepsis in man. Br J Surg 70:237–244

Ogletree M, Oates, J, Brigham K, Hubbard W (1982) Evidence of pulmonary release of 5-HETE during endotoxemia in shock. Prostaglandins 23:459–468

Riede UN, Joachim H, Hassenstein J. Sandritter P, Mittermayer C (1978) The pulmonary air-blood barrier in human shock lungs. Pathol Res Pract 162:41–72

Roy RS, McCord JM (1983) Superoxide and ischemia: conversion of xanthine dehydrogenase to xanthine oxidase. In: Greenwald RA, Cohen G (eds) Oxy radicals and their scavenger systems,

vol 2: cellular and medical aspects. Elsevier, New York, pp 145–153
Safar P (1984) Recent advances in cardiopulmonary-cerebral resuscitation. A review. Ann Emerg Med 13 (2):856–862
Schoenberg MH, Fredholm BB, Haglund U (1985) Studies on the oxygen radical mechanism involved in the small intestinal reperfusion damage. Acta Physiol Scand 124:581–589
Schrör K (1984) Prostaglandine und verwandte Verbindungen. Thieme, Stuttgart
Slater TF (1984) Free radical mechanism in tissue injury. Biochem J 222:1–15
Stirpe F, Della Corte E (1969) The regulation of rat liver xanthine oxidase. J Biol Chem 244(14):3855–3863
Tate RM, Vanbenthyusen KM, Shasby DM, McMurty I (1982) Oxygen radical mediated permeability edema and vasoconstriction in isolated perfused rabbit lungs. Am Rev Respir Dis 126:802–806
Tate RM, Morris HG, Schroeder WR, Repine JE et al. (1984) Oxygen metabolites stimulate thromboxane generation and cause vasoconstriction in isolated perfused rabbit lungs. J Clin Invest 74:608–613
Taylor AE, Martin D, Townsley MI (1985) Oxygen radicals and pulmonary edema. In: Said S (ed) Pulmonary circulation and pulmonary vascular injury. Futura, Mt Kisco, pp 307–320
Till GO, Johnson KJ, Kunkel R et al. (1982) Intravascular activation of complement and acute lung injury: dependency on neutrophils and toxic oxygen metabolites. J Clin Invest 68: 1126–1135
Traber DL, Adams T, Sziebert L (1985) Potentiation of lung vascular response to endotoxin by superoxide dismutase. J Appl Physiol 58: 1005–1009
Ward PA, Till GO, Hatherill JR, Annesley TA (1985) Systemic complement activation, lung injury and products of lipid peroxidation. J Clin Invest 76:517–527

Part 4:
Pulmonary Circulation

Regulation of the Pulmonary Circulation During Lung Injury

N.F. Voelkel, S. Chang, T. McDonnell, C. Chen, and J. Czartolomna

Adult respiratory distress syndrome (ARDS) [1] is not a disease but a disorder which is associated with many clinical states, the most frequent being sepsis, trauma, and aspiration of gastric contents [19]. Less frequently occurring situations are amniotic fluid embolization, acute pancreatitis, radiation lung injury, disseminated intravascular coagulation, and ARDS induced by certain drugs [13]. ARDS was described approximately 20 years ago, yet, since its description the overall mortality has remained stable, indicating that, although some aspects of this syndrome have been studied in various model systems [4–8, 11, 14, 15], the impact of these experiments on patient survival has been very small [2]. Conceptually, ARDS is a massive insult damaging the integrity of the lung membranes. The event which triggers a cascade of metabolic reactions is acute; occasionally the syndrome is rather transient, but most frequently the lung subsequently undergoes a chronic inflammatory phase which leads to cell proliferation and scar tissue formation [19]. The lung circulation is involved in the syndrome since the injurious agents, for example lipopolysaccharide or activated circulating cells, are often carried to the lung via the bloodstream. Pulmonary hypertension has been recognized as part of the syndrome in many patients, as described by Zapol and Snider in 1977 [20]. Morphological studies show obliteration of pulmonary arteries, perivascular edema, and compression of the microcirculation by edema fluid. Functionally, the lung circulation appears to be altered in that the vascular reactivity of the lung is impaired. A study by Newman et al. (1983) demonstrated a vast reduction in the pressure response to infusion of a prostaglandin H_2 analogue in chronically hyperoxic animals [15].

Figure 1 connects some of the injurious influences and mechanisms of impaired vascular tone regulation in acute lung injury. It is our impression that,

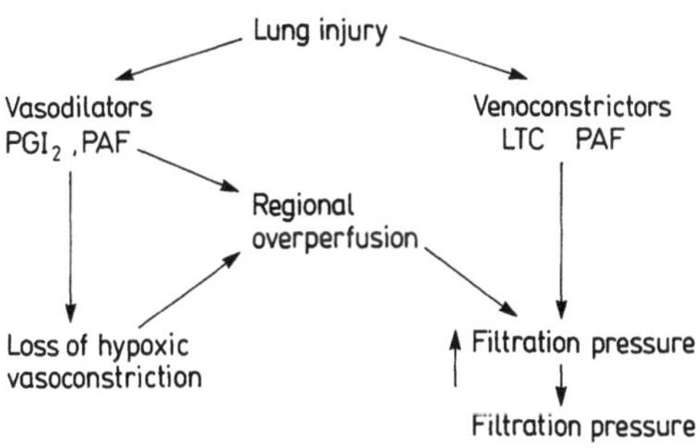

Fig. 1. Factors and mechanisms involved in impairment and regulation of vascular tone

in this highly regionally controlled organ, effects of vasodilators and vasocon strictors occur side by side in different lung regions or adjacent lung areas. Vasodilating mediators like prostacyclin or prostaglandin E prevent hypoxic vasoconstriction and cause regional overperfusion. In adjacent lung areas, the effect of venoconstrictors such as peptidoleukotrienes and platelet activating factor (PAF) may prevail. Venoconstriction increases hydrostatic stress and amplifies–because of an increase in filtration pressures–edema formation.

Mechanistically, vascular tone and vascular permeability may be regulated together. Mediators or other highly localized principles of injury (active oxygen species, proteases, cationic enzymes) meet a phalanx of defensive mechanisms which are part of the organization of the lung vessel wall (surface glycocalix with attached plasma proteins) or products of the metabolism of endothelial cells (Fig. 2). The endothelium is covered with a glycocalix which together with plasma proteins may form a protective coat. Endothelium can release several vasodilators, prostacyclin [18], PAF [3, 12, 16], and EDRF to name just a few. The endothelium can also produce oxidants, antioxidants, and probably antiproteases.

Our work has focused in recent years on the effect of mediators released in the lung microcirculation. Our own studies [10] and those by Hanley et al. [11] in the dog strongly indicate that in a model of *Pseudomonas* induced lung injury there is considerable release of vasodilative prostaglandin, which, in the above dog studies, caused a decrease in the arterial PO_2 indicative of inhibition of hypoxic vasoconstriction. Studies by Garrett and Thomas [9] convincingly showed that inhibition of vasodilative prostaglandins via cyclooxygenase blockers prevented the increase in shunt perfusion in the injured lung; we showed increased lung tissue levels of prostacyclin in *Pseudomonas* infected rats [10].

In our laboratory we have generated several models of acute lung injury using isolated rat lung preparations, which are perfused at constant flow and ventilated in a controlled manner. This preparation is well suited as an assay organ to probe the effects of lipid mediators [2, 3, 5, 14] and other injurious

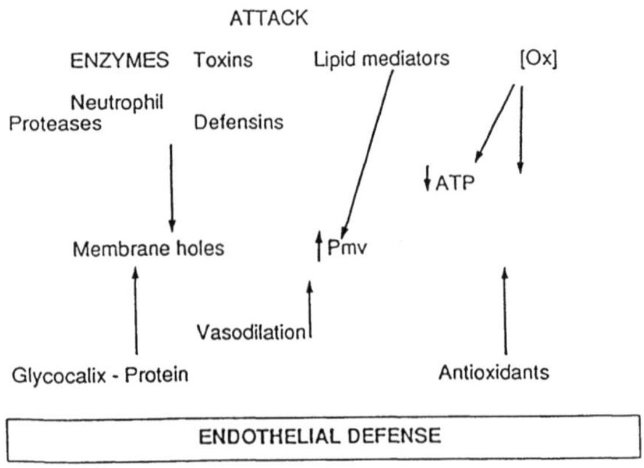

Fig. 2. Factors involved in acute vascular lung injury

stimuli [17] produced as a consequence of the interaction between activated circulating blood cells, e.g., neutrophils and monocytes, and the endothelial lining of the lung circulation. As indicated, hypoxic vasoconstriction is impaired in most situations of lung injury; we studied the effect of endotoxin in monitored rats and showed impairment of hypoxic vasoconstriction which was associated with a release of PAF into the bloodstream and with high lung tissue concentrations of PAF [5]. Several PAF antagonists were shown to inhibit the action of PAF in the rat, including the preservation of hypoxic vasoconstriction by CV 3988 [5]. These studies led us to the investigation of the mechanism of action of PAF in acute lung injury [17]. Conceptually, lipid mediators can affect lung vascular endothelial membranes directly and increase their permeability; they can also affect the microcirculation hemodynamically. Lung microvascular pressure can be assessed using the double clamp method. This measurement gives some indication of the hemodynamic stress in the lung microcirculation. Using isolated lungs, we studied the effects of injection of α-staphylotoxin (α-T) and found that the pulmonary artery pressure rise could be inhibited by indomethacin and by a 5-lipoxygenase synthesis blocker [7]. These studies show that, although pulmonary artery pressure increases, the relative increase in *microvascular pressure* may be much greater and more relevant for edema formation. We asked: How do lipid mediators affect the lung microcirculation? We used leukotriene (LTC_4) which increased pulmonary microvascular pressure and lung vascular leakage (Fig. 3). This action could be inhibited by pretreatment of the lungs with dibutyryl cAMP [17]. We concluded from these studies that α-staphylotoxin causes lung injury and mediator release and that mediators act in part by increasing lung microvascular pressure. Small increases in lung microvascular pressure in the injured lung have consequences for edema formation. Vasodilators which reduce microvascular pressure reduce edema formation [12].

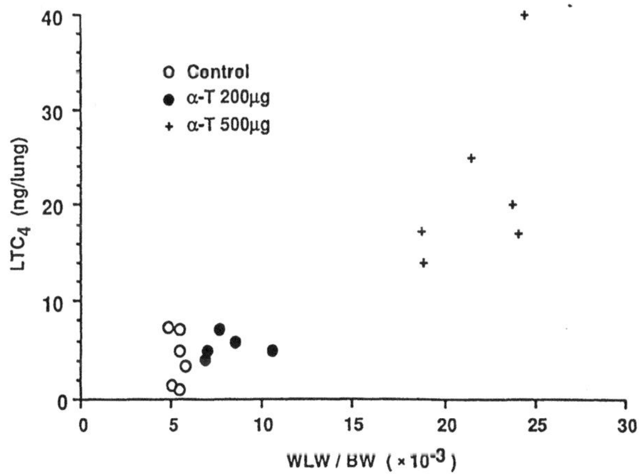

Fig. 3.

We next examined the effects of amphotericin B, a frequently used chemotherapeutic agent, whose fungicide action is due to production of oxygen radicals. In these experiments we showed that a LT antagonist inhibited the pulmonary artery pressure increase after amphotericin and reduced the albumin vascular leakage [14]. Figure 4 illustrates that amphotericin and endotoxin caused comparable vascular damage; however, only amphotericin stimulated LTC_4 synthesis. We therefore postulate that LTC_4 is derived from the epithelial injury which occurs with amphotericin, but not with endotoxin. Although lipid mediators are produced and released in acute lung injury, it is likely that they initiate synergistic effects and interact with other injurious principles. To model synergism between a lipid mediator and a cationic protein (for example a neutrophil derived cationic protein or defensin) we combined protamine [2], a commercially available cationic protein (used to reverse the action of heparin), and small amounts of PAF. We found vast potentiation of lung vascular injury when both agents were used in sequence, whereas each of the agents alone had relatively small effects in the lungs. We showed that the synergism between PAF and protamine is PAF receptor dependent and that the major mechanism of action of PAF in the synergism is through elevation of the microvascular pressure in the lung (Fig. 5). A variation of the synergism theme is illustrated by unpublished results of our group. It is known that oxidant stress leads to a reduction in intracellular ATP. To model this decrease in intracellular ATP in the lung we perfused isolated rat lungs with cyanide (which inhibits oxidative phosphorylation and leads to a decrease in ATP) and added PAF. We found that lungs which have decreased ATP levels are more susceptible to vascular injury triggered by small concentrations of PAF.

Lastly, we were interested in the concept that, in the microenvironment of the lung capillaries, one lipid mediator can lead to the production of another. Indeed, nanomolar concentrations of PAF caused enhancement of LTC_4 and to some degree also of thromboxane synthesis. It is postulated that PAF activates phospholipase A_2 leading to enhanced eicosanoid synthesis.

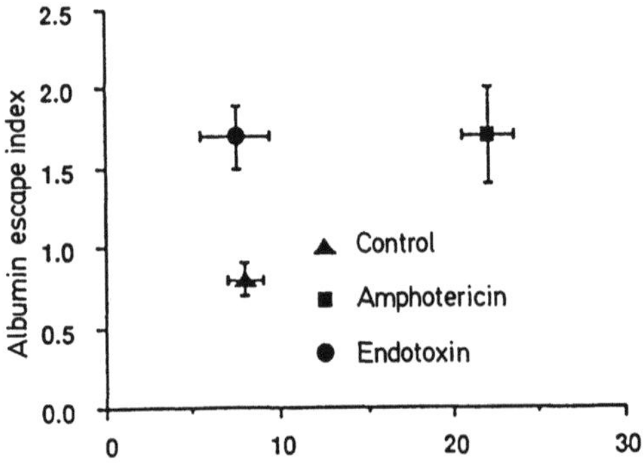

Fig. 4. Lung vascular leak

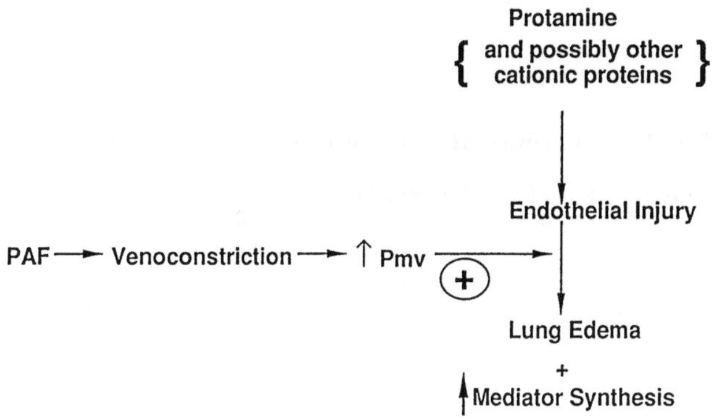

Fig. 5. Mechanism of action of PAF

Our work in the area of acute lung injury has recently led us to examine the question of genetic susceptibility to lung injury. We found that there are animal strain differences which can be used to examine basic mechanisms. In the comparative experiments, which were done in our laboratory, Fischer and Sprague Dawley rats, which are genetically different, were exposed either to hydrogen peroxide, elastase, or to ventilation with 95% oxygen for 3 h. These experiments, which are preliminary, demonstrated that the Fischer rat strain was more injury prone when exposed to oxidant stress than the Sprague Dawley strain. Although the exact mechanism of this susceptibility is not yet understood, experiments of this kind may pave the way to a better understanding of genetically controlled defense mechanisms in acute lung injury.

Eicosanoids and other lipid mediators are released during acute lung injury. PAF appears to be an important factor which amplifies the local vascular damage by its receptor-dependent venoconstriction. The concept of synergistic interactions between lipid mediators and other injurious molecules is important. This synergism can manifest itself in various ways. First, the combination of an injured endothelial surface and venoconstriction amplifies edema formation. Second, it can be demonstrated that the presence of relatively small concentrations of one mediator can lead to the synthesis of other lipid mediators. It follows that it is unrealistic that one mediator or one injurious principle alone dominates the battlefield of acute lung injury. More likely, and more difficult to study, are the many possible different interactions between the vascular wall, inflammatory cells, and their products. To isolate the particular interactions which are most relevant to the course of lung injury and its final results, healing or scar formation of the lung, is a task yet to be accomplished. Finally, it is important to begin work on the proliferative potential of lipid mediators. It is currently unknown whether LTs and PAF–in addition to their effects on vascular tone control and cell permeability–stimulate cell proliferation, thus contributing to fibrosis and scar tissue formation.

References

1. Asbaugh DG, Bigelow DB, Petty TL, Levine BE (1967) Acute respiratory distress in adults. Lancet 2:319–323
2. Bernard GR, Luce JM, Sprung CL, Rinaldo JE, Tate RM, Sibbald WJ, Kariman KK, Higgins S, Bradley R, Metz CA, Harris TR, Brigham KL (1987) High-dose corticosteroids in patients with the adult respiratory distress syndrome. N Engl J Med 317:1565–1570
3. Bussolino F, Camussi G, Baglioni C (1988) Synthesis and release of platelet-activating factor by human vascular endothelial cells treated with tumor necrosis factor or interleukin I. J Biol Chem 263:11856–11861
4. Chang S, Voelkel NF (1989) Charge related lung microvascular injury (state of the art). Am Rev Respir Dis 139:534–545
5. Chang S, Feddersen CO, Henson PM, Voelkel NF (1987) Platelet activating factor mediates hemodynamic changes and lung injury in endotoxin treated rats. J Clin Invest 79:1498–1509
6. Chang S, Westcott JY, Pickett WC, Murphy RC, Voelkel NF (1989) Endotoxin-induced lung injury in the rat: the role of eicosanoids. J Appl Physiol 66:2407–2418
7. Chang S, Czartolomna J, Voelkel NF (1990) Role of eicosanoids in staphylococcal α-toxin induced lung injury in the rat. J Appl Physiol (to be published)
8. Chang S, Fernyak S, Voelkel NF (1990) Post-treatment with WEB 2086, a platelet activating factor antagonist, decreases lung injury in endotoxin-treated rats. Am J Physiol 258 153–158, 1990
9. Garrett RC, Thomas HM III (1983) Meclofenamate uniformly decreases shunt fraction in dogs with lobar atelectasis. J Appl Physiol 54:284–289
10. Graham LM, Vasil A, Vasil ML, Voelkel NF, Stenmark KR (1990) Decreased pulmonary vasoreactivity in an animal model of chronic pseudomonas pneumonia. Am Rev Resp Dis 142, 221–229, 1990
11. Hanley PJ, Sienko A, Light RB (1988) Role of prostacyclin and thromboxane in the circulatory changes of acute bacteremic pseudomonas pneumonia in dogs. Am Rev Respir Dis 137:700–706
12. Lewis MS, Whatley RE, Cain P (1988) Hydrogen peroxide stimulates the synthesis of platelet-activating factor by endothelium and induces endothelial-cell dependent neutrophil adhesion. J Clin Invest 82:2045–2055
13. McDonnell TJ, Voelkel NF, Petty TL (1987) Adult respiratory distress syndrome and its management. Comprehensive Therapy 13(7):33–40
14. McDonnell TJ, Chang SW, Westcott JY, Voelkel NF (1988) Role of oxidants, eicosanoids, and neutrophils in amphotericin B lung injury in rats. J Appl Physiol 65(5): 2195–2206
15. Newman JH, Loyd JE, English DK, Ogletree ML, Fulkerson WJ, Brigham KL (1983) Effects of 100% oxygen on lung vascular function in awake sheep. J Appl Physiol 54:1379–1368
16. Prescott CM, Zimmerman GA, McIntyre TM (1987) The production of platelet-activating factor by cultured human endothelial cells: regulation and function. In: Snyder F (ed) Platelet -activating factor and related lipid mediators. Plenum, New York, pp 323–340
17. Sakai A, Chang S, Voelkel NF (1989) The importance of vasoconstriction in lipid mediator induced pulmonary edema. J Appl Physiol 66, 2667–2674, 1989
18. Van Grondelle A, Worthen GS, Ellis D et al. (1984) Altering hydrodynamic variables influences PGI_2 production by isolated lungs and endothelial cells. J Appl Physiol 57:388–395
19. Voelkel NF (1990) The adult respiratory distress syndrome. Klin Wochenschr 67, 559–567, 1989
20. Zapol W, Snider G (1977) Pulmonary hypertension in severe acute respiratory failure. N Engl J Med 296:476–480

Investigations of the Pathophysiology of the Pulmonary Microcirculation Using In-vivo Microscopy*

E. Rügheimer

Within the framework of earlier animal experimental research on the pathogenesis of vagus pneumonia, so-called, following high resection of the oesophagus, the consequences of high cervical dissection of the vagus were investigated [17]. On the basis of cine-angiographic records, the following phenomenon was observed at that time.

If, following high cervical vagotomy, a contrast medium is injected into a sub-segment of the lung, part of the contrast medium flows off via the venous system, while another part remains within the pulmonary microcirculation and can be observed over a period of hours as a "cloud" of contrast medium.

At the time, we interpreted this phenomenon as a constriction of the muscular component of the pulmonary arteries brought about by a predominance of sympathetic activity, subsequently followed by a local chemical effect. We assumed that a role is also played by tissue hormones that exert a profound effect on the functional activity of the microcirculation, and are responsible for the development of a permeability oedema.

The investigations thus ended in the paradox so typical of science. Although cine-angiography revealed evidence that something must have happened in the pulmonary circulation, this evidence was indirect and unspecific, and merely provided food for conjecture. Ever since, we have been applying ourselves to the question as to how the processes in the pulmonary microcirculation might be observed and measured.

The spectrum of available investigative methods for defining the dynamics of the microcirculation is wide. Table 1 shows a list of the measuring procedures that might be employed. If, however, the parameters measurement site, course and resolution are differentiated, it becomes apparent that only in-vivo microscopy permits a direct and continuous observation and measurement, and is suitable for the study of individual capillaries.

On the occasion of the first Shock Symposium held in Vienna in October 1978, Watts Webb, a surgeon at the Tulane University School of Medicine in New Orleans, presented a film showing in-vivo microscopic views of the lungs [25]. The technical facilities available at that time did not permit any long-term continuous observation of the fixed lung area. This explains why most of the scientists who within the last 40 years have been concerned with in-vivo microscopy of the lungs (Table 2), abandoned this approach again after only

* Supported by the German Research Society (Grant No. Ru 325-3)

Table 1. Measuring methods for determining blood flow in the microcirulation.

Technique	Measurement mode	Course	Resolution
Tissue surface pO_2	indirect	continuous	Hemisphere: diameter 50 µm
H_2 clearance	indirect	discontinuous	Hemisphere: diameter 65 µm
Reflexion-spectrophotometry	direct	discontinuous	Club-shaped: depth 100–500 µm
Radioctive microspheres	indirect	discontinuous	detector-dependent: of the order of mm
Laser Doppler	direct	continuous	Volume of crossed beams: diameter 5–10 µm
In-vivo microscopy	direct		better than 1 µm

Table 2. In-vivo microscopic quantification of the pulmonary microcirculation.

Authors	Parameter	Visualisation	Documentation
Vogel, 1947	Blood flow velocity	Indian ink	High-speed film
Burrage et al., 1953	Vessel diameter		Photograph
Knisely, 1960	Vessel diameter	Transillumination	
Schlosser and Bartels, 1965	Blood flow velocity, Transit times		Film
Daly et al., 1973	Alveolus diameter		Video
Webb et al., 1974	Alveolus diameter		Film
Sohara et al., 1982	Blood flow velocity	Dye	Video
Götz et al., 1984	Blood flow velocity, Vessel diameter	Erythrocytes	SIT Video
Wagner et al., since 1963	Recruitment Transit times	Dye	Film, Video
Nieman et al., since 1981	Alveolus diameter, Recruitment		Photograph

a short time. It was shown that a quantification of ventilation and perfusion parameters in the observable areas of the lung by means of objective measurement was simultaneously possible for only a few parameters.

To enable our goals to be achieved, a thoracic window was developed that was capable of being implanted air-tight over the long-term (Fig. 1). To date, the longest period of observation we have achieved was 3 days, with no deterioration in quality. With the aid of a special suction manifold, it proved possible to fix the lung surface at a relatively large distance from the point of observation, while at the same time preserving the movements of respiration, so that no impairment of the measured results was to be expected. Histological-morphological studies performed on conclusion revealed no changes in pulmonary ultra-structure in the area under observation.

Although in-vivo microscopy is ideal for observing the microcirculation, it is, nevertheless difficult to perform a quantitative analysis with this technique. Following other investigators, one of the first attempts at quantification involved the use of FITC-labelled erythrocytes (e.g. 9). By using incident light

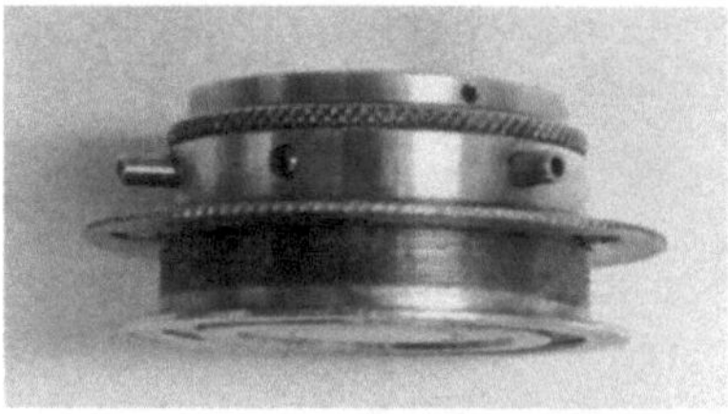

Fig. 1. Thoracic window with lens adapter and device for fixing the working distance for observation

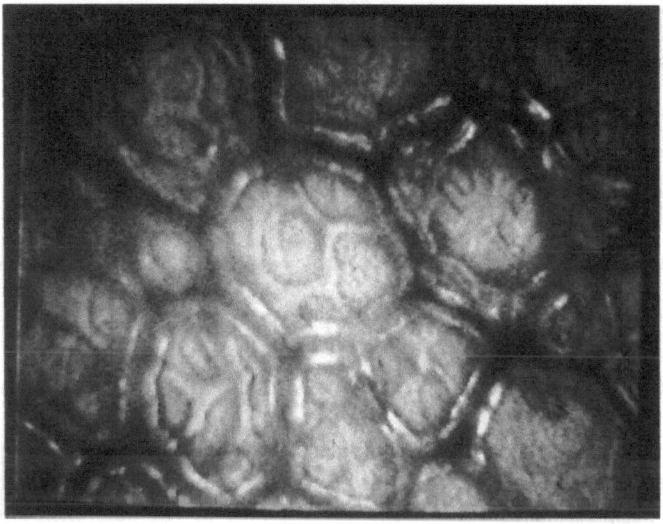

Fig. 2. In-vivo microscopic videorecording of the surface of the lung with FITC-labelled erythrocytes (recorded) with an SIT camera

illumination with an appropriate wavelength (488 nm), excitation of these "fluorochromes" proved possible, and the signal was then measured with the aid of a silicon intensifier target image tube (SIT) camera. During measurements, ventilation was stopped at the end of inspiration in order to exclude interference due to movements (Fig. 2).

It was discovered that stopping ventilation for 20 seconds had an influence on capillary flow. It was not possible in view of the small number of labelled erythrocytes involved to determine dynamic redistributions, changes in velocities or alveolar changes. Since FITC labelling of all of the erythrocytes is not possible, a further experiment was made after staining the plasma with Na fluorescein (Fig. 3).

Although at first glance this permits excellent visualisation of the capillary flow, the alveoli are only unclearly discernible, and the so-called photodynamic effect results in stagnation of the flow after only a short period of observation.

On the basis of these and numerous other preliminary experiments carried out over the past years, and utilising present-day technologies, we developed

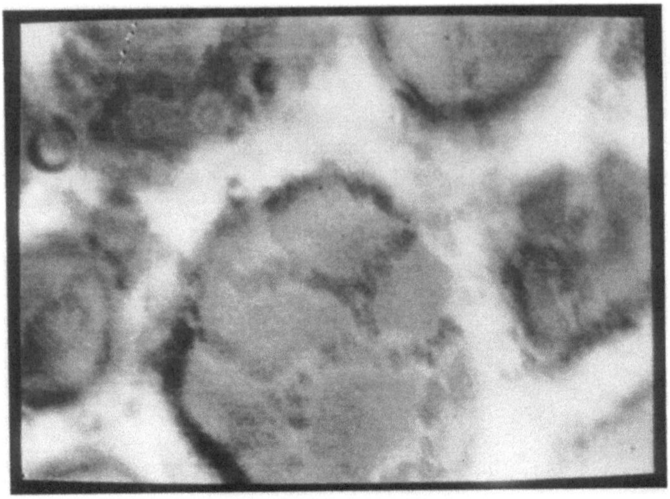

Fig. 3. In-vivo microscopy recording of the capillary network on the surface of the lung. The plasma has been stained with Na-fluorescein

a concept for the quantitative analysis of in-vivo microscopic observations [2, 3].

Image acquisition was done with a highly sensitive videocamera. In order not to have the erythrocytes appear on the monitor screen as "comet tails", which invariably happens when the images are exposed at the conventional video rate of 50 Hz for 20 milliseconds and then represented using the interlaced raster scanning technique in pairs simultaneously, a CCD camera with a sensor is employed, the light-sensitive cells of which can be exposed in parallel. Slaaf et al. [19] described the possibilities of such image acquisition for the first time in 1984. This makes it possible to read an entire image using the so-called frame transfer facility. Movement unsharpness is virtually eliminated by using a stroboscope flashlamp triggered by the video signal and having an exposure time of 2 microsecs. The flickering caused by the interlaced scanning method can be completely eliminated with the aid of digital image processing. In this way, dynamic processes can be "split up" into the sharp individual views that a quantitative analysis requires.

In order to obtain as three-dimensional a view of the structures as possible, oblique illumination from the side is employed, either via a dark-field lens, or via light guides that direct the light onto the observation field. The obliquely incident light throws the three-dimensional structures such as erythrocytes or alveoli into sharp relief. In this way, erythrocytes with differing velocities can be detected. The blood flow is no longer impaired through the use of marker substances. The video images are then digitised and stored in a raster containing 512 × 512 picture elements. Each picture element can define any of 256 different intensity steps. This resolution is much higher than that of the human eye, which, against a uniform gray background, can differentiate only about some 30 different shades of gray.

Figure 4 shows a single video image. Two alveoli lying close together can be recognised. The bright spot below on the left, has been produced by the light reflected at the confluence of several small venous vessels.

Using special image processing techniques, contrast is enhanced, contours sharpened, and the effects of non-uniform illumination corrected. In Fig. 5, the contours of the erythrocytes have been particularly strongly emphasized.

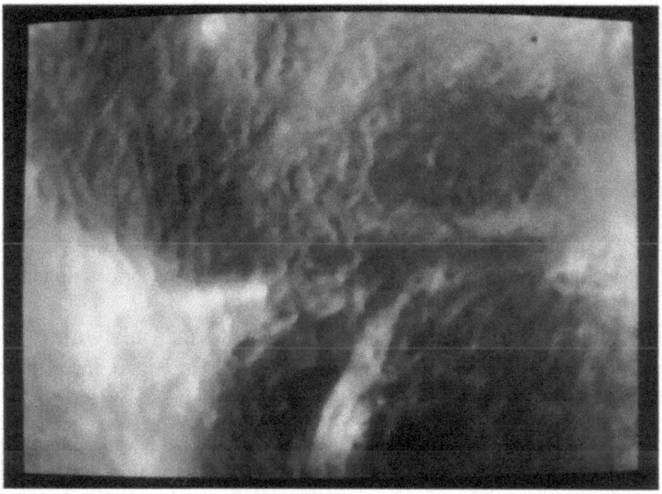

Fig. 4. Digitized video image of the surface of the lung (see text for description)

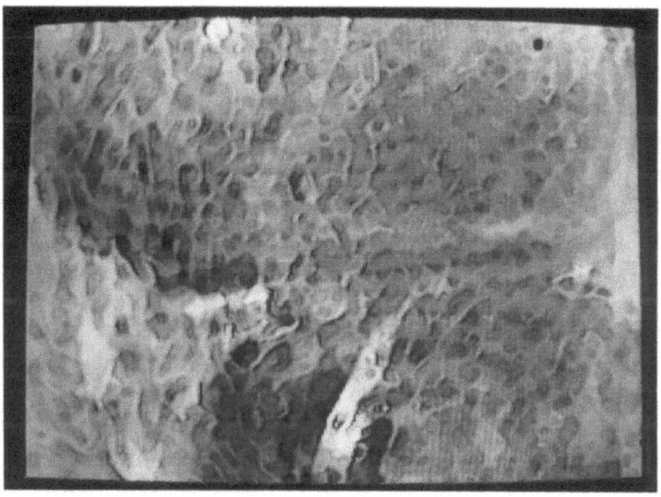

Fig. 5. Figure 4 after processing. The errors due to non-uniform illumination have been corrected and the contours of the erythrocytes enhanced

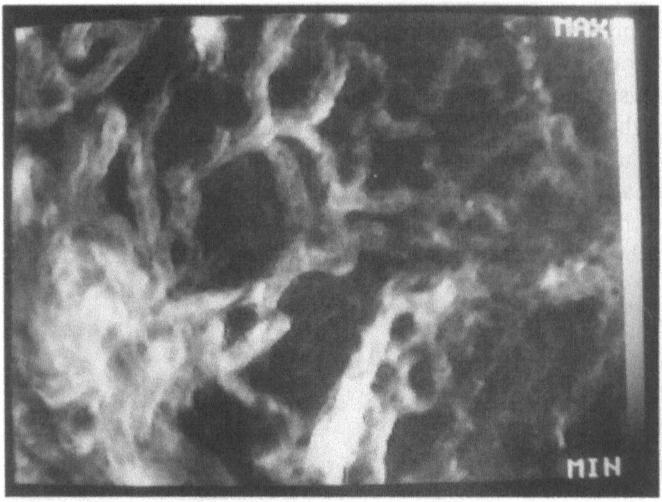

Fig. 6. Reconstruction of the capillary network from an image series lasting 2.5 seconds. The gray shade bar indicates the velocity distribution within this period of time (see text for description)

The capillaries, which are often not recognisable, or at least only with great difficulty, can be reconstructed from a short image sequence. In Fig. 6, the course of individual capillaries (above, right) to the confluence of the venules (below, left) can be recognised.

Of particular interest is the velocity distribution within the vessels. In this figure, the differing flow velocities of the erythrocytes in the reconstructed vessels are marked by gray levels. The bar on the right hand side serves as a measure of the velocity. The dark shade of gray (below) signifies a very low, a light shade (above) a very high velocity. As is to be expected, velocity increases from the capillaries to the venules.

Digital image processing offers ideal possibilities for quantitative analysis. Known analogous procedures for acquiring measured data [10, 20, 24] can be employed in the form of a program, and offer even greater application possibilities. Examples are the "dual window technique" and the spatial correlation technique for determining flow velocities. The digital version of these methods eliminates the restriction of measurement to straight capillary segments, permitting selection of almost any number of measuring sites [8]. Within the framework of the present study, the measured values were obtained through the use of "frame-to-frame analysis", so-called [7].

In-vivo microscopy thus permits direct observation of the current dynamic situation of the pulmonary microcirculation within the limits of resolution defined by light microscopy. We compensated for this restriction through the use of lung biopsies that are obtained at defined points in time and submitted to histological work-up. Quantification is, however, possible only with the methods of morphometry and stereology – proven, but very labour-intensive methods. Random sampling, however, does permit information about the

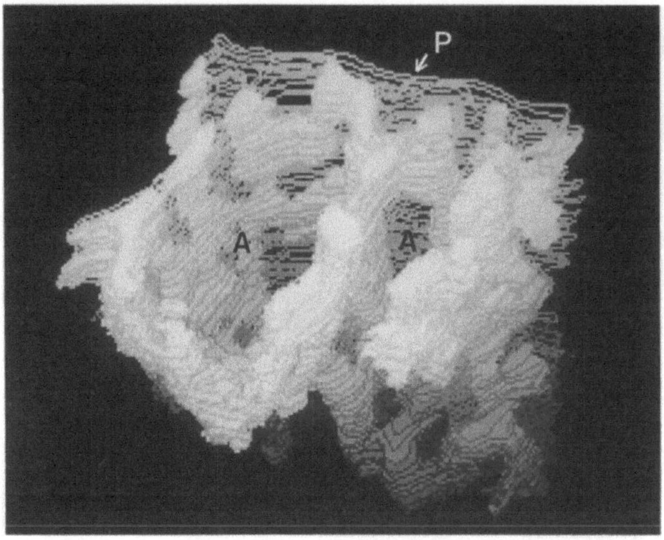

Fig. 7. Three-dimensional reconstruction of a subpleural alveolus

current state of certain histological or cytological structures to be extrapolated to the entire lungs. Recently, computer-supported three-dimensional reconstructions have become possible. Figure 7 shows the 3-D display of an alveolar region close to the pleura which was obtained by Duncker an Kriete (13) in Gießen. For the present, the contours of the underlying images have to be input interactively, although TV image feed-in is already possible.

Even under physiological conditions, the microcirculation is not homogeneous. On the contrary: its inhomogeneity is a physiological characteristic that results from the temporal and spatial activity changes observed in most organ systems. To accomplish this, accurate local feedback mechanisms must exercise a control effect aimed at ensuring local supply. The physiological situation is, consequently a need- adapted controlled heterogeneity. In the pathophysiological situation, this regulation is disordered, due either to a generalised change in vascular tone, or to a dissociation of the vascular function and tissue metabolism. The resulting heterogeneity is thus determined by the unequal distribution of the supply rather than by the demand.

Contributions to the Objectification of Pathophysiological Current Images in the Pulmonary Microcirculation

A scanning electron micrograph might serve to give the reader an idea of what can be recognised when the lung is observed (Fig. 8):

- Beneath the pleura alveoli of varying size with a mean diameter of about 70 µm under conditions of mid-expiratory level expansion are to be seen, which optimally fill the space like a dense mass of spheres.

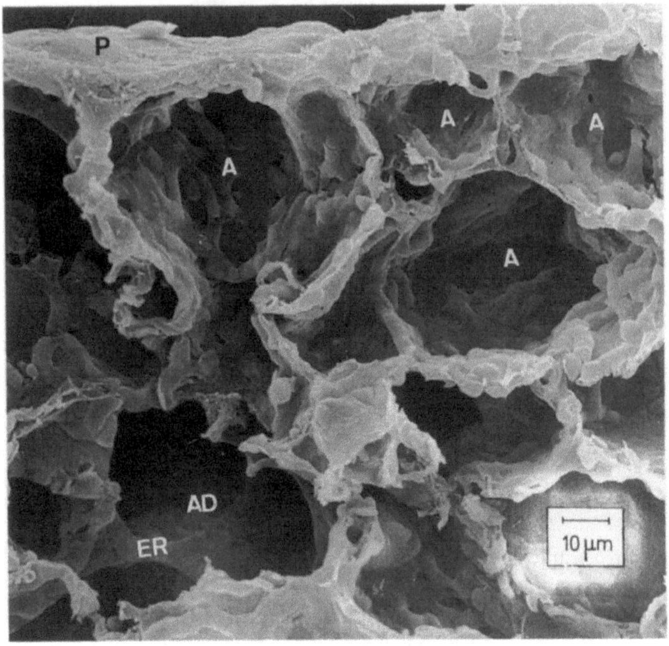

Fig. 8. Scanning-electron micrograph of the most peripheral "gas-exchange parenchyma" in logitudinal section. P = pleura, A = alveolus, AD = Alveolar duct, ER = Entrance ring (500 ×)

Between the alveoli, the interalveolar septa present as a very thin connective tissue septum, the capillary network it carries, and a thin lining of epithelium.

This picture can readily be correlated with the in-vivo microscopic images.

Details as to the processes occurring in the microcirculation in the initial phase of acute pulmonary failure are now documented in selected observational images in so-called septic shock, hypovolaemic shock and after vagotomy.

The investigations were performed in anaesthetised rabbits weighing 4 to 5 kg. Ventilation was carried out via an endotracheal tube, haemodynamic monitoring via a right-sided femoral catheter and a pulmonary catheter. The observation window was implanted after partial resection of the 4th and 5th ribs.

The Lungs in Endotoxic Shock

Clinical and Pathophysiological Aspects

In terms of frequency and mortality, sepsis is the most severe of the post-operative complications.

The onset of the sepsis syndrome can be traced back to a few basic events. Pathogenic bacteria from a septic focus, breach the body's own defence mechanisms, either because they are too numerous, or because there are defects in the body's defence system. The release of endotoxin and other mediators associated with the bacterial invasion has an effect on blood vessels, myocardium, immune system and metabolism. Of the numerous pathomechanisms that contribute to the ischaemic hypoxic and toxic metabolic injury to the endothelium and various organ cells, extending even to cell destruction, we consider only a few that, on the basis of our in-vivo microscopic observations, may need to be re-considered and interpreted anew.

Disturbances in the circulatory regulation in the case of sepsis are usually divided into a hyperdynamic and a hypodynamic phase, with a morphological reaction pattern similar to that of haemorrhagic shock, although much more deleterious in the end-phase.

Following initial application of the endotoxin, our own in-vivo microscopic observations revealed a completely unexpected course.

In-vivo Microscopic Observations

Under physiological conditions, alveolar structure and perfusion reveal a characteristic pattern that depends upon respiratory movements (Fig. 9a). The alveoli, covered with a close-meshed alveolar capillary network, are separated from one another by their septa, and are readily discernible. A well-regulated microcirculation permits optimal gas exchange. Figure 10a shows an enlarged section. In the interalveolar septum seen running from the left, above, to the right, below, a large, homogeneously perfused alveolar vessel can be recognised. Owing to the dense erythrocyte column that has formed, individual erythrocytes cannot be differentiated. A sectioned alveolus can be seen at each image margin.

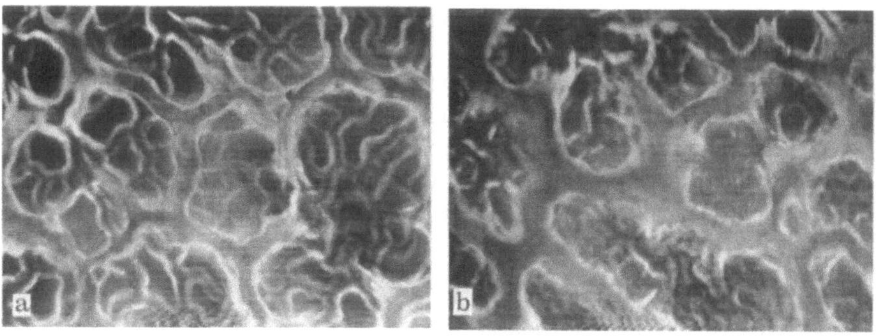

Fig. 9. a. In-vivo microscopic overview of the surface of the lung: The readily differentiable subpleural alveoli are visualized together with their clearly recognisable capillary network (objective: dark-field 12.8 ×). **b.** In-vivo microscopic overview of the surface of the lung after 5 hours of haemorrhagic shock (MAP 40 mmHg): In comparison with figure 9a, the alveolar septa are clearly thickened in consequence of interstitial oedema. (objective: dark-field 12.8 ×)

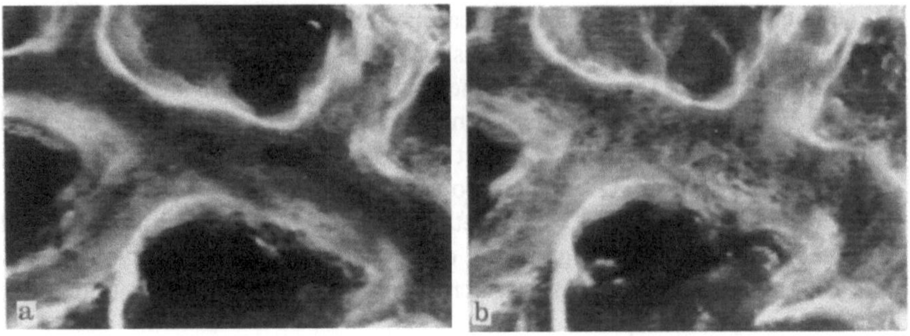

Fig. 10. a. Enlarged in-vivo microscopic detail. Within the interalveolar septum, which can be seen running from above, left to below, right, a large, homogeneously perfused alveolar vessel can be seen (objective: dark-field 20 ×). **b.** Enlarged in-vivo microscopic detail obtained 10 sec. after the application of *E. coli* endotoxin. The blood within the interseptal vessel has stopped flowing. Reversible aggregation of the erythrocytes has occurred, and the number of cell-free zones of plasma have increased. (objective: dark-field 20 ×)

Some 10 seconds after application of *E. coli* endotoxin, the blood flow is arrested (Fig. 10b). In the interseptal vessels, a wide band of plasma containing only a few erythrocytes can be seen. The latter move back and forth in rhythm with the respiratory cycle. The reversible aggregation of erythrocytes makes the blood column appear to be interrupted by cell-free areas of plasma. This effect is reproducible and occurs immediately after administration of endotoxin. We have since obtained evidence that this is a direct effect of the mediator thromboxan on the endothelium of the capillaries. At this point in time, mechanical occlusion caused by granulocytes, as can be observed in the end phase, does not occur. This effect was observed for the first time in our own investigations, since previously no continuous observation of the pathogenesis had been undertaken.

The following "hyperdynamic phase", so-called, is characterised by a rapid flow within the large interseptal vessels, while the capillary flow is impaired by the adhesion of leukocytes–initially only a few in number – to the capillary endothelium.

In the end stage, blockage by neutrophil leukocytes becomes more and more pronounced, and capillary flow is reduced almost to a standstill. In the septa, rouleau-like aggregates are to be seen. The alveolar walls are appreciably thickened due to oedematous swelling, and the surface film has been destroyed. Severe impairment of the gas exchange is the result.

Quantitative Analysis and Histology

Figure 11 shows the course of the erythrocyte flow velocity in the capillaries (above, left) of the visible alveolar surfaces (adjacent, right), of the septal width as indicator of the development of oedema (below, left), and of perfusion (below,

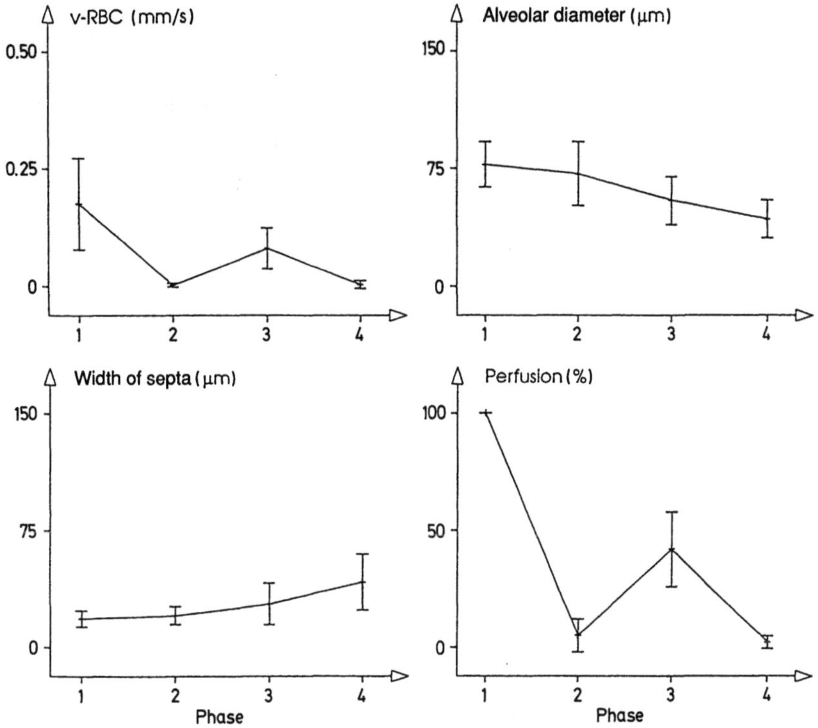

Fig. 11. Endotoxin shock – quantitative analysis (see text for explanation)

right), by which is meant the percentage of perfused capillaries in relation to the initial situation.

Phase 1 shows the initial situation, phase 2 the acute phase, phase 3 the hyperdynamic phase, so-called, and phase 4 the final state. The erythrocyte flow velocity (above, left), and perfusion (below, right) decrease to zero in the acute phase (phase 3), increase again in the so-called hyperdynamic phase – but only to about one-half of the initial values – and decrease again to zero in the final state. The thickening of the alveolar septa indicates the presence of oedema.

As the histological evaluation shows, the rapid onset of the effect of endotoxin results in dramatic changes at the cellular level (panel I). The capillaries are dilated and filled with damaged erythrocytes and granulocytes (panel Ia). The number of macrophages increases rapidly, and they are found, aggregated to a varying extent, in the alveoli close to the septa (panel Ia).

The high-resolution electron micrographs reveal the ultrastructural aspects of these changes (panel Ib–f). Massive interstitial oedema filled with cellular detritus (panel Ib) distend the alveolar septa. Granulocytes have passed into the interstitium and are "squeezing" themselves past thick bundles of collagen fibres (panel Ie). The inhomogeneity of their cytoplasm and the, in part empty, granules, indicate that they are undergoing lysis (panel Id, e).

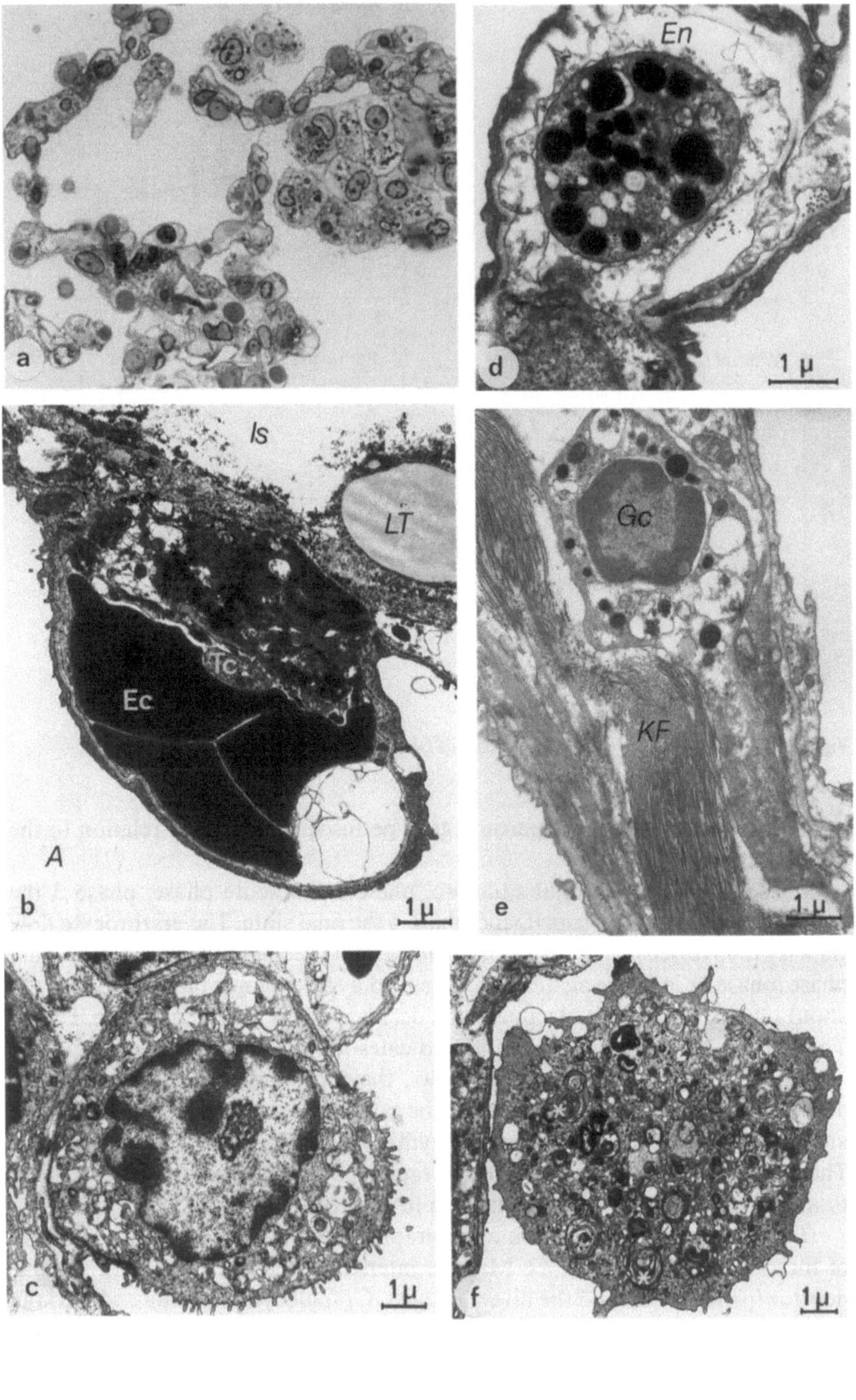
a
En
d
1 µ
ls
LT
Tc
Ec
A
b
1µ
Gc
KF
e
1µ
c
1µ
f
1µ

The erythrocyte stagnation seen in panel Ib is so marked that the erythrocytes appear to be fused with one another and with the surrounding endothelial cell. As a result, oxygen transportation is massively impaired and irreversible cell damage occurs. The cytoplasm of the endothelial cells which is disintegrating and giving rise to vesicles (panel Ib, d) promotes this stagnation and thus the damage being done to the trapped blood cells.

Type II epithelial cells develop more microvilli, but only a few lamellar bodies (panel Ic). Within a short period of time this change leads to the collapse of the surfactant system in the lungs. The macrophages, which are quite numerous (panel Ia), contain dense "packages" of phagolysomes with a variety of different cell constituents within the cytoplasm. Some contain complete lamellar bodies (*).

The Lungs in Hypovolaemic Shock

Clinical and Pathophysiological Aspects

One of the most common complications met with in emergency care medicine and in the operating room is hypovolaemic shock. A reduction in the circulating blood volume may be due to the loss of blood, plasma or extracellular fluid. If hypovolaemia overwhelms the body's compensatory mechanisms, this condition leads to effects in the lungs which, depending upon duration, show a characteristic evolution.

Hypovolaemia was experimentally induced by the removal of 150 ml of blood and a reduction in MAP to 30–40 mm/Hg for a period of about 6 hours.

←

Panel I. Endotoxin

a. Light micrograph of an alveolar section obtained after induction of endotoxin shock. The capillaries are dilated and, for the most part filled with granulocytes or devitalised erythrocytes. The alveolar space contains individual or groups of (alveolar) macrophages.

b–f. Transmission electron micrographs (TEM)

b. The capillary is crammed full of erythrocytes (Ec), the disintegrating endothelial lining is restricting the lumen still further. In part, erythrocytes and endothelium are pressed so close together that the two cells appear to be fused. Ec = erythrocytes, Is = interstitium, LT = lipid drops, TC = thrombocyte.

c. Type II epithelial cell with increased microvilli formation and a few lamellar bodies.

d. Capillary cross-sectioned. The cytoplasm of the endothelial cell (En) has almost completely disintegrated and is swollen. En = endothelial cell.

e. A granulocyte (Gc) that has entered the interstitium. Note the "pseudopodium". The interstitium also contains increased numbers of collagen fibres (KF).
Gc = granulocyte, KF = collagen fibres.

f. Alveolar macrophage. The cytoplasm is densely packed with phagolysosomes containing abundant cell constituents and lamellar bodies.

In-vivo Microscopic Observations

In the initial state, a rapid flow of erythrocytes can be observed in all blood vessels (Fig. 9a). Occasional leukocytes also pass through the capillaries.

During the bleeding, the flow is reduced in all vessels. As a result, the transparency of the alveolar septa increases. In addition, the number of perfused capillaries decreases.

After about 5 hours of haemorrhagic shock, the capillaries of the alveoli are almost completely shut down (Fig. 9b). The venules are dilated and, depending upon the flow velocity are blocked to varying degrees by erythrocytes aggregates. Oedematous swellings have increased and the septa are clearly widened; the compliance of the alveoli is reduced. If no treatment is forthcoming, shock now becomes irreversible and the cells will die. Only timely blood replacement can prevent these events. In future, we may still have a chance even at this stage. With the aid of so-called hyperoncotic, hyperosmotic solutions, an attempt is presently being undertaken to "suck back", as it were, into the capillary network the water that has already been lost, and to re-start blood flow. These solutions are presently being investigated experimentally. After administration of a hyperoncotic hyperosmotic solution, perfusion increases, initially in the interseptal vessels, and – at a later stage – also in the capillaries.

Quantitative Analysis and Histology

Phase 1 in Fig. 12 again shows the initial situation; phase 2 the situation during bleeding, phase 3 immediately thereafter (40 mmHg MAP), phase 4 after 5 hours of shock, and phase 5 after treatment.

The results are not surprising: the velocity of the erythrocytes decreases continuously during bleeding, and even after treatment no longer attains to the initial level. On account of the oedema that develops, the visible surface of the alveoli also decreases. The thickening of the septa behaves accordingly. As expected, perfusion also decreases, but 5 hours after bleeding (phase 3) reveals a wide range of scatter. After treatment it also increases, but attains to a maximum of 50% of initial levels. The changes in the ultrastructure in the end phase of hypovolaemic shock are similar, but even more dramatic.

In panel II the changes at the cellular level in the alveolar region after hypovolaemic shock are illustrated. Already in light microscopic sections, it can be seen that hypovolaemic shock leads to an increase in granulocytes within the capillaries (table IIa). Also the number of macrophages is clearly increased. These occur in part more frequently in the alveolar space (panel IIa, e). The alveolar septa are thickened as a result of interstitial oedema and increased formation of collagen fibres (panel IIb, c).

The increase in the formation of pinocytotic vesicles in the endothelial and type II epithelial cells forces swelling of the cells, and thus impairs gas exchange (panel IIb, c, d). The changes in the ultrastructure are, in part, irreversible.

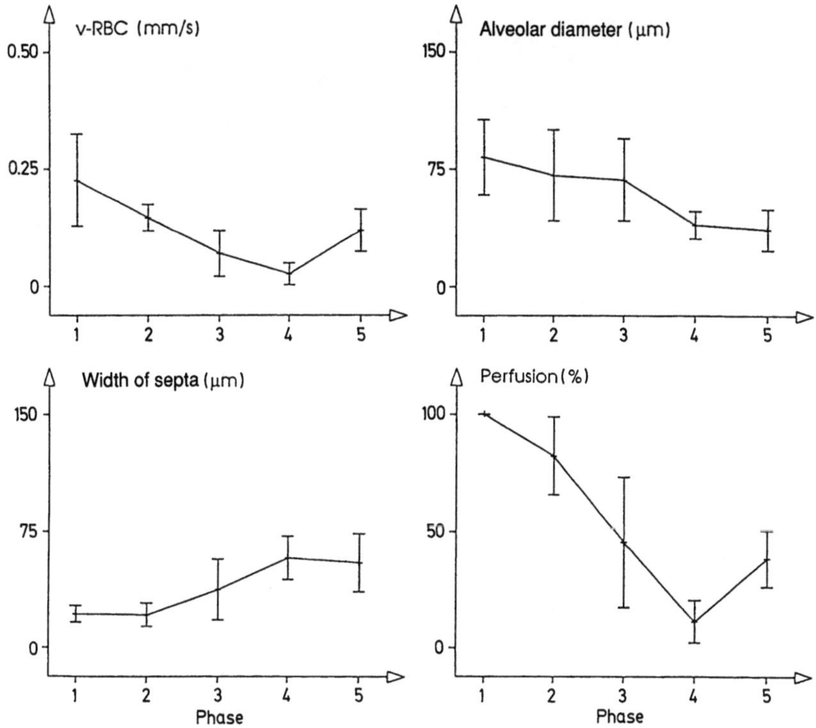

Fig. 12. Hypovolemic shock – quantitative analysis (see text for explanation)

Lysis of the endothelial cells is in part, so far advanced that the membranes rupture and release cytoplasm in the form of vesicles into the capillary lumen (panel IIc). This process also leads to insular cytoplasmic sectional profiles with well preserved contents that are occasionally to be seen. (panel IIb, c, d). Owing to stricturing of the capillary lumen, stasis-induced damage to the blood cells is unavoidable. The oxygen supply to the tissue is progressively restricted and gradually leads to irreversible damage. In these malperfused segments, granulocytes and erythrocytes no longer show sharp contours (panel IIb, c).

The Lungs After Vagotomy

Clinical and Pathophysiological Preconditions

Our in-vivo microscopic observations in the lungs following surgical vagotomy prompted us to take up again the question as to the actual processes going on in the microcirculation that arose out of our earlier studies [17].

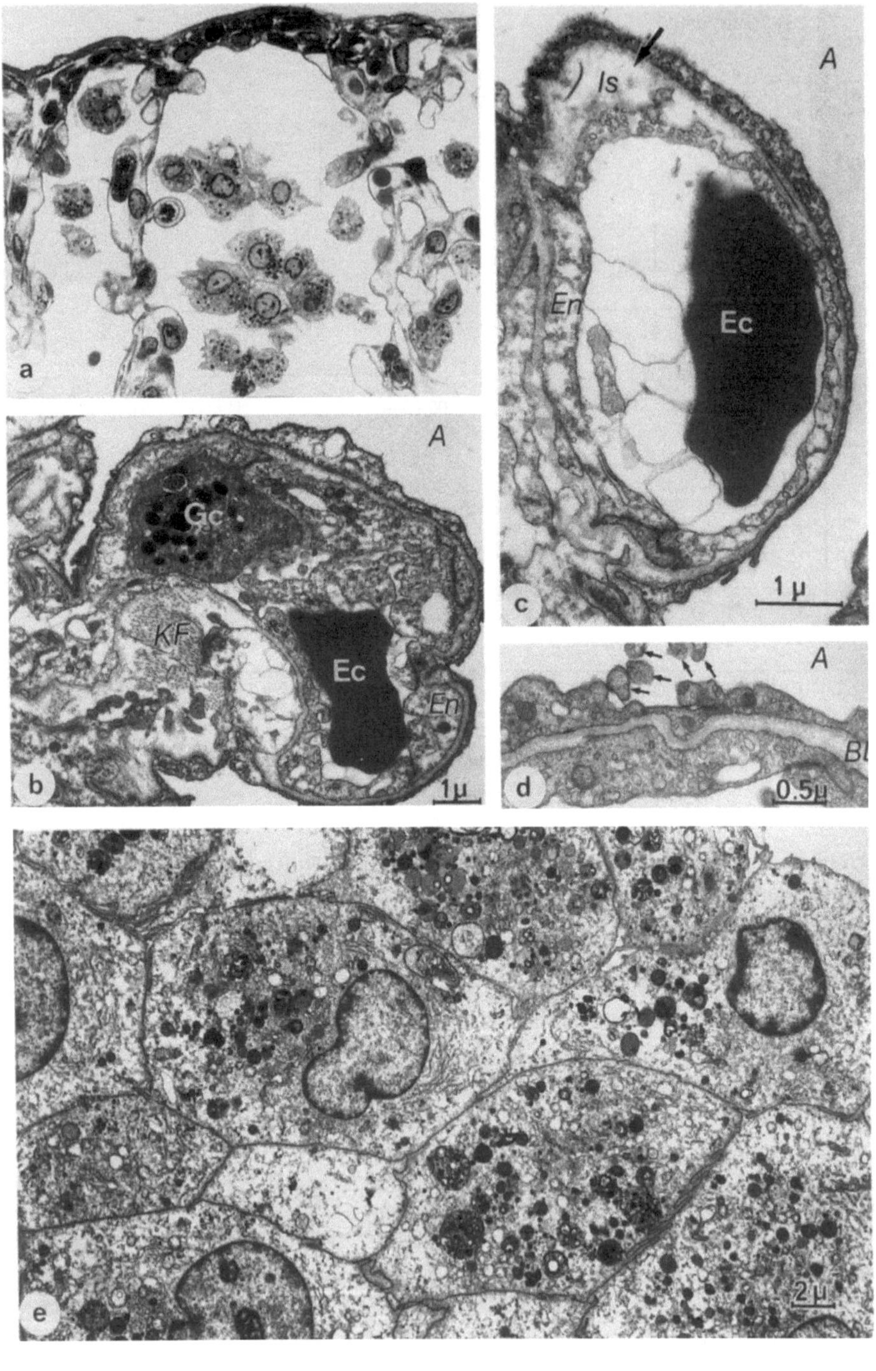
a
A
Is
En
Ec
c
1μ
A
Gc
KF
Ec
En
b
1μ
A
Bl
d
0.5μ
e
2μ

The reason for performing these animal experimental studies was the disturbing fact that surgery of the oesophagus is burdened by a high rate of pulmonary complications, and that the incidence of such complications is all the greater, the higher the level of the surgical intervention.

Prospective clinical investigations [14, 16] have also been able to show that even during the operation, changes occur in the pulmonary circulation that are of definitive pathogenetic significance for the development of respiratory failure.

The significance of the parasympathetic nerve for the numerous functional interactions between the various neural, cellular and humoral systems is not yet completely understood. Although – even in oesophageal extirpation – no surgeon divides the cervical vagus nerve in toto, irritation and affection of both afferent and efferent vagal fibres always occurs, and this is, in the last resort, responsible for the resulting clinical symptomatology. Admittedly, the significance of this has still not been definitively clarified. From the teleological point of view, sensors that "taste" the blood and "smell" the breath must be postulated [6]. And indeed, corresponding morphological structures have been identified, namely the neuroepithelial bodies with their function as peripheral O_2 sensors for the regional adaptation of ventilation. These are located close to the surface in the bronchial mucosa, and are connected via synapses with afferent and efferent parasympathetic fibres. Morphologically and anatomically, they are largely identical with the peripheral chemoreceptors of the carotid sinus. When the oxygen partial pressure is low, they secrete substances with a bronchoconstrictory effect into the capillary system. After denervation, swelling of the cellular structures occurs, together with atrophy of the neuroepithelial bodies.

A noteworthy observation is the interstitial and intra-alveolar oedema that occurs soon after vagotomy. In addition, a loss of compliance indicating a surfactant disorder has been measured.

←

Panel II. Haemorrhage

a. Light micrograph of a region adjacent to the pleura. The capillaries contain numerous cut granulocytes. The alveolar space contains increased numbers of macrophages.

b–e. Transmission electron micrographs (TEM).

b. Section of capillary. The lumen of a capillary is greatly narrowed by a swollen endothelial cell. It is undergoing lysis, and reveals isolated, insular cytoplasmic sectional profiles. Embedded completely within the disintegrating cytoplasm are a granulocyte and an erythrocyte.

c. Capillary showing marked interstitial oedema (arrow). The endothelial cell has formed numerous large pinocytotic vesicles that are in the process of "dissolving" the cell into individual cytoplasm vesicles.

d. Greater magnification of the gas exchange barrier. The numerous pinocytotic vesicles within the cytoplasm have produced swelling of the endothelial and epithelial cells, resulting in an increase in the resistance to gas exchange. Insular cytoplasmic profiles (arrow).

e. TEM micrograph of alveolar exudate. The alveolar space is filled with closely packed granulocytes, macrophages and cell fragments.

In-vivo Microscopy Observations

Prior to transecting the vagus nerve, a homogeneously perfused capillary bed with occasional leukocyte transit can be observed.

Some 15 minutes following division of the vagus nerve, the capillary flow increases considerably as a result of the predominance of the sympathetic tone.

After a period of 4 hours, thickened septa with interstitial oedema, a decreased capillary perfusion with pulsatile flow, and a considerable decrease in the number of capillaries perfused are observed. A number of alveoli are seen to have collapsed. Erythrocyte aggregates can be seen, in particular in the septal vessels.

After 36 hours, perfusion of the capillaries can no longer be observed. In the septal vessels, flow has slowed down considerably. Leukostasis is apparent and alveolar oedema has developed.

Quantitative Analysis and Histology

Erythrocyte flow rate (Fig. 13) is largely preserved during dissection (phase 2); the maximum values of perfusion (below, right) are in excess of 100%. In the further

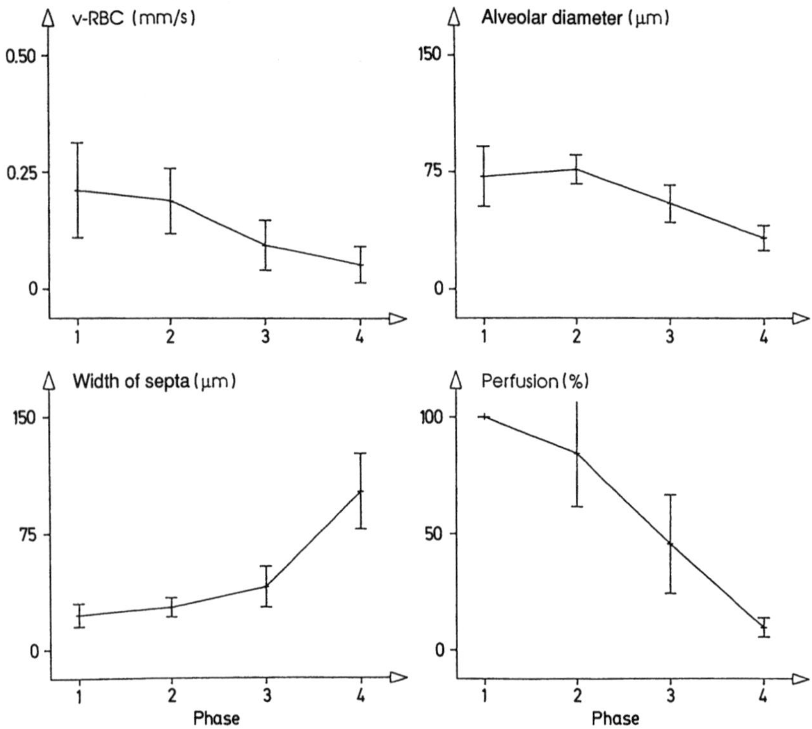

Fig. 13. Vagotomy quantitative analysis (see text for explanation)

evolution, however, both parameters decrease progressively. Another interesting observation is the very marked widening of the septa suggestive of interstitial oedema.

Not only does bilateral vagotomy give rise to an in-vivo microscopic appearance that is similar to that seen after bleeding, but it also has an effect at the cell level which is similar to that seen in the shock model already discussed above (panel III). After 8 hours, however, the damage is not so marked.

In the capillaries, granulocytes occur in increased quantities, leading in some segments to occlusion, and displacing the erythrocytes to the marginal zones (panel IIIa, b).

Macrophages also occur in increased numbers within the alveolar space, although no aggregation has been found (panel IIIa, b). An increase in the formation of vesicles within the cytoplasm leads initially to a "serpentine" folding (arrows) of the endothelial cell, and thus to an impairment of gas exchange (panel IIId). In a more advanced stage, cytoplasmic vesicles are pinched off, leading in turn to a thinning of the endothelium (panel IIIb). Cell organelles also undergo pathological changes. When swollen mitochondria in the markedly thinned endothelial cell burst, they may also rupture the surrounding thin zone of endothelial cytoplasm (panel IIIe).

Type II epithelial cells increase considerably in number and produce more lamellar bodies. The secretion of these surfactant-containing lamellar bodies, now often no longer takes place in a "dosed" manner, but in "spurts".

We hope that the examples given will illustrate how in-vivo microscopy of the lungs, although an extremely difficult method, is also extremely useful for obtaining objective functional- morphological information on pathophysiological states of the pulmonary microcirculation and its response to therapeutic

---

Panel III. Vagotomy

a. Light micrograph showing enlarged detail of an alveolar section following vagotomy. Note the numerous granulocytes in the capillaries and the small number of aggregated erythrocytes. The alveolar space contains an increased number of macrophages.

b–e. Transmission electron micrographs (TEM):

b. Granulocyte (Gc) in a capillary. Here, too, the increase in vesicle formation in the cytoplasm has led to the pinching off cytoplasmic vesicles which, in turn, have led to a thinning of the endothelium (arrow).
Gc = granulocyte, A = alveolar space

c. Type II epithelial cells are increased in number, and form more lamellar bodies. Inset: in many cases, surfactant material is released "in spurts"
C = capillary, A = alveolar space, LB = lamellar bodies, EpII = type II epithelial cells.

d. TEM micrograph of a longitudinally sectioned capillary. The numerous granulocytes (Gc) have displaced the erythrocytes (Ec) to the marginal zones. Increased vesicle formation in the endothelial and epithelial cells has led to "serpentine" folding (arrow). Some of the granulocytes are seen to have pseudopodia (double arrow), as an expression of their activation.
Gc = granulocytes, Ec = erythrocytes, A = alveolar space

e. Massively swollen mitochondria that finally burst, can lead to rupture of the thin surrounding zone of epithelial cytoplasm. C = capillary, A = alveolar space, M = mitochondria

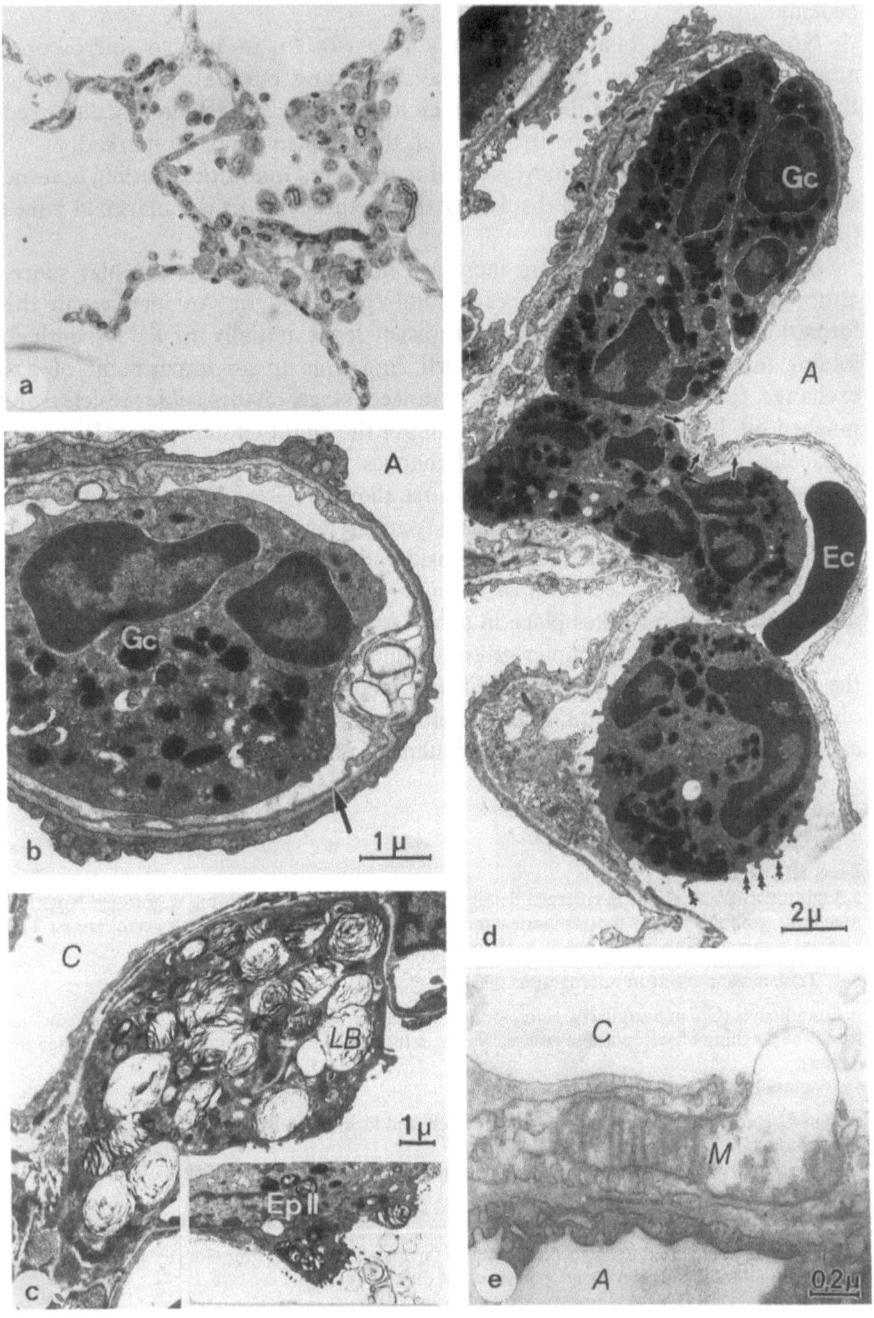
a
A
Gc
b
1 μ
C
LB
1μ
Ep II
c
Gc
A
Ec
2μ
d
C
M
A
e
0,2μ

approaches. Admittedly, the complex "method network" of which in-vivo microscopy is an integral part, can no longer be mastered by any single individual. Rather, a well-harmonized team of physicians, biologists, computer experts and technicians working in close interdisciplinary cooperation with anatomists, biochemists, pathologists, pharmacologists and physiologists is required, and many discussions leading to innumerable small advances and modifications are needed to finally concretise and implement the project.

Literatur

1. Ahnefeld FW, Bergmann H, Burri C, Dick W, Halmágyi M, Hossli G, Rügheimer E (Hrsg) (1979) Akutes Lungenversagen. Springer-Verlag, Berlin Heidelberg New York
2. Brunner M, Ittner W (1988) Viper: a general purpose digital image-processing system applied to video-microscopy. Comp Meth Prog Biomed 26:167–182
3. Brunner M, Ittner W (1988) Vitalmicroscopy of the lung: acquisition and processing of video-microscopy images. Int J Microcirc 7:169
4. Burrage WS, Irwin JW (1953) Microscopic observations of the pulmonary arterioles, capillaries, and venules of living mammals before and during anaphylaxis. J Allergy 24:289–296
5. Daly BDT, Edmonds CH, Norman JC (1973) In vivo alveolar morphometrics with positive and expiratory pressure. Surg Forum 24:217–219
6. Duhm J (1988) Die pulmonale Zirkulation. In: Peter K, Lawin P, Jensen U, Martin E (eds) Schock. Intensivmedizin, Notfallmedizin, Anaesthesiologie, Bd 63. Thieme, Stuttgart, pp. 91–105
7. Ellis CG, Fraser S, Hamilton G, Groom AC (1984) Measurement of the lineal density of red blood cells in capillaries in vivo, using a computerized frame-by-frame analysis of video images. Microvasc Res 27:1–13
8. Ellis CG, Tyml K, Burgess W (1987) Quantification of red cell movement in microvessels: a new application of interactive computergraphics. Microvasc Res 33:428–432
9. Götz A, Conzen PFM, Brendel W (1984) Red blood cell velocities and capillary transit times in the intact rat lung. Int J Microcirc 3:346
10. Intaglietta M, Tompkins WR (1972) On-line measurement of microvascular dimensions by television microscopy. J Appl Physiol 32:506–511
11. Intaglietta M, Silverman NR, Tompkins WR (1975) Capillary flow velocity measurements in vivo and in situ by television methods. Microvasc Res 10:165–179
12. Knisely WH (1960) In vivo architecture of blood vessels supplying and draining alveoli. Am Rev Resp Dis 81:735–736
13. Kriete A (1989) 3-D image processing with image analyzing systems. Europ J Cell Biol 48 (Supplement 25) 76–80
14. Murakami T (1978) Studies on pulmonary complications after surgery for esophageal cancer: especially the relationship between the vagus nerve and the pulmonary complication. Arch Jap Chir 47:413–426, 48:135–159
15. Niemann GF, Bredenburg CE, Clark WR, West NR (1981) Alveolar function following surfactant deactivation. J Appl Physiol: Resp Env Exerc Physiol 51(4):895–904
16. Pasch T, Brandl M, Feistel G, Kamp HD, Rügheimer E (1981) Postoperative Probleme und Intensivtherapie nach Ösophagusexstirpation. In: Häring R (ed) Chirurgie des Ösophaguskarzinoms. Edition Medizin, Weinheim Deerfield Beach (FL) Basel, pp. 113–122
17. Rügheimer E (1964) Folgen der hohen Vagusdurchtrennung. Langenbecks Arch Chir 308:880–885
18. Schlosser D, Heyse E, Bartels H (1965) Microcinematographic measurement of the erythrocyte flow rate in lung capillaries. Bibl Anat 7:106–108
19. Slaaf DW, Jeurens TJM, Alewijnse MA, Tangelder GJ, Reneman RS, Arts T (1984) The use of a CCD-camera for red cell velocity measurements based on spatial correlation. Microvasc Res 29:251

20. Slaaf DW, Jeurens TJM, Tangelder GJ, Reneman RS, Arts T (1986) Methods to measure blood flow velocity of red blood cells in vivo at the microscopic level. Ann Biomed Eng 14:175–186
21. Sohara Y, Mitsui K, Hori M (1982) Blood flow velocity in the small pulmonary arteries and arterioles. Nippon Kyobu Geka Gakkai Zasshi 30(7):1250–1256
22. Vogel H (1947) Die Geschwindigkeit des Blutes in den Lungenkapillaren. Helv Physiol Acta 5:105–121
23. Wagner WW, Filley GF (1963) Cinemicrography of the in vivo Lung. Isr J Exp Med 11:112
24. Wayland H, Johnson PC (1967) Erythrocyte velocity measurement in microvessels by a two-slit photometric method. J Appl Physiol 22:333–337
25. Webb WR, Wax SD, Kusajima K, Kamiyama TM (1974) Microscopic studies of the pulmonary circulation in situ. Surg Clin North Am 54:1067–1076

Pulmonary Capillary Transit Times in Fully Recruited Networks

W.W. Wagner, Jr.

I must begin this presentation by congratulating Professor Rugheimer and his excellent research team for their work on the pathophysiology of the pulmonary microcirculation in the adult respiratory distress syndrome. In vivo microscopy of the pulmonary microcirculation is an extremely difficult area, since it is fraught with many technical obstacles. Their persistance and clever solutions to the formidable problems with this technique deserve special recognition.

The data that I will present have also been obtained using in vivo microscopy of the pulmonary microcirculation. This presentation will focus on some aspects of the mechanism of gas exchange reserve in the normal lung. These mechanisms are certainly used when we go from the resting state to exercise. Also of importance, however, is how these mechanisms may be disrupted by diseases and also by the treatment of diseases.

There are two principal ways in which the pulmonary capillaries can alter blood perfusion characteristics to increase surface area for gas exchange. The first is capillary recruitment. In that process, more capillary segments are perfused and surface area is increased. The second mechanism is not so apparent. It involves capillary transit time. Normally, venous blood entering the pulmonary capillaries is rapidly saturated with oxygen. The best calculations we have at the present time (Wagner 1977) suggest that saturation is complete in no more than 0.25 s. Since the average time for a red cell to cross the capillary bed is about 1 s during resting conditions, red cells become fully saturated long before they leave the capillaries. Thus, there is a reserve in capillary length that can be recruited simply by speeding up the flow rate of the erythrocytes. Both the recruitment of length through decreased transit time and recruitment of new capillary segments effectively increase gas exchange surface area.

An additional aspect of capillary transit time that needs to be considered. There is a dispersion of capillary transit times about the mean. The 1 s capillary transit time that is often discussed is the mean transit time. Because the capillary network is so complex, the red cells are presented with a large variety of pathways to traverse. This causes a variation not only of resistance between segments but also a variation of path lengths that the red cells can follow. This combination leads inevitably to a dispersion of capillary transit times about the mean and will cause some red cells to transit the capillary bed more rapidly than the mean and many other cells to travel more slowly than the mean time. The fast cells are in potential danger of crossing the capillaries too rapidly to become saturated with oxygen. The slow cells are inefficient because they waste time by spending needless time in the capillaries after they are loaded with oxygen.

Capillary perfusion patterns change with exercise when cardiac output and pulmonary arterial pressure are elevated. Capillary volume increases. This change has been well documented by measuring the diffusing capacity of the lung for carbon monoxide (Johnson et al. 1960). Whether the increased volume is accounted for by recruitment or distension, however, has been a hotly debated issue for three decades. Almost certainly both occur. In the lower lung, where the capillary bed is nearly fully recruited during rest (Fig. 1A), distension must be important. In the upper lung, where most of the gas exchange reserve lies, recruitment is important, although recruitment without distension is obviously

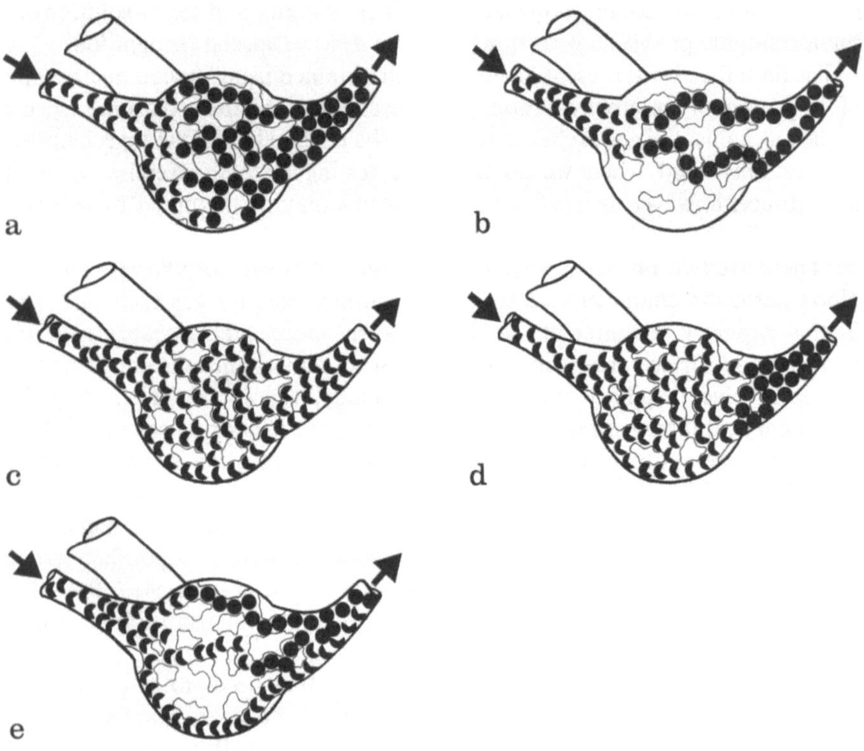

Fig. 1A–E. Blood enters the alveolar capillaries from the *left* through an arteriole and exits to the *right* through a venule. Erythrocytes load up with oxygen as they cross the capillaries and become completely saturated (*solid circles*). **A** In a fully recruited bed, such as in the lower lung during rest, the slowly flowing cells saturate with oxygen at about the first third of the way across the capillaries. **B** In slowly perfused, derecruited networks in the upper lung, the erythrocytes also saturate soon after they enter the capillaries. **C** If the capillary flow rate is too rapid, the cells cross before they become completely saturated. **D** Under optimal conditions, all capillaries are recruited and the flow rate is such that the cells just saturate as they leave the capillaries. This kind of homogeneous perfusion loads the maximal number of red cells per unit time. **E** In reality, the capillary network is complex and provides a variety of path lengths and resistances which inevitably cause a distribution of transit times. This kind of heterogeneous distribution can lead to hypoxemia if some of the pathways are sufficiently rapid impossible. Figure 1B shows that the capillary bed in the upper lung is, by comparison, relatively unrecruited. I will not focus further on this mechanism for increasing surface area but, following Professor Rugheimer's request, will concentrate on capillary transit times.

Red blood cells passing through a fully recruited, slowly perfused capillary bed rapidly saturate (Fig. 1A). If the cardiac output and pulmonary arterial pressure rise to very high levels, then the blood may cross the capillaries too rapidly to become saturated with oxygen (Fig. 1C). Under ideal conditions, the blood would become fully saturated with oxygen just as it left the capillary network (Fig. 1D). This combination of a fully recruited capillary bed and rapid homogeneous transit times would provide maximum utilization of gas exchange surface area reserve. Since there are reasons to suspect a dispersion of transit times at rest, there must likewise be a dispersion of transit times when cardiac output and pressure increase during exercise. This is illustrated in Fig. 1E where three different transit times through the capillary network are shown. In the slowest pathway, the red cells immediately saturate with oxygen. In the next fastest pathway, saturation is complete about half way across. In the very rapid pathway, saturation is incomplete. This last pathway would contribute to hypoxemia. Ideally, all cells would have the same transit time and become fully saturated just as they exit the capillary network as shown in Fig. 1D.

The transit times depicted in Fig. 1 are imaginary since they have not yet been directly measured. Recently, we have managed to make direct measurements both of the mean and the distribution of capillary transit times not only during rest but also when cardiac output was elevated. The measurements were made via a transparent window implanted in the chest wall of dogs. After aspirating the pneumothorax, we can observe the surface of the lung through the window. By using a surface illuminating microscope, it is possible to record microcirculatory events. For many years we attempted to use high-speed motion pictures to quantify the rate of blood flow across the capillaries. That technique, however, did not provide information about the range of transit times. All we were ever able to measure was red cell velocity through a few capillaries.

More recently, with the advent of extremely sensitive television cameras, it is possible to record the passage of a dye such as fluorescein as it traverses the microcirculation. If a photodetector is placed over an arteriole, the passage of the dye can be recorded as a dye dilution curve on a chart recorder. Once the dye enters the venule, draining the capillary bed fed by that arteriole, a venular dye dilution curve can be recorded as well. These two curves (Fig. 2) can be treated as the input and output to a given capillary bed. There is much information contained in these curves. By subtracting the time-weighted means of the curves, we can calculate mean capillary transit time. The venular curve is always more dispersed than the arteriolar curve indicating that there is a distribution of transit times across the capillary bed. The increased dispersion is of particular interest. One way to do that is with a mathematical technique called deconvolution which computes what happens to the input function as it passes through the

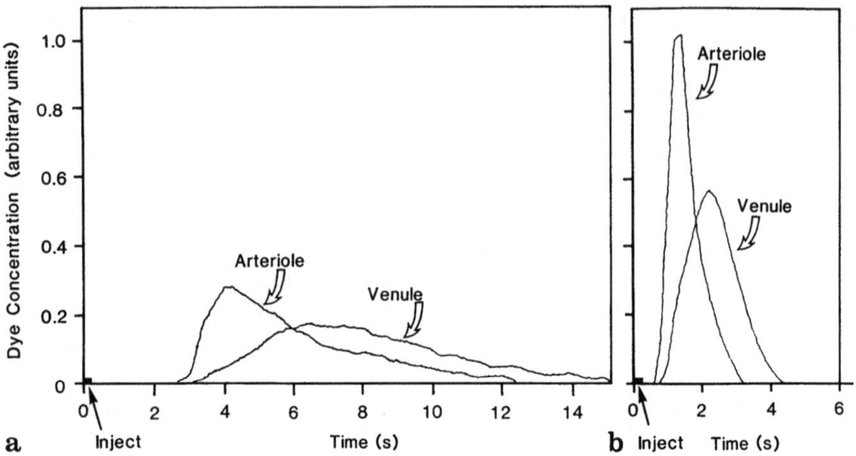

Fig. 2A. Dye dilution curves from a pulmonary arteriole and venule that feed and drain a common capillary bed. Fluorescent dye was injected into the lobar artery. The dye took about 10 s to clear; **B** Dye dilution curves from the same vessels when cardiac output was tripled. The curves are left-shifted, having much more rapid mean times and less dispersion

capillaries and disperses before it exits. By this computation the entire distribution of transit times through the capillary bed can be calculated.

The technique permitted us to attempt to answer some interesting questions about pulmonary microcirculatory function. The first question was whether there is a vertical gradient of capillary transit times. It is known from classical measurements that whole lung mean capillary transit time is equal to about 1 s. We also know from the work of West (1979) that most capillaries are open in the lower lung. In the upper lung, however, far fewer capillaries are perfused. This causes a vertical gradient for capillary recruitment with heavy recruitment in the lower lung and not so much recruitment in the upper lung. It is not straightforward to predict whether there is also a vertical gradient for transit times. Although there are fewer capillaries open in the upper lung, there is less flow. This combination could result in a 1 s transit time. On the other hand, the lower driving pressure could result in longer transit times. We lack sufficient data to make credible predictions.

To determine the distribution of mean transit times throughout the lung, we made direct observations in animals through windows placed in three positions, so that transit times could be measured in the upper lung the mid-lung, and the lower lung. The upper lung transit times were surprisingly long, 10–12 s on average with some times above 20 s (Fig. 3). In the mid-lung position, the transit times were faster, around 3 s. In the lower lung, we found more familiar numbers of about 1.5 s. Simultaneous measurements of recruitment showed the expected gradient (Fig. 3). These measurements demonstrated for the first time that vertical gradients exist both for capillary recruitment and transit times (Wagner et al. 1982, 1986). Since then the vertical gradient for microcirculatory

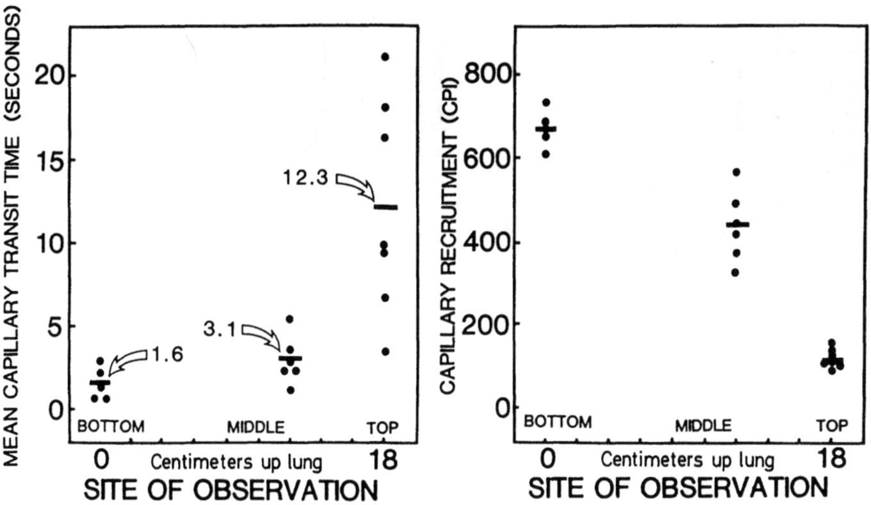

Fig. 3. Mean capillary transit time decreased as the observation site was moved from the upper lung to the lower lung (*left panel*). There was also a vertical gradient for capillary recruitment (*right panel*)

transit times has been confirmed by others (Hogg et al. 1988) using different methods.

In our next studies we concentrated on the lower lung, since that is where most of the blood flow goes. We were curious about the effect of increasing cardiac output (Capen et al. 1990). A beta agonist, isoproterenol, plus a fluid load of dextran were used to elevate cardiac output. This produced an increase in cardiac output from about 3 liters/min control to nearly 10 liters/min.

The dye dilution curves from an arteriolar and venular pair during control conditions are shown in Fig. 2A. At time zero, the dye was injected and these rather sluggish dye dilution curves resulted. Even though the measurements were made in the heavily perfused lower lung, dye was still being cleared 12 or 14 s later. The mean capillary transit time was 4–5 s. Curves from the same vessels when cardiac output was elevated are shown in Fig. 2B. All the dye appeared much more rapidly after the injection. The arteriolar curve rose briskly and fell to zero about 3 s later. The venular curve was brisk as well. The arteriolar curve during high cardiac output had returned to baseline at about the same time that the arteriolar curve started during control conditions. The same was true for the venular curve. There was a dramatic left shift of these curves towards more rapid transit times. From these kinds of curves we can compute the mean capillary transit time.

In Fig. 4A cardiac output is plotted against mean capillary transit time. Output was regularly increased to 10–12 liters/min. The capillary transit times started at 2–4 s and, as output increased, the times immediately decreased to about 1 s and then down to 0.5 s. On average, the control times were 2 s and decreased to 0.8 s at high cardiac output. Since blood can become completely saturated with oxygen in about 0.25 s, the measurement for mean time of 0.8 s,

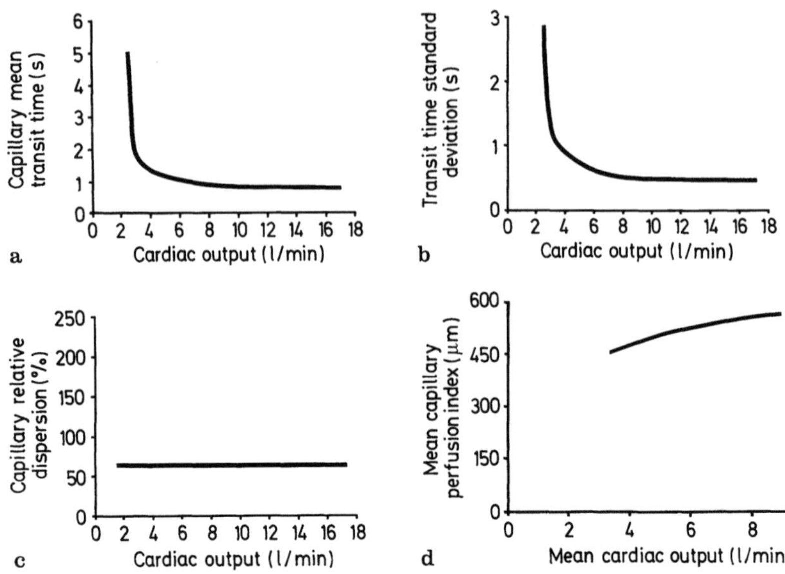

Fig. 4. A Mean capillary transit time fell rapidly as cardiac output was initially elevated, but then leveled off. **B** A similar relationship existed for the width of the distribution of transit times. The distribution narrowed as soon as output rose, but then did not change further. **C** The result of these variables changing in such similar ways was that the relative dispersion did not change, indicating that the capillaries were perfused homogeneously whether the flow was high or low. **D** One explanation for the unchanging relative dispersion is that in the lower lung, where our measurements were made, the capillaries were fully recruited under all flow conditions so that the transit times through individual pathways varied in unison as flow rates changed

even though it was rapid, was still well above the minimum time required for complete saturation.

By deconvolving the arteriolar and venular curves, the distribution of capillary transit times was obtained. The distribution of transit times appeared similar to a dye dilution curve, i.e., a right skewed curve. The width of the curve can be approximated by computing its standard deviation. Wide standard deviations indicate wider distribution of times. In Fig. 4B the capillary transit time standard deviation is plotted against cardiac output. Under control conditions the standard deviation is reasonably wide, around 1 s. With increased output it becomes narrow. For this group of animals the standard deviation was 1.2 s control and decreased to 0.5 s with increased output. This means that the absolute dispersion of these curves became smaller, indicating that all pathways across the capillary network were perfused more rapidly.

There is another measure of dispersion called relative dispersion, which is calculated by dividing the variance of the distribution of transit times by the mean time. It permits comparison of the dispersions about the mean of groups of objects, such as red cells, moving at different rates. From that calculation, we can determine whether the capillaries are perfused more homogeneously or heterogeneously when cardiac output changes. More homogeneous perfusion would be indicated by a decreased relative dispersion, while the reverse would be true for increased heterogeneity. In Fig. 4C the relative dispersion is plotted against cardiac output. As cardiac output increased, the relative dispersion did not change; it was 64% during low cardiac output and 61% during increased cardiac output. Thus, the homogeneity of capillary perfusion did not change as cardiac output increased, i.e., the same percent of capillaries were perfused more rapidly than the mean and the same percent were perfused more slowly than the mean, regardless of cardiac output. At first thought, this is quite surprising. It means that the capillary bed was perfused at the same level of homogeneity despite large changes in flow.

Part of the explanation for the consistent homogeneity is that the observations were made in the lower lung where the capillaries were fully recruited during low cardiac output. Therefore there was little change in capillary recruitment as cardiac output was raised. This is demonstrated in Fig. 4D, which shows that the total length of all perfused capillaries in a given alveolus did not change much as blood flow was increased. With a capillary bed that is always fully open increased blood flow is likely to increase evenly throughout the network, and therefore the homogeneity of perfusion would remain constant.

In summary, in the zone 3 dependent lung, increased cardiac output causes: a decrease in mean time, decreased standard deviation (absolute dispersion), but relative dispersion is constant, which means there is no change in capillary perfusion homogeneity since there is little capillary recruitment. This raises the interesting question about what happens in zone 2 in the upper lung where there are recruitable capillaries. Those measurements are being made at present and should provide insight not only into the way the pulmonary gas exchange vessels increase their surface area under normal circumstances, but also may have implications for understanding hypoxemia in patients and in normal people living at high altitude.

Acknowledgements. The author thanks A.B. Wagner for skillful preparation of the artwork.

References

Capen RL, Hanson WL, Latham LP, Dawson CA, Wagner WW Jr. (1990) Distribution of pulmonary capillary transit times in recruited net works J Appl Physiol 69:473–478

Hogg JC, McLean T, Martin BA, Wiggs B (1988) Erythrocyte transit time and neutrophil concentration in the dog lung. J Appl Physiol 65:1217–1225

Johnson RL Jr, Spicer WS, Bishop JM, Forster RE (1960) Pulmonary capillary blood volume, flow, and diffusing capacity during exercise. J Appl Physiol 15:893–902

Wagner PD (1977) Diffusion and chemical reaction in pulmonary gas exchange. Physiol Rev 57:257–312

Wagner WW Jr, Latham LP, Gillespie MN, Guenther J, Capen RL (1982) Red cell transit times across pulmonary capillaries. Science 218:379–380

Wagner WW Jr, Latham LP, Hanson WL, Hofmeister SE, Capen RL (1986) Vertical gradient of pulmonary capillary transit times. J Appl Physiol 61:1270–1274

West JB (1979) Respiratory physiology. Williams and Wilkins, Baltimore

New Drugs for the Treatment of Pulmonary Hypertension Associated with the Adult Respiratory Distress Syndrome*

P. Radermacher, B. Santak, K.J. Falke, and J. Tarnow

Acute pulmonary hypertension due to diffuse vasoconstriction and microembolization is a common event in patients with adult respiratory distress syndrome (ARDS) [1, 2]. Why should pulmonary artery hypertension be treated?

Pulmonary hypertension represents an increase of one of the determinants of right ventricular afterload, and it may lead to right ventricular dysfunction. Using gated radionuclide angiography Sibbald and coworkers found a negative correlation between the mean pulmonary artery pressure and the right ventricular ejection fraction [3]. Moreover, acute pulmonary hypertension increases the intravascular hydrostatic capillary pressure in the lung, which results in increased microvascular filtration pressure and, hence, abnormal accumulation of extravascular lung water [4]. In patients with ARDS even a small rise in the intravascular hydrostatic pressure may be important, since in this situation the difference between the interstitial and plasmatic oncotic pressure becomes negligibly small due to the increased capillary permeability. Under these circumstances, changes in the microvascular filtration pressure then only depend on variations in the intravascular hydrostatic pressure, because the interstitial hydrostatic pressure hardly varies [4]. The analysis of the pressure decay curve in the pulmonary artery after balloon occlusion allows one to estimate the intravascular hydrostatic capillary pressure, generally termed "effective pulmonary capillary pressure" [4].

Due to these potentially noxious consequences, reducing pulmonary hypertension is regarded as an important therapeutical maneuver in the treatment of ARDS [5]. After hydrochloric acid aspiration in a canine model of ARDS, Gottlieb and coworkers demonstrated that infusing sodium nitroprusside was associated with a reduction of extravascular lung water [6]. The clinical use of sodium nitroprusside, however, was associated with a deterioration of pulmonary gas exchange [2] caused by an increase of the intrapulmonary right-to-left shunt [7]. Therefore new drugs are currently under investigation which, apart from their vasodilative abilities, could act on the pathophysiologic mechanisms of ARDS.

Serotonin, a broncho- and vasocontrictor, is released by activated platelets. Since platelet entrapment is reported in patients with ARDS, serotonin is regarded as a putative mediator of ARDS [8]. Therefore, ketanserin, a competitive antagonist of serotonin, has been proposed for the treatment of pulmonary hypertension associated with ARDS [9].

---

* Supported by the Deutsche Forschungsgemeinschaft (grant Fa 139/1–2)

We compared the pulmonary hemodynamic and gas exchange effects of ketanserin and sodium nitroprusside in patients with severe ARDS after a comparable reduction of the mean systemic arterial pressure had been achieved [7]. Although ketanserin induced a slight but significant fall in the pulmonary artery pressure, it was less efficient than sodium nitroprusside. In contrast to sodium nitroprusside, ketanserin infusion did not induce alterations in pulmonary gas exchange (Fig. 1), which is likely due to its moderate effect on pulmonary hemodynamics. Because of the minor effect on pulmonary hemodynamics compared to the systemic vasodilation, ketanserin will probably not play an important role in the treatment of pulmonary hypertension in ARDS.

Thromboxane is regarded to be an important mediator in the development of ARDS since it is a potent pulmonary vasoconstrictor with platelet aggregating abilities. Vasodilative prostaglandins like prostaglandin E_1 (PGE_1) and prostacyclin (PGI_2) inhibit platelet aggregation and macrophage and granulocyte activation, possible mechanisms contributing to the development of ARDS. Infusing these substances improved the survival of animals in different

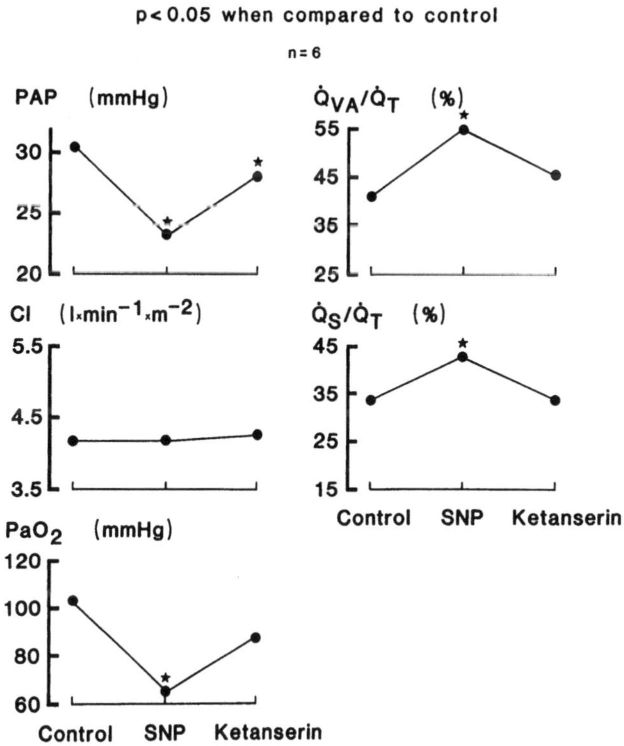

Fig. 1. Hemodynamic and gas exchange effects of ketanserin and sodium nitroprusside (*SNP*) in patients with severe ARDS ($n = 6$). *PAP*, mean pulmonary artery pressure; *CI*, cardiac index; *PaO_2*, arterial PO_2; $\dot{Q}_{VA}/\dot{Q}_T$, venous admixture; $\dot{Q}_S/\dot{Q}_T$, intrapulmonary right-to-left shunt. *Asterisks* denote significant differences between the control and the vasodilator infusion ($p < 0.05$)

experimental shock models [10, 11]. In a prospective clinical study infusing PGE_1 for 1 week, Holcroft and coworkers reported an improved survival of the treated patients [12]. Two multicenter studies in Europe and North America, however, failed to confirm these results.

In ten patients with moderate to severe ARDS we compared the hemodynamic and gas exchange alterations induced by PGE_1 and nitroglycerin after achieving comparable systemic vasodilation [13]. The two drugs induced an equivalent fall in pulmonary artery pressure, which, together with the decreased pulmonary artery wedge pressure, resulted in a comparable reduction of the effective pulmonary capillary pressure (Fig. 2). Confirming animal data reported by Kadowitz and Hyman [14, 15] neither of the drugs caused a change in the contribution of the venous resistance to the total pressure drop over the pulmonary vascular bed.

Right ventricular function parameters, namely ejection fraction and end diastolic volume, which were determined by using the thermodilution technique, remained unchanged during the drug infusions [16]. It has to be noted, however, that the control values were within the normal range, which made it unlikely that further changes due to vasodilator infusions would occur.

In contrast to data reported by Shoemaker and Apple [17], PGE_1 as well as nitroglycerin caused the PaO_2 to fall due to increased intrapulmonary right-to-left shunt (Fig. 2). These data reproduce results recently reported by Melot [18] and Anjou-Lindskog [19], respectively, on the effects of PGE_1 in patients

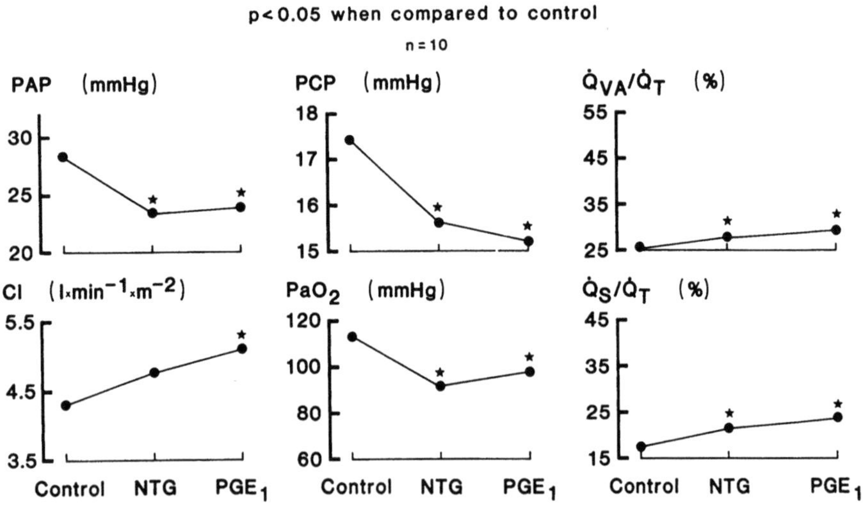

Fig. 2. Hemodynamic and gas exchange effects of nitroglycerin (*NTG*) and prostaglandin E_1 (PGE_1) in patients with ARDS ($n = 10$). *PAP*, mean pulmonary artery pressure; *CI*, cardiac index; *PCP*, effective pulmonary capillary pressure; PaO_2, arterial PO_2; $\dot{Q}_{VA}/\dot{Q}_T$, venous admixture; $\dot{Q}_S/\dot{Q}_T$, intrapulmonary right-to-left shunt. *Asterisks* denote significant differences between the control and the vasodilator infusion ($p < 0.05$)

with ARDS [18] and nitroglycerin in patients after coronary bypass grafting [19].

Despite the fall in PaO_2, PGE_1 infusion induced increased oxygen delivery because of the increased cardiac index (Fig. 2). Therefore, PGE_1 may be superior to nitroglycerin in the treatment of pulmonary hypertension in ARDS.

Since pulmonary endothelium is injured in ARDS and prostacyclin is a natural vasodilator produced by endothelial cells with antiplatelet-aggregating abilities, it should perhaps replace other drugs in the treatment of ARDS. Moreover, in an bovine model of acute pulmonary hypertension infusing prostacyclin induced the most pronounced increase in cardiac index compared to PGE_1 and nifedipine [20]. Bihari and coworkers reported that prostacyclin not only increases oxygen delivery in patients with septic acute respiratory failure, but also improves oxygen distribution as documented by increased uptake [21]. Because of these potentially beneficial effects, we studied the central hemodynamic and gas exchange effects of infusing prostacyclin in nine patients with severe ARDS after a 20% reduction of the mean systemic arterial pressure had been achieved. Prostacyclin induced a small significant rise in the right ventricular ejection fraction, as assessed by thermodilution, suggesting improved global right ventricular function (Table 1). This result was underscored by a significant relationship between the fall in pulmonary vascular resistance and the rise in the right ventricular ejection fraction. The decreased pulmonary vascular pressures resulted in a reduction of the effective pulmonary capillary pressure (Table 1) without a change in the contribution of the venous resistance to the total pulmonary vascular resistance. Similar to other vasodilator drugs, PGI_2 caused a marked deterioration of the matching of ventilation and perfusion, as documented by the substantial increase in intrapulmonary right-to-left shunt, measured by inert gas elimination technique (Table 1). In this group of

Table 1. Hemodynamic and gas exchange effects of prostacyclin (PGI_2) infusion in patients with ARDS ($n = 9$)

	Control	PGI_2
PAP (mm Hg)	36 ± 6 b.	29 ± 5**
CI ($l\ min^{-1}\ m^{-2}$)	4.2 ± 1.4	5.8 ± 1.3**
PVRI ($mm\ Hg\ min\ m^2\ l^{-1}$)	5.1 ± 2.2	2.5 ± 1.0**
PCP (mm Hg)	22.9 ± 3.2	19.7 ± 3.0**
RVEF (%)	47 ± 11	52 ± 10**
PaO_2 (mm Hg)	94 ± 22	90 ± 29 ns
$\dot{Q}_S/\dot{Q}_T$ (%)	29 ± 10	39 ± 14*
$\dot{D}O_2$ ($ml\ min^{-1}\ m^{-2}$)	657 ± 175	894 ± 160**

PAP, mean pulmonary artery pressure; CI, cardiac index; PVRI, pulmonary vascular resistance index; PCP, effective pulmonary capillary pressure; RVEF, right ventricular ejection fraction; PaO_2, arterial PO_2; $\dot{Q}_S/\dot{Q}_T$ intrapulmonary (inert gas) right-to-left shunt; $\dot{D}O_2$, oxygen delivery
Asterisks denote significant differences between the control period and PGI_2 influsion; *, $p < 0.05$; **, $p < 0.01$

patients the PaO_2, however, remained unchanged due to the considerable rise in the cardiac index, resulting in an improved oxygen delivery (Table 1). This increased oxygen delivery is especially important in patients with ARDS, because in this situation tissue oxygen extraction is disturbed [22] causing a rise in critical oxygen delivery, below which oxygen uptake is linearly dependent on oxygen delivery.

In summary, it may be concluded that pulmonary hypertension associated with ARDS causes an increased microvascular filtration pressure and may lead to right ventricular dysfunction. Therefore, reducing pulmonary artery pressure is especially important in the management of patients with ARDS. The new agents either have only moderate effects on pulmonary hemodynamics (ketanserin) or, similar to conventional vasodilators, cause a marked deterioration of the matching of ventilation and perfusion which results in only minor alterations of PaO_2 as seen during the infusion of prostacyclin. Since oxygen delivery is improved during the infusion of prostacyclin, it may be beneficial for the treatment of pulmonary hypertension in patients with ARDS. Further investigation is warranted as to whether long-term treatment improves survival in these patients.

References

1. Zapol WM, Snider MT (1977) Pulmonary hypertension in severe acute respiratory failure. N Engl J Med 196:476–480
2. Zapol WM, Snider MT, Rie MA, Frikker M, Quinn DA (1985) Pulmonary circulation during adult respiratory distress syndrome. In: Zapol WM, Falke KJ (eds) Acute respiratory failure. Dekker, New York, pp 241–273
3. Sibbald WJ, Driedger AA, Myers ML, Short AIK, Wells GA (1983) Biventricular function in the adult respiratory distress syndrome. Chest 84:126–134
4. Grimbert FA (1988) Effective pulmonary capillary pressure. Eur Respir J 1:297–301
5. Bernard GR, Brigham KL (1986) Pulmonary edema. Chest 89:594–600
6. Gottlieb SS, Wood LDH, Hansen DE, Long R (1987) The effect of nitroprusside on pulmonary edema, oxygen exchange, and blood flow in hydrochloric acid aspiration. Anesthesiology 67:203–210
7. Radermacher P, Huet Y, Pluskwa F, Hérigault R, Mal H, Teisseire B, Lemaire F (1988) Comparison of ketanserin and sodium nitroprusside in patients with severe ARDS. Anesthesiology 68:152–157
8. Huval WV, Lelcuk S, Sherpo D, Hechtman HB (1984) Role of serotonin in patients with acute respiratory failure. Ann Surg 200:166–172
9. Vincent JL, Degaute JP, Domb M, Simon P, Berre J, Vendersteene A (1984) Ketanserin, a serotonin antagonist. Chest 85:510–513
10. Lefer AM, Tabas J, Smith EF (1980) Salutary effects of prostacyclin in endotoxic shock. Pharmacology 21:206–212
11. Lewitt MA, Lefer AM (1987) Beneficial effects of prostaglandin E_1 infusion in experimental traumatic shock. Crit Care Med 15:769–773
12. Holcroft JW, Vassar MJ, Weber CJ (1986) Prostaglandin E_1 and survival in patients with the adult respiratory distress syndrome. Ann Surg 203:371–378
13. Radermacher P, Santak B, Becker H, Falke KJ (1989) Prostaglandin E_1 and nitroglycerin reduce pulmonary capillary pressure but worsen ventilation-perfusion distributions in patients with adult respiratory distress syndrome. Anesthesiology 70:601–606
14. Hyman AL (1969) The active responses of the pulmonary veins in intact dogs to prostaglandin $F2_{\alpha}$ and E_1. J Pharmacol Exp Ther 165:267–273

15. Kadowitz PJ, Nandirwada P, Gruetter CA, Ignarro LJ, Hyman AL (1981) Pulmonary vasodilator responses to nitroprusside and nitroglycerine in the dog. J Clin Invest 67:893–902
16. Radermacher P, Santak B, Assmann R, Falke KJ (1989) Prostaglandin E_1 and right ventricular function in ARDS. Intensive Care Med 15:146–147
17. Shoemaker WC, Appel PL (1986) Effects of prostaglandin E_1 in adult respiratory distress syndrome. Surgery 99:275–282
18. Mélot C, Lejeune P, Leeman M, Moraine JJ, Naeije R (1989) Prostaglandin E_1 in the adult respiratory distress syndrome. Am Rev Respir Dis 139:106–110
19. Anjou-Lindskog E, Broman L, Holmgren A (1982) Effects of nitroglycerin on central hemodynamics and $\dot{V}_A/\dot{Q}$ distributions early after coronary bypass surgery. Acta Anaesthesiol Scand 26:489–497
20. Prielipp RC, Rosenthal MH, Pearl RG (1988) Hemodynamic profiles of prostaglandin E_1, isoproterenol, prostacyclin, and nifedipine in vasoconstrictor pulmonary hypertension in sheep. Anesth Analg 67:722–729
21. Bihari D, Smithies M, Gimson A, Tinker J (1987) The effects of vasodilation with prostacyclin on oxygen delivery and uptake in critically ill patients. N Engl J Med 317:397–403
22. Kariman K, Burns SR (1985) Regulation of tissue oxygen extraction is disturbed in the adult respiratory distress syndrome. Am Rev Respir Dis 132:109–114

Part 5:
Gas Exchange

Effects of Mechanical Ventilation and Cardiac Output upon Perfusion in Hypoxic Lung Areas

H. Burchardi

Coordination between pulmonary ventilation and perfusion is controlled and optimized by two essential reflex mechanisms: hypocapnic bronchoconstriction and hypoxic pulmonary vasoconstriction (HPV).

HPV controls perfusion in hypoxic lung areas: A decrease in alveolar oxygen concentration leads to pulmonary vasoconstriction. This physiological reflex mechanism acts not only in the lung as a whole, as in the case of general hypoxic breathing, but also regulates regional perfusion in case of atelectasis or local alveolar hypoxia.

Under clinical conditions this is an important and effective compensatory mechanism. In lung areas with atelectasis or a low ventilation-perfusion ratio ($\dot{V}_A/\dot{Q}$ ratio) so-called "slow compartments", the HPV reflex is able to reduce shunt significantly (about 30%–60%). Therefore, pulmonary gas exchange often remains effective even in cases of mismatching.

The efficiency of this powerful mechanism can, however, be impaired in various pathophysiological conditions as well as by many pharmacological influences:

The HPV reflex is known to be reduced or even eliminated by:

- Pharmacological vasodilation
- Most of the inhalation anesthetics (namely nitrous oxide, isoflurane, fluroxene and possibly also halothane, but not by intravenous agents like opioids)
- Pulmonary hypertension
- Pulmonary infections as well as systemic sepsis and endotoxemia

Influence of Cardiac Output

During acute respiratory failure the physiological connection between cardiac output and intrapulmonary perfusion often becomes obvious: A decrease in cardiac output (e.g., during shock) generally also reduces intrapulmonary shunt. This has already been shown experimentally by Steenblock et al. [16], who found a fall in shunt during hemorrhagic shock in spontaneously breathing dogs with normal lungs; arterial pO_2 consequently remained constant. In patients Wolff et al. [17] found a significant correlation between an increase in the arteriovenous difference in oxygen content ($avDO_2$) (decrease in cardiac output) and decrease of shunt.

It must, however, be taken into account that a low mixed venous pO_2 of course enhances the negative effect of shunt upon the pulmonary oxygenation. Lynch et al. [10] analyzed this correlation using dogs with oleic acid-induced hemorrhagic lung edema. Here, cardiac output was reduced either by a barbiturate infusion at high cardiodepressive dosage or by blocking venous return with a balloon catheter in the vena cava inferior and superior. Both mechanisms reduced cardiac output by approximately 50%, and intrapulmonary shunts by 30%–37% or 25%, respectively. Similar results were found by Smith et al. [15].

This correlation between a decrease in shunt and in cardiac output seems logical. Reduction in total lung perfusion may mainly be effective in diseased lung areas where HPV leads to regional vasoconstriction. This then decreases the shunt ratio. Dantzker et al. [4] even postulated that the effect of positive end-expiratory pressure (PEEP) upon intrapulmonary shunts may be due to reduction in cardiac output. Restoring a depressed cardiac output to control levels also raised the intrapulmonary shunt (even above this range [10]).

The correlation between increasing cardiac output and increasing shunt is somewhat more complex. Clinically, this phenomenon is often found: Increased cardiac output (e.g., with fluid administration, or with catecholamines, like isoprenaline, dopamine, dobutamine) is often accompanied by an increased intrapulmonary shunt. However, the pathomechanisms still seem to be uncertain [5, 6, 14].

We looked experimentally at this problem in a working group at Oxford [3]: During barbiturate anesthesia in 14 dogs, the left upper and middle lobes were resected via thoracotomy and electromagnetic flow probes were placed in the pulmonary arterial trunk and left lower lobe artery. A double-lumen endotracheal tube enabled selective ventilation of the left lower lobe (LLL), either with a hypoxic (7% O_2) or a hyperoxic (50% O_2) gas mixture or, alternatively, lobar collapse to exclude LLL from ventilation. The effect of HPV could then be quantified by the ratio of regional to total perfusion ($\dot{Q}_l/\dot{Q}_t$). Total perfusion, acid-base equilibrium, and body temperature were kept normal and constant during the whole procedure.

Under lobar hypoxia, regional perfusion was significantly reduced by the HPV mechanism by about 35% or 41% (Fig. 1). During lobar collapse, shunt was reduced by 42%. This reduction in regional perfusion is somewhat smaller than it has been demonstrated in other studies [1, 11, 12] with reductions of 45%–55%. Nevertheless, it is within a similar range.

We then increased cardiac output intermittently, either by opening arteriovenous fistulae (prepared between a. and v. femoralis and a. carotis and v. jugularis as well) or by adding fluid volume (Haemaccel) or by a combination of both.

These measures increased cardiac output significantly: by about 29%–47% with arteriovenous fistulae, about 48%–69% by volume loading, and about 115%–133% by combining both. However, this considerable rise in cardiac output did not change the regional perfusion ratio ($\dot{Q}_l/\dot{Q}_t$) significantly, even though volume loading increased pulmonary artery pressure by about 6–7 mmHg.

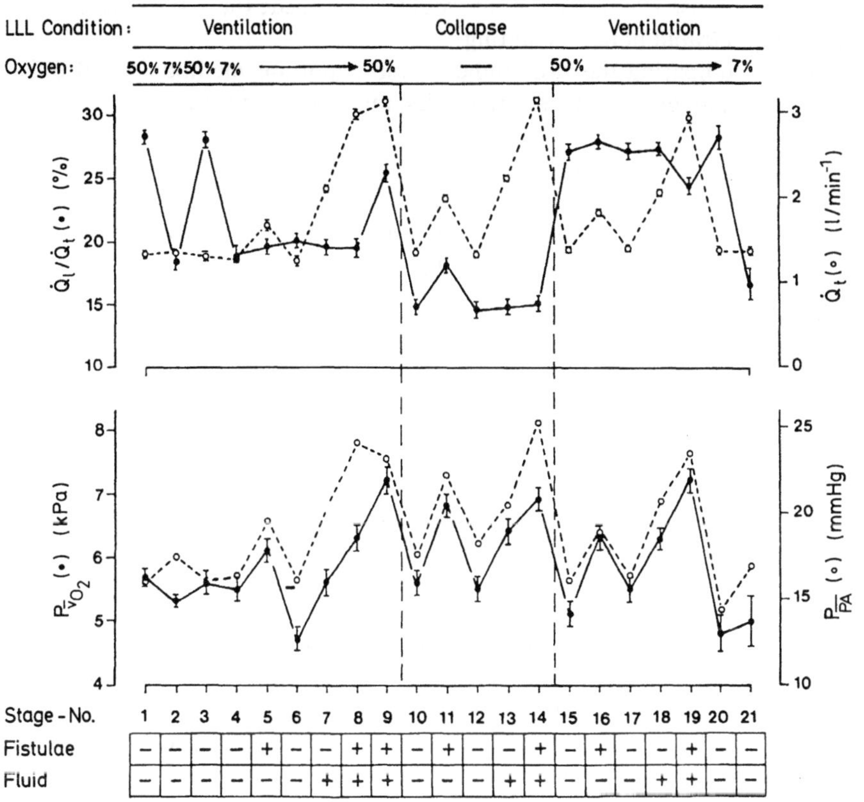

Fig. 1. Changes in cardiac output ($\dot{Q}_t$), lobar-to-total blood flow ratio ($\dot{Q}_l/\dot{Q}_t$), mixed venous oxygen tension ($P_{\bar{v}O_2}$), and mean pulmonary artery pressure ($P_{\bar{A}P}$) under 21 different experimental conditions: regional ventilation with 50% or 7% oxygen, and left lower lobe (LLL) collapse. Increase in cardiac output (+) by arteriovenous fistulae, by fluid administration, or by combination of both. For details, see text. [From 3]

Thus, an increase in cardiac output does not influence the HPV mechanism, provided that no pathological or pharmacological effects interfere and the pressure rise in the pulmonary circuit remains moderate.

This seems to contradict the current clinical impression that increase in cardiac output always results in an increase in intrapulmonary shunt. This has also been suggested by Schumacker et al. [14] from their studies in dogs with left lung collapse. However, when their results are examined more closely, two different reactions can be recognized: In a group of six animals the increase in cardiac output by about 60% indeed raised shunt perfusion from 24.0% ± 3.3% to 42.0% ± 2.0%. On the other hand, in a second group of four animals shunt remained stable even though cardiac output had been increased considerably by about 85%. In this group, however, the initial shunt ratio was already rather high (46.0% ± 6.5%). Therefore, the authors concluded that the HPV mechanism was only intact initially when shunt was low. Increasing pulmonary artery pressure by a rise in cardiac output would then impede the HPV reflex, hereby increasing intrapulmonary shunting.

When comparing the two studies, some important methodological differences, that may explain the discrepancies, must be considered:

1. In contrast to our experiments, the Schumacker study [14] was performed under closed chest conditions. Shunt was measured by the six inert gas technique, which determines the total intrapulmonary shunt fraction. It is, therefore, possible that shunts from parts of the lungs outside the collapsed lobe reacting to the increase in cardiac output are also included.
2. It is well known that redistribution of pulmonary perfusion by the HPV mechanism is less effective when large lung areas become hypoxic [11]. As in the Schumacker study, the whole left lung was collapsed, the HPV mechanism may have been less effective.
3. In mechanical ventilation under closed chest conditions the distribution of intrathoracical pressure is quite different to open chest conditions. In the Schumacker study, therefore, overdistension of the right lung may have occurred, resulting in a shift of perfusion into the collapsed left lung.

Based on our results, we are convinced that an increase of cardiac output per se does not affect intrapulmonary shunt distribution as long as the HPV mechanism remains intact. However, this still needs a final confirmation.

All experimental results discussed until now were performed in basically healthy animals. Under pathological conditions or during acute respiratory failure, however, other supplementary effects may play a role. It is well known that pulmonary infections or endotoxins can impair the HPV mechanism. Hutchison et al. [8] studied the influence of endotoxin upon the HPV mechanism in chronic instrumented conscious sheep. Under spontaneous breathing, alternating between air and a hypoxic mixture (12% O_2), they determined (among other parameters) the pulmonary vascular resistance (PVR). Before endotoxin, the HPV reflex was intact and PVR raised. However, endotoxin (*E. coli* endotoxin, 0.2–0.5 μg) blocked the HPV mechanism. Under hypoxic breathing PVR remained unchanged or even decreased.

Some authors suggest that products of arachidonic acid metabolism may affect the HPV mechanism. It has been demonstrated by Hutchison et al. [8] that at least vasodilating metabolites, like prostacyclin or prostaglandin E_1, may be able to damp or even eliminate the HPV reflex. However, blocking the cycloxygenase pathway by meclofenamate did not improve the HPV reaction. The authors therefore concluded that arachidonic acid metabolites do not affect the HPV reaction. On the other hand, studies in dogs by Hales et al. [7] showed that indomethacin (another cycloxygenase blocker) indeed inhibited the effects of endotoxin upon the HPV mechanism. Concerning this question, then, the experimental data remain controversial.

Catecholamines like dopamine and dobutamine are well known to decrease the efficiency of the HPV reaction and, thus, to increase intrapulmonary shunt.

Dobutamin acts by directly influencing the HPV reflex [12], dopamine (at least in higher dosage of 20–30 µg/kg min) rather by increasing vasoconstriction under normoxic conditions [5, 6].

Whenever the HPV reaction is significantly damped or even eliminated (no matter by what mechanism), then an increase in cardiac output will, of course, increase intrapulmonary shunt. Pulmonary perfusion will then be redistributed, possibly by the increase of pulmonary artery pressure. In hypoxic lung areas vessels will be reopened, regional shunt perfusion will rise, and gas exchange will deteriorate.

In clinical conditions this unfavorable course certainly often occurs. Therefore, regarding intensive care patients, the correlation between cardiac output and shunt often becomes obvious.

Lemaire et al. [9] found a significant correlation between cardiac output and intrapulmonary shunt in 28 adult respiratory distress syndrome patients. However, shunt only correlated with pulmonary artery pressure when pulmonary vascular resistance was low. They therefore concluded that an increase in shunt with unstable hemodynamics may result from redistribution of pulmonary perfusion, and may not necessarily indicate pulmonary deterioration.

In intensive care medicine these special conditions have to be taken into account when diagnosing and monitoring acute respiratory failure.

Influence of Mechanical Ventilation

Hyperventilation seems to reduce the efficiency of the HPV mechanism; this has been shown by both experimental [13] and clinical studies.

Bindslev et al. [2] found, in eight healthy men, that decrease in arterial pCO_2 damps the HPV reaction: Low pCO_2 increases shunt perfusion through atelectatic or hypoxic alveolar regions and diminishes the efficiency of pulmonary gas exchange. Therefore, in the case of acute respiratory failure, hyperventilation should be avoided.

Studies concerning the influence of airway pressure upon HPV are scarce. In dogs with healthy lungs and a closed chest a PEEP of 10 cmH_2O has no influence upon HPV [1]. Intrathoracic pressure is well distributed within the lungs. However, under open chest conditions a selective PEEP in the non-hypoxic lung redistributes blood into the hypoxic areas and hereby reduces the efficiency of HPV significantly.

Under clinical conditions, the same limitations as for the influence of cardiac output apply: In contrast to healthy lungs, in intensive care patients with respiratory diseases airway pressure (as well as many other influences like pulmonary infections, pharmacological effects) may also damp the HPV reaction considerably. This may cause a redistribution of pulmonary perfusion and result in a significant deterioration of pulmonary gas exchange.

Conclusion

Influences of Cardiac Output

1. During acute respiratory failure the mechanism of hypoxic pulmonary vasoconstriction (HPV) diminishes the degree of pulmonary gas exchange.
2. Under certain conditions the amount of intrapulmonary shunt depends on the cardiac output:
   a) A decrease in cardiac output reduces intrapulmonary shunt.
   b) The appropriate correlation for increasing cardiac output seems not so evident. However, under special conditions the HPV mechanism is apparently suppressed, so that shunt will increase: increase in pulmonary artery pressure, pharmacological effects (e.g., catecholamines), pathological influences (pulmonary infections, endotoxins, etc.).
3. In healthy lungs without pharmacological influences the HPV mechanism remains active in various situations.

Influences of Mechanical Ventilation

1. The regional alveolar CO_2 concentration influences the HPV reaction:
   a) Regional hypocapnia increases regional perfusion (and thereby intrapulmonary shunt)
   b) Regional hypercapnia reduces regional perfusion.
2. Regional perfusion may be redistributed by intrathoracic pressure. Therefore, under mechanical ventilation PEEP and airway pressure influence shunt perfusion.

References

1. Benumof JL, Rogers SN, Moyce PR, Berryhill RE, Mahrenbrock EA (1979) Hypoxic pulmonary vasoconstriction and regional whole-lung PEEP in the dog. Anesthesiology 51:503–507
2. Bindslev L, Jolin-Carlsson A, Santesson J, Gottlieb I (1985) Hypoxic pulmonary vasoconstriction in man: effects of hyperventilation. Acta Anaesthesiol Scand 29:547–551
3. Cannon D, Kalso EJ, Burchardi H, Sykes MK (1988) Effects of increased cardiac output on pulmonary blood flow distribution during lobar ventilation hypoxia and collapse. Br J Anaesth 60:430–438
4. Dantzker DR, Lynch JP, Weg JG (1980) Depression of cardiac output is a mechanism of shunt reduction in the therapy of acute respiratory failure. Chest 77:636–642
5. Furman WR, Summer WR, Kennedy TP, Sylvester JT (1982) Comparison of the effects of dobutamine, dopamine, and isoproterenol on hypoxic pulmonary vasoconstriction in the pig. Crit Care Med 10:371–374
6. Gardaz J-P, McFarlane PA, Sykes MK (1986) Mechanisms by which dopamine alters blood flow distribution during lobar collapse in dogs. J Appl Physiol 60:959–964
7. Hales CA, Sonne L, Peterson M, Kong D, Miller M, Watkins WD (1981) Role of thromboxane and prostacyclin in pulmonary vasomotor changes after endotoxin in dogs. J Clin Invest 68:497–505

8. Hutchison AA, Ogletree ML, Snapper JR, Brigham KL (1985) Effect of endotoxemia on hypoxic pulmonary vasoconstriction in unanesthetized sheep. J Appl Physiol 58:1463–1468
9. Lemaire F, Gastine H, Régnier B, Teisseire B, Rapin M (1978) Perfusion changes modify intra-pulmonary shunting (QS/QT) in patients with adult respiratory distress syndroms (ARDS). Am Rev Respir Dis 117:144
10. Lynch JP, Mhyre JG, Dantzker DR (1979) Influence of cardiac output on intrapulmonary shunt. J Appl Physiol 46:315–321
11. Marshall BE, Marshall C, Benumof J, Saidman LJ (1981) Hypoxic pulmonary vasoconstriction in dogs: effects of lung segment size and oxygen tension. J Appl Physiol 51:1543–1551
12. McFarlane PA, Mortimer AJ, Ryder WA, Madgwick RG, Gardaz J-P, Harrison BJ, Sykes MK (1985) Effects of dopamine and dobutamine on the distribution of pulmonary blood flow during lobar ventilation hypoxia and lobar collapse in dogs. Eur J Clin Invest 15:53–59
13. Noble WH, Kay JC, Fisher JA (1981) The effect of PCO_2 on hypoxic pulmonary vasoconstriction. Can Anaesth Soc J 28:422–430
14. Schumacker PT, Newell JC, Saba TM, Powers SR (1981) Ventilation-perfusion relationships with high cardiac output in lobar atelectasis. J Appl Physiol 50:341–347
15. Smith G, Cheney FW, Winter PM (1974) The effect of change in cardiac output on intrapulmonary shunting. Br J Anaesth 46:337–342
16. Steenblock U, Mannhart H, Wolff G (1976) Effect of hemorrhagic shock on intrapulmonary right-to-left shunt (QS/QT) and dead space (VD/VT). Respiration 33:133–142
17. Wolff G, Grädel E, Claudi B, Rist M, Schwab T (1972) Der Einfluß des akut erniedrigten Herzminutenvolumens auf den intrapulmonalen Rechts-Links-Shunt. Schweiz Med Wochenschr 102:198

Determination of Lung Water Content and Distribution by Nuclear Magnetic Resonance*

A.G. Cutillo,[1] A.H. Morris, D.C. Ailion, C.H. Durney, and K. Ganesan

Introduction

Pulmonary edema is a common consequence of experimental and clinical lung injury. The importance of pulmonary edema explains the considerable effort made to develop methods for the measurement of lung water content [1–3]. Unfortunately, most of the available methods have limitations (e.g., they are destructive or invasive, subject to errors from various sources, or involve exposure to ionizing radiation), which reduce their sensitivity and accuracy and prevent their widespread application. The accurate but destructive gravimetric technique remains the reference standard in basic lung water research [1]. The evaluation of the chest roentgenogram is the only approach generally applied to the clinical assessment of pulmonary edema; this evaluation is mostly nonquantitative or semiquantitative, although quantitative criteria have recently been proposed [4, 5]. It seems likely that substantial progress in the measurement of lung water will be made possible by the recent application of new techniques, among which proton nuclear magnetic resonance (proton NMR) appears to be particularly promising.

Basic Principles of NMR

A detailed discussion of the basic principles of NMR is beyond the scope of this paper and can be found in recent publications [6–11]. Unless otherwise specified, the term NMR in this article refers to proton NMR, which has generally been used for lung water studies. Briefly, since hydrogen nuclei (protons) have a magnetic dipole moment, they tend to align preferentially in the direction of an externally applied magnetic field H_0, resulting in a net magnetization M. The magnetic moments of the individual protons precess around the axis of H_0 at a specific angular frequency ω_0 (Larmor frequency), determined by the magnitude of H_0. In order to detect the NMR behavior of the specimen studied, it is necessary to irradiate the specimen with a radiofrequency (rf) magnetic field H_1, at the same frequency as its proton precession frequency ω_0. The magnetization M is tilted away from the axis of H_0 and nutates around the axis of H_1 at

* Our work was supported in part by National Heart, Lung and Blood Institute, grant HL31216 and National Cancer Institute, grant CA44972.

a frequency proportional to H_1. The resulting precessing magnetization M induces an electromotive force (EMF) in a receiver coil tuned to the Larmor frequency ω_0. The EMF is then amplified, demodulated, usually digitized, and finally displayed. If the rf magnetic field H_1 is suddenly turned off (thereby forming a pulse), the amplitude of the NMR signal decays with time (free induction decay, FID). In an ideal, perfectly homogeneous, external magnetic field the NMR signal decays because of precessing proton dephasing induced by local magnetic field variations due to interactions between neighboring nuclei. This NMR signal decay is irreversible and is characterized by the decay constant T_2 (the spin-spin relaxation time). In actual external magnetic fields, inhomogeneity may result in a greater signal loss characterized by a decay time T_2^*. In contrast to the irreversible T_2 signal loss, the signal loss due to external magnetic field inhomogeneity can be recovered using the NMR spin-echo technique. An additional recoverable signal loss is present in lungs but only when they are inflated. This signal loss is due to the alveolar air/tissue interface, which produces an internal (tissue-induced) magnetic field inhomogeneity (see NMR Lung Properties and State of Inflation). The time required for the re-establishment of thermal equilibrium (i.e., the time required for realignment of M along H_0) following the rf pulse is characterized by another time constant T_1 (the spin-lattice relaxation time). NMR pulse sequences are usually repeated in order to improve the signal-to-noise ratio. The repetition time should be at least several times T_1 in order to prevent errors arising from loss of NMR signal due to incomplete recovery of the nuclear magnetization M between pulse sequences.

Spatial resolution of the precessing protons, required for NMR imaging, can be achieved by superimposing linear magnetic field gradients (i.e., magnetic fields whose strength varies linearly with position) on the main field H_0 in various directions across the specimen. Because of these gradients, the protons in various positions in the specimen will experience magnetic fields of different strength and thus precess at different frequencies. Spatial position is thus frequency encoded. Since the contributions of protons at different spatial locations are then distinguishable from one another by Fourier analysis, images of proton density at each location in the specimen can be obtained.

NMR Determination of Lung Water Content and Distribution

NMR can be used to quantify lung water because, under appropriate measurement conditions, the NMR signal is proportional to proton (water) density. Compared with other methods for measuring lung water content, NMR techniques, especially NMR imaging, have important advantages because NMR measurements are noninvasive, relatively rapid, easily repeatable, and, with proper safety precautions, without known harmful effects. NMR imaging techniques are particularly suitable for the assessment of lung water distribution because the image contains spatial information. In addition, NMR techniques are remarkably versatile because the NMR signal is affected by numerous factors (e.g., proton density, relaxation times, blood flow) [6–11]. Therefore, when appropriately used, NMR can provide additional information which is, potentially, of pathophysiologic and clinical interest (see below).

NMR imaging studies performed on excised rat lung specimens have shown that absolute lung water content can be determined accurately from NMR signal intensity [12], as demonstrated by the good agreement observed between NMR and gravimetric measurements. However, the measurement of absolute lung water content requires special technical procedures (e.g., to prevent or correct for the T_1 and T_2 signal losses), which may increase the measurement time. Fortunately, recent studies on various animal species have shown that standard NMR techniques, which detect only a fraction of the total lung volume and use uncorrected NMR signal intensity data, can adequately quantify relative changes in lung water content. Relative lung water changes, measured by NMR imaging or spectroscopy from the NMR signal intensity, have been studied in various experimental models of pulmonary edema (intrabronchial saline instillation, left atrial balloon inflation, oleic acid injection, rapid saline infusion) in sheep, rabbits, and rats (excised lungs, intact, dead or living animals) [13–18]. Although uncorrected NMR signal intensity measurements result in an underestimation of the true lung water content [18], a good correlation has been observed between such NMR measurements and gravimetric lung water data [15, 16, 18]. Recent data obtained in intact living rats [18] suggest that NMR methods can be as sensitive as the gravimetric technique to changes in lung water content and can provide easily repeatable measurements to follow the time course of experimental lung injury.

Nonproton NMR (sodium NMR imaging) has been used in combination with proton imaging to estimate lung sodium content in rats with normal and edematous lungs [19]. The sodium signal intensity has been found to correlate with gravimetric lung water content. Compared with proton imaging, sodium imaging has poorer resolution and is more time consuming; however, it has potential for distinguishing intravascular from extravascular sodium when coupled with an intravascular NMR contrast agent [19].

Since, in animal tissues, the relaxation times T_1 and T_2 vary with water content, lung T_1 and T_2 measurements have often been used to quantify relative lung water changes. Lung T_1 and T_2 have been studied in various animal species, using several experimental models of pulmonary edema (e.g., pulmonary edema induced by steam inhalation, alloxan or oleic acid injection, rapid saline infusion, endotracheal saline lavage) [15, 16, 20–24] and other models of lung injury (oxygen-induced injury, chemical or bacterial inflammation, hemorrhage, bleomycin- or radiation-induced fibrosis) [25–30]. These studies have confirmed that T_1 and T_2 increase with lung water content, their values being correlated with gravimetric lung water data. However, recent experimental data suggest that, as in other tissues, lung T_1 and T_2 may depend not only on water content, but also on other factors (see below).

An important advantage of the NMR imaging techniques is their ability to assess the spatial distribution of lung water. Investigations conducted on living sheep, dogs, and rats with normal or edematous lungs [12, 14, 23, 31] have provided regional measurements of relative lung water content and have documented the effects of gravity on lung water distribution. Studies of the distribution of absolute lung water content in small (0.76 ml) excised rat lung specimens have demonstrated the accuracy and the excellent spatial resolution achievable by NMR imaging [12].

The conventional spatial approach to the assessment of lung water distribution is complemented by a new nonspatial method [18] which uses the NMR signal intensity data to generate a distribution of fractional lung volume, V_f, as a function of lung water density, ρH_2O; fractional lung volume is the fraction of the total lung volume having a given water density. Analysis of the V_f vs ρH_2O distribution provides the average ρH_2O (reflecting the lung water content) and a measure of the lung water distribution nonuniformity. As shown by studies on excised rat lungs and on living rats [18], the distribution changes markedly with lung edema. The changes reflect both the increased lung water content and the nonuniformity of the injury.

Limited measurements of lung water content and distribution have been obtained in normal living human subjects [14, 32–34] and in excised human lungs [35]. These preliminary measurements suggest that the NMR methods more extensively used in animal research are also applicable to experimental and clinical studies in humans.

Characterization of Lung Injury

Although relaxation time (T_1 and T_2) measurements have often been used to quantify relative changes in lung water, T_1 and T_2 depend not only on water content, but also on other factors such as interactions between water and macromolecules [8, 9, 36–38]. These interactions can be described by simple two-state models, which distinguish two fractions of water in biologic tissues: free water and water bound to macromolecules. A two-state model which also assumes a fast exchange between the free water compartment and the bound-water compartment has been used to explain the behavior of T_1 and predicts that T_1 will vary with the ratio of free water to bound water.

Lung water is partly free and partly bound to the macromolecules that constitute the lung matrix, such as collagen, elastin and proteoglycans, and other extracellular and intracellular molecules (including plasma proteins) [39–41]. On the basis of these concepts, recent experimental evidence suggests that measurements of relaxation times, in addition to proton density, may ultimately contribute valuable information for the characterization of lung injury, including pulmonary edema. For instance, the T_1 of sheep lung lymph (which reflects the composition of the interstitial lung fluid) has been found to differ between hydrostatic and increased permeability edema, being inversely related to the lymph/plasma protein ratio [42]. This finding is important because it could provide a means of distinguishing between these two pathogenetic types of pulmonary edema by lung NMR relaxation time measurements on the basis of differences in protein content (and therefore in the bound water fraction) of the edema fluid. Protein content is higher in increased permeability pulmonary edema (in which there is marked transcapillary protein leakage) than in high pressure pulmonary edema. Variations in the lung free water and bound water fractions may also partly account for the T_1 and T_2 changes observed during the course of oleic acid-induced pulmonary edema (in cats) [24] and other models of experimental lung injury (in rats, intratracheal bleomycin instillation or exposure to 80% oxygen) [26, 30]. However, these findings and the results of other studies [16, 21, 27, 29] show inconsistencies which need to be explained. Although of great interest, the role of T_1 and T_2 measurements in the characterization of lung injury requires further investigation.

NMR Lung Properties and State of Inflation

It has been shown that the NMR FID is much shorter (the NMR signal decreases more rapidly) in inflated lungs than in collapsed (airless) lungs [43]. This loss of signal associated with lung inflation is due to the presence of internal (tissue-induced) magnetic field inhomogeneity caused by the alveolar air-tissue interface (because of the different magnetic susceptibilities of water and air). The air-tissue interface effect has been explained using phantoms and theoretical models [44, 45]. The signal loss due to the alveolar air-tissue interface effect can be measured as the NMR signal intensity difference between a pair of images obtained using standard and modified NMR pulse sequences [43, 46, 47]. Since this difference-signal is produced only by lung water exposed to the alveolar air-tissue interface effect, its measurement has interesting pathophysiologic and clinical implications. Data obtained from normal excised rat lungs at various levels of inflation [48] suggest that, under appropriate technical conditions, the difference-signal is very sensitive to alveolar recruitment but relatively insensitive to volume changes occurring in already open alveoli. Therefore, NMR difference-signal measurements might be used to assess the relative role of alveolar recruitment and alveolar distention in the pressure-volume behavior of lungs. These measurements might detect the loss of alveolar air-tissue interface caused by alveolar flooding and collapse in lung injury, as suggested by data obtained in edematous lungs [49]. When combined with lung volume data, NMR difference-signal measurements might provide a means of distinguishing between alveolar recruitment and alveolar overdistention as the volume of injured lungs increases in response to the application of positive airway pressure. This information is of clinical interest because it has been suggested that regional alveolar overdistention due to high positive airway pressures may be an important determinant of iatrogenic lung damage in adult respiratory distress syndrome patients [50]. Further research is needed to test the sensitivity of difference-signal measurements to regional lung volume changes.

Limitations and Problems

Several problems still remain to be solved in the application of NMR to the measurement of lung water, including the relatively weak proton NMR signal from normal lung; effects of respiratory motion; stringent requirements for measuring absolute lung water content; lack of discrimination between intravascular and extravascular lung water; other potential causes of increased proton density (in addition to pulmonary edema); interactions between the magnetic field and monitoring or supportive equipment such as electrocardiographs, ventilators, and infusion pumps; and the complexity and lack of mobility of the NMR instrumentation [7–9, 51]. These problems are especially important in the clinical applications of NMR, for instance, in critically ill patients. The use of NMR for human studies requires precautions for the effect of the magnetic field on metallic implants [7–9, 51]. Progress has been made toward the solution of some of the above problems, particularly the effects of respiratory motion and interactions between magnetic field and monitoring or supportive equipment [7–9, 51–55]. It has been suggested that gadolinium-diethylenetriaminepentaacetic acid (Gd-DTPA), a paramagnetic contrast agent which enhances the NMR lung signal by decreasing T_1, might be helpful for distinguishing the intravascular from the extravascular lung compartment [56, 57]. However, further research is needed to test these and other possible approaches to the solution of problems posed by the application of NMR to the study of lung water.

Conclusions

NMR is a reliable and convenient method for detecting and monitoring changes in lung water content and distribution in experimental lung injury. The measurement of absolute lung water content by NMR is more complex and time consuming. Preliminary data indicate that NMR methods can be used for human studies, suggesting that the clinical evaluation of pulmonary edema by NMR should also be feasible. Relaxation time measurements and the quantitation of the alveolar air-tissue interface effect may increase the information provided by NMR images by further characterizing pulmonary edema and by clarifying the contributions of alveolar distention and recruitment to lung volume changes. Several technical problems require solution before the application of NMR to the assessment of lung water becomes routine.

Acknowledgement. We thank Jerri Duncan-Goff for her excellent secretarial assistance.

References

1. Casaburi R, Wasserman K, Effros RM (1978) Detection and measurement of pulmonary edema. In: Lung water and solute exchange, vol 7. Dekker, New York
2. Staub NC (1986) Clinical use of lung water measurements: report of a workshop. Chest 90:588–594
3. Cutillo AG (1987) The clinical assessment of lung water. Chest 92:319–325
4. Pistolesi M, Miniati M, Milne ENC, Giuntini C (1985) The chest roentgenogram in pulmonary edema. Clin Chest Med 6:315–344
5. Milne ENC, Pistolesi M, Miniati M, Giuntini C (1985) The radiologic distinction of cardiogenic and noncardiogenic edema. AJR 144:879–894
6. Budinger TF, Margulis AR (eds) (1986) Medical magnetic resonance imaging and spectroscopy. A primer. Society of Magnetic Resonance in Medicine, Berkeley
7. Higgins CB, Hricak H (eds) (1987) Magnetic resonance imaging of the body. Raven, New York
8. Stark DD, Bradley WG Jr (eds) (1988) Magnetic resonance imaging. Mosby, St Louis
9. Partain CL, Price RR, Patton JA, Kulkarni MV, James AE Jr (eds) (1988) Magnetic resonance imaging. Saunders, Philadelphia
10. Oldendorf W, Oldendorf W Jr (1988) Basics of magnetic resonance imaging. Nijhoff, Hingham
11. Young SW (1988) Magnetic resonance imaging. Basic principles. Raven, New York
12. Cutillo AG, Morris AH, Blatter DD, Case TA, Ailion DC, Durney CH, Johnson SA (1984) Determination of lung water content and distribution by nuclear magnetic resonance. J Appl Physiol 57:583–588
13. Hayes CE, Case TA, Ailion DC, Morris AH, Cutillo A, Blackburn CW, Durney CH, Johnson SA (1982) Lung water quantitation by nuclear magnetic resonance imaging. Science 216:1313–1315
14. Carroll FEJ, Loyd JE, Nolop KB, Collins JC (1985) MR imaging parameters in the study of lung water. A preliminary study. Invest Radiol 20:381–387
15. Schmidt HC, McNamara MT, Brasch RC, Higgins CB (1985) Assessment of severity of experimental pulmonary edema with magnetic resonance imaging: effect of relaxation enhancement by Gd-DTPA. Invest Radiol 20:687–692
16. Schmidt HC, Tsay D, Higgins CB (1986) Pulmonary edema: an MR study of permeability and hydrostatic types in animals. Radiology 158:297–302
17. Siefkin AD, Nichols BG (1986) Noninvasive lung water quantitation by ^{1}H nuclear magnetic resonance spectroscopy. Am Rev Respir Dis 134:509–512
18. Cutillo AG, Morris AH, Ailion DC, Case TA, Durney CH, Ganesan K, Watanabe F, Akhtari M (1988) Assessment of lung water distribution by nuclear magnetic resonance. A new method for quantifying and monitoring experimental lung injury. Am Rev Respir Dis 137:1371–1378
19. Kundel HL, Shetty A, Joseph PM, Summers RM, Kassab EA, Moore B (1988) Sodium NMR imaging of lung water in rats. Magn Reson Med 6:381–389
20. Lauterbur PC (1976) Feasibility of NMR zeugmatographic imaging of the heart and lungs. Presented at the Engineering Foundation conference on comparative productivity of techniques for noninvasive medical diagnosis, New England College, Henniker, New Hampshire, 15–20 Aug 1976
21. Huber DJ, Adams DF (1984) Proton NMR of acute pulmonary edema and hemorrhage. Invest Radiol 19:S21
22. Skalina S, Kundel HL, Wolf G, Marshall B (1984) The effect of pulmonary edema on proton nuclear magnetic resonance relaxation times. Invest Radiol 19:7–9
23. Wexler HR, Nicholson RL, Prato FS, Carey LS, Vinitski S, Reese L (1985) Quantitation of lung water by nuclear magnetic resonance imaging. A preliminary study. Invest Radiol 20:583–590
24. Phillips DM, Allen PS, Man SFP (1989) Assessment of temporal changes in pulmonary edema with NMR imaging. J Appl Physiol 66:1197–1208

25. Huber DJ, Kobzik L, Melanson G, Adams DF (1985) The detection of inflammation in collapsed lung by alterations in proton nuclear magnetic relaxation times. Invest Radiol 20:460–464
26. Vinitski S, Pearson MG, Karlik SJ, Morgan WKC, Carey LS, Perkins G, Goto T, Befus D (1986) Differentiation of parenchymal lung disorders with in vitro proton nuclear magnetic resonance. Magn Reson Med 3:120–125
27. Inch WR, Prato FS, Butland TS, Frei JV (1986) Use of nuclear magnetic resonance to monitor lung injury by X-radiation: a preliminary study. Respir Care 31:388–394
28. Huber DJ, Kobzik L, Solorzano C, Melanson G, Adams DF (1987) Nuclear magnetic resonance spectroscopy of acute and evolving pulmonary hemorrhage. An in vitro study. Invest Radiol 22:632–637
29. Taylor CR, Sostman HD, Gore JC, Smith GW (1987) Proton relaxation times in bleomycin-induced lung injury. Invest Radiol 22:621–626
30. Shioya S, Haida M, Tsuji C, Ohta Y, Yamabayashi H, Fukuzaki M, Kimula Y (1988) Acute and repair stage characteristics of magnetic resonance relaxation times in oxygen-induced pulmonary edema. Magn Reson Med 8:450–459
31. Cutillo AG, Morris AH, Ganesan K, Ailion DC, Case TA, Durney CH, Watanabe F (1989) Regional effects of repetition time on NMR quantitation of water in normal and edematous lungs. Magn Reson Med 12:137–144
32. Lallemand DP, Brasch RC, Gooding CA, Wesbey GE, Higgins CB (1984) NMR imaging of lung parenchyma. Magn Reson Med 1:190–191
33. MacLennan FM, Foster MA, Smith FW, Crosher GA (1986) Measurement of total lung water from nuclear magnetic resonance images. Br J Radiol 59:553–560
34. Ailion DC, Case TA, Blatter DD, Morris AH, Cutillo AG, Durney CH (1986) New imaging techniques for lung and fat. In: New developments in nuclear magnetic resonance and magnetic resonance and quantum electronics. CIP Press, Bucharest
35. Johnston PW, MacLennan FM, Simpson JG, Smith FW (1985) Nuclear magnetic resonance imaging of pulmonary infarction and oedema in excised cadaver lungs. Magn Reson Imaging 3:157–161
36. Mathur-De Vre R (1984) Biomedical implications of the relaxation behaviour of water related to NMR imaging. Br J Radiol 57:955–976
37. Bottomley PA, Foster TH, Argersinger RE, Pfeifer LM (1984) A review of normal tissue hydrogen NMR relaxation times and relaxation mechanisms from 1–100 MHz: dependence on tissue type, NMR frequency, temperature, species, excision, and age. Med Phys 11:425–448
38. Bottomley PA, Hardy CJ, Argersinger RE, Allen-Moore G (1987) A review of ^{1}H nuclear magnetic resonance relaxation in pathology: are T_1 and T_2 diagnostic? Med Phys 14:1–37
39. Prockop DJ (1979) Collagen, elastin, and proteoglycans: matrix for fluid accumulation in the lung. In: Pulmonary edema. American Physiological Society, Bethesda
40. Taylor AE, Parker JC, Kvietys PR, Perry MA (1982) The pulmonary interstitium in capillary exchange. Ann NY Acad Sci 384:146–165
41. Turino G (1985) The lung parenchyma—a dynamic matrix. Am Rev Respir Dis 132:1324–1334
42. Podgorski GT, Carroll FE, Parker RE (1986) MR evaluation of pulmonary interstitial and intravascular fluids. Invest Radiol 21:478–482
43. Morris AH, Blatter DD, Case TA, Cutillo AG, Ailion DC, Durney CH, Johnson SA (1985) A new nuclear magnetic resonance property of lung. J Appl Physiol 58:759–762
44. Case TA, Durney CH, Ailion DC, Cutillo AG, Morris AH (1987) A mathematical model of diamagnetic line broadening in lung tissue and similar heterogeneous systems: calculations and measurements. J Magn Reson 73:304–314
45. Durney CH, Bertolina J, Ailion DC, Christman R, Cutillo AG, Morris AH, Hashemi S (1989) Calculation and interpretation of inhomogeneous line broadening in models of lungs and other heterogeneous structures. J Magn Reson 85:554–570
46. Ailion DC, Case TA, Blatter DD, Morris AH, Cutillo AG, Durney CH, Johnson SA (1984) Applications of NMR spin imaging to the study of lungs. Bull Magn Res 6:130–139
47. Blatter DD, Morris AH, Ailion DC, Cutillo AG, Case TA (1985) Asymmetric spin echo sequences: a simple new method for obtaining NMR ^{1}H spectral images. Invest Radiol 20:845–853
48. Cutillo AG, Ganesan K, Ailion DC, Morris AH, Durney CH, Symko SC, Christman RA (1991) Alveolar air-tissue interface and nuclear magnetic resonance behavior of lung. J Appl Physiol 70:2145–2154

49. Cutillo AG, Morris AH, Ailion DC, Ganesan K, Durney CH, Symko SC, Watanabe S, Kolem H (1989) Nuclear magnetic resonance (NMR) behavior of edematous lungs as a function of inflation. Am Rev Respir Dis 139:A417
50. Gattinoni L, Pesenti A, Mascheroni D, Marcolin R, Fumagalli R, Rossi F, Iapichino G, Romagnoli G, Uziel L, Agostoni A, Kolobow T, Damia G (1986) Low-frequency positive-pressure ventilation with extracorporeal CO_2 removal in severe acute respiratory failure. JAMA 256:881–886
51. Cutillo AG, Morris AH, Ailion DC, Durney CH, Ganesan K (1988) Quantitative assessment of pulmonary edema by nuclear magnetic resonance methods. J Thorac Imaging 3:51–58
52. Dunn V, Coffman CE, McGowan JE, Ehrhardt JC (1985) Mechanical ventilation during magnetic resonance imaging. Magn Reson Imaging 3:169–172
53. Ramsay JG, Gale L, Sykes MK (1986) A ventilator for use in nuclear magnetic resonance studies. Br J Anaesth 58:1181–1184
54. Hedlund LW, Deitz J, Nassar R, Herfkens R, Vock P, Dahlke J, Kubek R, Effmann EL, Putman CE (1986) A ventilator for magnetic resonance imaging. Invest Radiol 21:18–23
55. Rokey R, Wendt RE, Johnston DL (1988) Monitoring of acutely ill patients during nuclear magnetic resonance imaging: use of a time-varying filter electrocardiographic gating device to reduce gradient artifacts. Magn Reson Med 6:240–245
56. Montgomery AB, Paajanen H, Brasch RC, Murray JF (1987) Aerosolized gadolinium-DTPA enhances the magnetic resonance signal of extravascular lung water. Invest Radiol 22:377–381
57. Schmiedl U, Ogan M, Paajanen H, Marotti M, Crooks LE, Brito AC, Brasch RC (1987) Albumin labeled with Gd-DTPA as an intravascular, blood pool-enhancing agent for MR imaging: biodistribution and imaging studies. Radiology 162:205–210

Volumetric Evaluation of Diaphragm Motion

S. Krayer

Introduction

Although the natural shape of the lungs and thoracic cavity are different, they conform to each other at any time. Therefore, the pattern of chest wall motion should reflect lung expansion. Alterations in lung ventilation may be detected by changes in chest wall motion. It was suggested that the diaphragm, as a major part of the chest wall, could be an important determinant of lung volume and intrapulmonary distribution of ventilation.

Froese and Bryan [4] described diaphragm position and motion during tidal breathing in men lying supine. The authors employed cross-table X-ray cineradiography to study the lateral silhouette of the diaphragm during spontaneous breathing while awake and during mechanical ventilation while anesthetized-paralyzed. In awake men most diaphragm motion was found to occur in dependent diaphragm regions. This pattern of diaphragm motion corresponds to a distribution of ventilation with largest ventilation of the dependent lung regions [10, 15, 16]. The small radii of curvature in the dependent diaphragm regions, produced by the hydrostatic pressure gradient in the abdomen, facilitate pressure development in these regions corresponding to the law of LaPlace, $\Delta P = T \times (1/r_1 + 1/r_2)$, in which ΔP is the pressure development of the diaphragm, T is the diaphragm tension, and r_1 and r_2 are the principal radii of diaphragm curvature. Furthermore, concomitant distension of the dependent diaphragm regions may have increased their pressure generation because stretching of the diaphragm fibers produces a more favorable length-tension relationship [1].

After induction of anesthesia, the diaphragm was displaced into the thorax [4]. Again, the hydrostatic pressure gradient, produced by the weight of the abdominal contents, displaced predominantly dependent diaphragm regions, thus reducing resting lung volume. This cephalad diaphragm shift after induction of anesthesia with or without paralysis was widely accepted as the major mechanism of the observed reduction of functional residual capacity [8].

Froese and Bryan [4] found that, during mechanical ventilation, the pattern of diaphragm motion is reversed compared to spontaneous breathing: most motion occurs in the nondependent diaphragm regions. They argued that a relatively uniform increase in airway pressure will thus displace the diaphragm preferentially in those regions where the opposing abdominal pressure is least, namely in nondependent areas [4]. This pattern of diaphragm motion during mechanical ventilation corresponds to the distribution of inspired gas, i.e., maximum ventilation of nondependent lung regions [16].

Froese and Bryan [4] also suggested that the hydrostatic pressure gradient in the abdomen largely determines position and motion of the diaphragm. If the position and motion of the diaphragm is in fact a function of abdominal pressure, the above observations should be dependent of body position, because the hydrostatic pressure gradient in the abdomen is gravity related. Krayer et al. [13] tested this hypothesis, that the position and motion of the diaphragm in recumbent men is gravity dependent. They examined the lower thorax, including the diaphragm, of six healthy young volunteers first during spontaneous breathing while awake and again after induction of anesthesia-paralysis and mechanical ventilation. Three subjects were studied while they were lying supine and the other three while they were lying prone.

In that study, three-dimensional X-ray computerized tomography (Dynamic Spatial Reconstructor, DSR [12, 18]) was employed to examine diaphragm position and motion in vivo [13]. Based on the principles of conventional computerized tomography, the DSR is a rapid scanner that simultaneously records multiple projection images in about 300 ms, permitting the reconstruction of a three-dimensional, i.e., cubic, array of X-ray densities in computer memory. From such data sets, a detailed description of the diaphragm surface can be obtained.

Spontaneous Breathing

Diaphragm motion during spontaneous breathing while awake was found to be nonuniform in both the supine and prone body positions (Figs. 1 and 2). There was a significant ventrodorsal gradient in displacement, with most motion of dorsal diaphragm regions, i.e., in dependent regions in supine and nondependent regions in prone body positions. The observation in supine position confirmed the findings of Froese and Bryan [4]. In contrast, the hypothesis that dependent diaphragm regions move the most also in the prone position was not confirmed.

It is recognized that the diaphragm consists of two muscles (crural and costal) [3] that may not share the same tension [2]. In this case, the distribution of pressure development of the diaphragm does not depend on curvature alone (see LaPlace's law). Furthermore, crural and costal diaphragm regions may have different length-tension relationships and compliances [19].

There was also a difference in displaced volume between the right and left hemidiaphragm with on the average 9% ± 8% (SD) more displacement of the right hemidiaphragm than the left hemidiaphragm [13]. The dome of the right hemidiaphragm always remained more cephalad than the dome of the left hemidiaphragm. Differences in the mechanical properties of the two hemidiaphragms, in phrenic innervation, in the preload and afterload, or in some combination of these may produce right-to-left differences of motion.

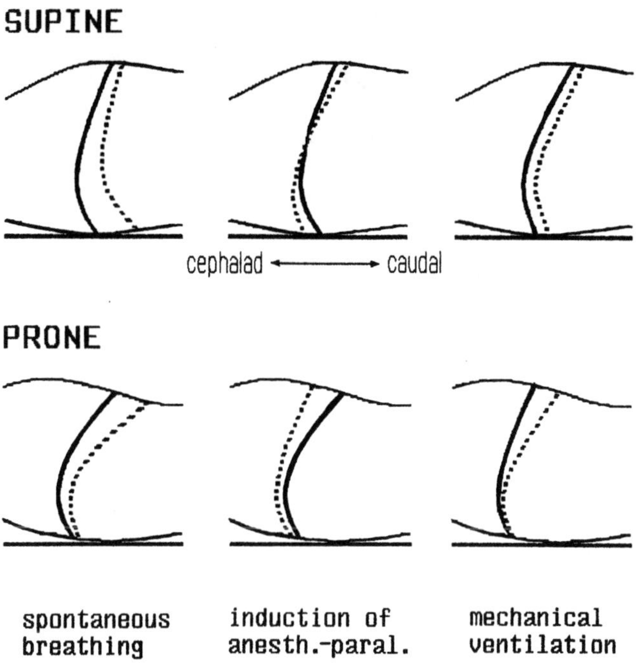

Fig. 1. Lateral views of diaphragm position for supine (*top*) or prone (*bottom*) subjects. *Solid lines* represent end-expiratory diaphragm positions during spontaneous breathing while awake (*left* and *center panels*) and during mechanical ventilation while anesthetized-paralyzed (*right panel*). *Broken lines* represent end-inspiratory diaphragm position (*left* and *right panels*) and end-expiratory position after induction of anesthesia-paralysis (*center panel*), respectively. (Adapted from [13])

Induction of Anesthesia-Paralysis

After induction of anesthesia-paralysis the end-expiratory diaphragm position was altered (Fig. 1). In the subjects lying supine the volume shift of the diaphragm was small and the direction was not consistent. This observation confirms previous findings [12] that a cephalad diaphragm shift after induction of anesthesia-paralysis contributes little to the reduction of resting lung volume. By contrast, a consistent and large cephalad volume shift of the diaphragm (316 to 1213 ml) occurred in the subjects lying prone, suggesting a major mechanism for the reduction of resting lung volume after induction of anesthesia-paralysis in subjects lying prone [17]. Regardless of body position, dorsal diaphragm regions always shifted cephalad after induction of anesthesia-paralysis. This observation cannot be explained by the hydrostatic pressure gradient in the abdomen acting on the paralyzed diaphragm, but suggests that, in awake subjects, dorsal diaphragm regions may have different anatomic and/or functional properties than ventral regions.

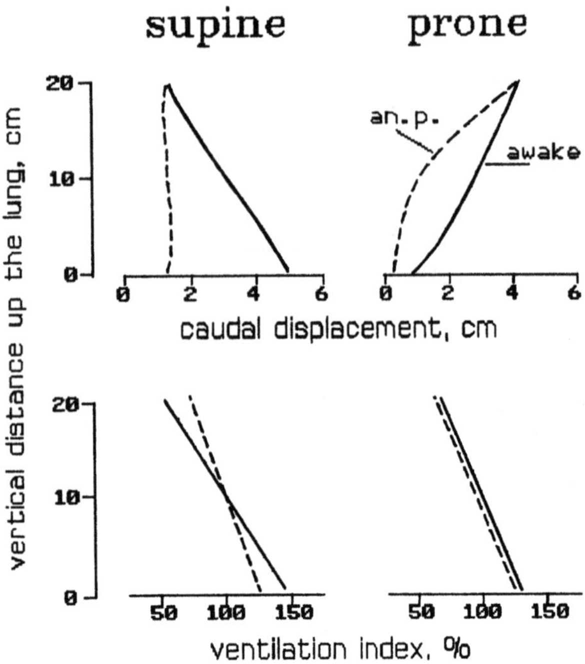

Fig. 2. Average diaphragm motion at any given vertical height (*top*) and intrapulmonary inspired gas distribution as a function of vertical distance (*bottom*) for supine and prone subjects. *Solid lines* indicate spontaneous breathing while awake and *broken lines* indicate mechanical ventilation during anesthesia-paralysis. (Adapted from [13] and [17])

Mechanical Ventilation

During mechanical ventilation, while anesthetized-paralyzed in supine or prone position, diaphragm motion was reduced in dependent regions (Figs. 1 and 2). In supine position, diaphragm displacement became more uniform without ventrodorsal or right-left gradients as compared to spontaneous breathing. Although the relative motion of nondependent diaphragm areas increased with mechanical ventilation, their absolute motion did not increase. This observation does not completely satisfy the hypothesis of Froese and Bryan [4]. In prone position, the decrease of motion in dependent diaphragm areas during mechanical ventilation produced an increased ventrodorsal gradient of motion with more relative motion of the nondependent diaphragm areas. The different diaphragm motions between supine and prone body positions during mechanical ventilation suggest that the paralyzed diaphragm does not behave as a homogeneous membrane and that its motion does not only depend on the distribution of transdiaphragmatic pressure. Other factors include the distribution of passive tension in the diaphragm, the principle radii of diaphragm curvature, and the thoracoabdominal anatomy that couples the diaphragm to its neighboring structures.

Diaphragm Volume Displacement

Until recently it has been thought that, because of the noncompressibility of the abdominal contents, diaphragm displacement results in an equal displacement of the ventral abdominal wall [5, 11]. Based on the assumption that the chest wall moves as a system with two degrees of freedom [11], tidal volume was partitioned into rib cage and diaphragm contributions using sensors to detect the motion of the body surface. Measuring the motion at mammillary and umbilical levels, some investigators [6, 7, 9, 20, 21] have estimated that the rib cage contributes between 15% and 40% to the tidal volume during spontaneous breathing in awake supine humans. However, it is now recognized that the rib cage contributes to the abdominal displacement [14] because it forms part of the abdomen in the area of diaphragm apposition. Thus, surface measurements may have overestimated rib cage contribution to tidal volume [11]. Whitelaw [22] employed conventional X-ray computerized tomography to estimate diaphragm volume displacement. In one awake subject he found the diaphragm contribution to be 68% of tidal volume. The diaphragm was scanned repeatedly during breath holding with the glottis open. This maneuver might have produced a different diaphragm position than during continuous breathing. Krayer et al. [13] determined the volume displacement during continuous breathing using the DSR. Table 1 shows the volume contribution of the diaphragm to tidal volume (V_T) expressed as % of V_T. Tidal volumes were similar during spontaneous breathing and mechanical ventilation in both supine and prone positions. Note that, during spontaneous breathing in the supine position, the diaphragm displacement was as much as the V_T. Assuming that rib cage expansion also contributed to the increase in lung volume, the overall increase of the thoracic cavity was larger than V_T. Thoracic blood volume presumably increased during active inspiration. After induction of anesthesia-paralysis and mechanical ventilation, the volume displacement of the diaphragm was consistently reduced to about 50% of V_T. Latter observation agrees with measurements using body surface sensors [6, 7, 9, 20, 21].

Table 1. Diaphragm contribution to tidal volume (mean ± SD)

	Supine		Prone	
	Awake	Anesthetized paralyzed	Awake	Anesthetized paralyzed
V_T (ml)	865 ± 147	795 ± 128	707 ± 67	723 ± 47
% of V_T	101 ± 7	53 ± 5	82 ± 16	51 ± 10

Adapted from Krayer et al. [13]

Diaphragm Motion and Distribution of Ventilation

Figure 2 relates the vertical distribution of diaphragm motion [13] to the vertical distribution of ventilation [17] for subjects lying supine or prone. During spontaneous breathing in the supine position, dependent diaphragm regions move the most and dependent lung regions have the most ventilation per unit lung volume. After induction of anesthesia-paralysis and mechanical ventilation, the vertical gradients of both diaphragm motion and ventilation become more uniform in supine subjects. In contrast, diaphragm motion does not match the distribution of ventilation in prone subjects: nondependent diaphragm regions move the most during spontaneous breathing and mechanical ventilation, but dependent lung regions ventilate the most in both instances. The discrepancy between the similar vertical distribution of ventilation in supine and prone position and the different vertical distribution of diaphragm motion in these body positions suggests that regional ventilation cannot be determined by diaphragm motion alone. Although the underlying mechanism remains unknown, intrapulmonary distribution of inspired gas might be affected by slippage of lung lobes, by mechanical interdependence of lung parenchyma, or by both.

Summary

Anatomic features of the diaphragm seem to be a more important determinant of the pattern of diaphragm motion than the hydrostatic pressure gradient in the abdomen. One may think of anatomic differences between the crural and costal diaphragm regions [2, 3, 19]. During spontaneous breathing the dorsal (i.e., crural) diaphragm regions move generally more than the ventral (i.e., costal) regions, regardless of body position [13]. After induction of anesthesia-paralysis, the dorsal diaphragm regions are shifted cephalad at end-expiration [13]. In prone body position, this cephalad diaphragm shift reduces resting lung volume, whereas in the supine position it may be of less importance for lung volume [12, 13].

Mechanical ventilation reduces the volume displacement of the paralyzed diaphragm predominantly in dependent regions, producing a different pattern of diaphragm motion between supine and prone positions. In prone subjects the vertical distribution of ventilation does not match the vertical distribution of diaphragm motion.

References

1. Braun NMT, Arora NS, Rochester DF (1982) Force-length relationship of the normal human diaphragm. J Appl Physiol 53:405–412

2. Decramer M, De Troyer A, Kelly S, Macklem PT (1984) Mechanical arrangement of costal and crural diaphragms in dogs. J Appl Physiol 56:1484–1490
3. De Troyer A, Sampson M, Sigrist S, Macklem PT (1981) The diaphragm: two muscles. Science 213:237–238
4. Froese AB, Bryan AC (1974) Effects of anesthesia and paralysis on diaphragmatic mechanics in man. Anesthesiology 41:242–255
5. Grassino A, Goldman MD, Mead J, Sears TA (1978) Mechanics of the human diaphragm during voluntary contraction: statics. J Appl Physiol 44:829–839
6. Grimby G, Hedenstierna G, Löfström B (1975) Chest wall mechanics during artificial ventilation. J Appl Physiol 38:576–580
7. Hedenstierna G, Löfström B, Lundh R (1981) Thoracic gas volume and chest-abdomen dimensions during anesthesia and muscle paralysis. Anesthesiology 55:499–506
8. Hedenstierna G, Strandberg Å, Brismar B, Lundquist H, Svensson L, Tokics L (1985) Functional residual capacity, thoracoabdominal dimensions, and central blood volume during general anesthesia with muscle paralysis and mechanical ventilation. Anesthesiology 62:247–254
9. Jones JG, Faithfull D, Jordan C, Minty B (1979) Rib cage movement during halothane anaesthesia in man. Br J Anaesth 51:399–407
10. Kaneko K, Milic-Emili J, Dolovich MB, Dawson A, Bates DV (1966) Regional distribution of ventilation and perfusion as a function of body position. J Appl Physiol 21:767–777
11. Konno K, Mead J (1967) Measurement of the separate volume changes of rib cage and abdomen during breathing. J Appl Physiol 22:407–422
12. Krayer S, Rehder K, Beck KC, Cameron PD, Didier EP, Hoffman EA (1987) Quantification of thoracic volumes by three-dimensional imaging. J Appl Physiol 62:591–598
13. Krayer S, Rehder K, Vettermann J, Didier EP, Ritman EL (1989) Position and motion of the human diaphragm during anesthesia-paralysis. Anesthesiology 70:891–898
14. Mead J, Loring SH (1982) Analysis of volume displacement and length changes of the diaphragm during breathing. J Appl Physiol 53:750–755
15. Milic-Emili J, Henderson JAM, Dolovich MB, Trop D, Kaneko K (1966) Regional distribution of inspired gas in the lung. J Appl Physiol 21:749–759
16. Rehder K, Sessler AD, Rodarte JR (1977) Regional intrapulmonary gas distribution in awake and anesthetized-paralyzed man. J Appl Physiol 42:391–402
17. Rehder K, Knopp TJ, Sessler AD (1978) Regional intrapulmonary gas distribution in awake and anesthetized-paralyzed prone man. J Appl Physiol 45:528–535
18. Ritman EL, Robb RA, Harris LD (1985) Imaging physiological functions: experience with the dynamic spatial reconstructor. Praeger, New York
19. Road J, Newman S, Derenne JP, Grassino A (1986) In vivo length-force relationship of canine diaphragm. J Appl Physiol 60:63–70
20. Tusiewicz K, Bryan AC, Froese AB (1977) Contributions of changing rib cage-diaphragm interactions to the ventilatory depression of halothane anesthesia. Anesthesiology 47:327–337
21. Vellody VPS, Nassery M, Balasaraswathi K, Goldberg NB, Sharp JT (1978) Compliances of human rib cage and diaphragm-abdomen pathways in relaxed versus paralyzed states. Am Rev Respir Dis 118:479–491
22. Whitelaw WA (1987) Shape and size of the human diaphragm in vivo. J Appl Physiol 62:180–186

12. [illegible]

Part 6:
Mechanics of Breathing and Surfactant

Inflation and Atelectasis in a Topographical Model of the Lung*

Y.C. Fung

Introduction

Instability and atelectasis of the lung are discussed in this article. The word *instability*, like the word *disease*, has no unique meaning. Here I mean the tendency of a system toward returning to the initial state after an arbitrary infinitesimal perturbation: A system is *stable* if it would return, unstable if the return is not guaranteed.

The term *atelectasis* may also mean different things to different people. Here I mean the existence of some groups of completely collapsed alveoli in which there is no ventilation. In contrast, Wilson (1982) considered the pressure-volume curves (PV) of the lung and used positiveness of the bulk modulus of the parenchyma as a criterion for stability. Stamenovic (1986) generalized this concept and defined atelectasis as a coexistence of different phases of expansion, with each phase having a uniform volume expansion ratio. While their investigations threw new light on the phenomenon, their definitions are different from what follows in this paper.

Thus defined, atelectasis and instability are not the same thing. A lung which is stable with respect to small perturbations may become atelectatic by a "large" deformation. On the other hand, an atelectatic lung may be quite stable in the atelectatic state. However, it is most likely that atelectasis follows instability. Hence we investigate them both: the initial tendency toward instability and the persistent atelectatic plaque.

Atelectasis is often seen in surgery, trauma, disease, airway obstruction, high oxygen breathing, high acceleration, etc. To a patient or a physician, the most important question is how to reinflate the collapsed region. A related question is the inflation of a new born baby's liquid-filled lung. The answers are discussed below.

Physical Principles of Stability Analysis

Figure 1 shows the common concepts of equilibrium and stability. A ball in a dish will rest at the bottom and is stable there. Turn the dish over, the ball will

* The support of United States NIH and NSF in this research is gratefully acknowledged.

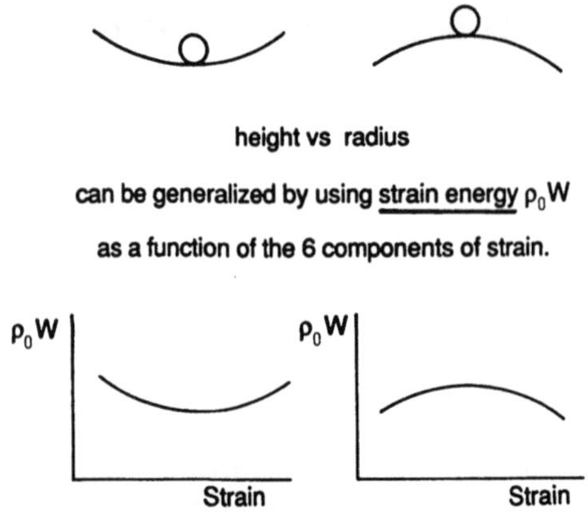

Fig. 1. The common concept of equilibrium and stability and its generalization to a complex elastic structure

be in equilibrium at the top but unstable there. This concept is expressed mathematically by saying that the potential energy of the ball is at a relative minimum at the stable equilibrium position and at a relative maximum at the unstable equilibrium position. The potential energy of the ball, derived from gravitation, is equal to the product of the mass of the ball and the height. The relative maximum or minimum is examined against variation of the radial distance from the equilibrium position.

This concept can be generalized to an elastic system by the method of calculus of variation (see, for example, Fung 1965, Chap. 10). One examines the variation of the potential energy of the system against all possible strains. If the first variation of the potential energy function is zero at a certain state of strain, then that state is in equilibrium. If the second variation of the potential energy is positive at the equilibrium state, then that state is stable. If the second variation of the potential energy is negative, then that state of equilibrium is unstable. This is illustrated in the lower half of Fig. 1. In this generalization, the slope of the dish is replaced by the first variation and the curvature of the dish is replaced by the second variation of the potential energy.

From the general theory of thermodynamics we recognize the existence of internal energy. For the lung, the internal energy per unit volume is designated as $\rho_0 W$, and it consists of two parts: (1) the strain energy in the tissue and (2) the surface energies of the liquid-gas interfaces of the alveolar walls. As to the external forces acting on the lung, some, like gravity, are conservative and have a potential function; others, like aerodynamic forces in airways and viscous shear forces in blood vessels, are nonconservative. All external forces multiplied by the corresponding displacements are equal to the work done, which has the same dimension as energy. When the lung deforms a little in an arbitrary way, the displacement of the lung can be described by a continuous vector field δu. This displacement causes a change of strain δE_{ij}, a change of stress δS_{ij}, a change of internal energy per unit volume $\delta(\rho_0 W)$, a work done by body force X_i equal to $X_i \times \delta u_i$, and work done by surface force T_i equal to $T_i \times \delta u_i$. Then a rigorous analysis yields the result (see, e.g., Fung 1965 p. 450):

$$S_{ij} = \frac{\partial \rho_0 W}{\partial E_{ij}} \tag{1}$$

$$\delta^2(\rho_0 W) > 0\text{: stable} \tag{2}$$

$$\delta^2(\rho_0 W) < 0\text{: unstable} \tag{3}$$

The critical condition of instability is:

$$\delta^2(\rho_0 W) = 0 \tag{4}$$

Here $\delta^2(\rho_0 W)$ is the second variation of $\rho_0 W$, i.e., the second order term of the change of $\rho_0 W$ due to the small variations of displacement δu_i.

Applying this theorem to the lung, we must allow δu_i to be completely arbitrary (subject only to the restrictions at the boundary of pleura). This is illustrated in Fig. 2, in which a model of an alveolar duct is shown on the left, with each alveolus represented by a 14-sided polyhedron, ventilated to the duct bounded by heavy lines at the center. A disturbed configuration is shown on the right, in which every wall and every edge is deformed in an arbitrary manner. In the theoretical examination of the critical condition of stability, the tendency to collapse is examined against any possible (accidental or otherwise) small perturbations. If the lung is stable, then any small transient disturbance will die away. If it is unstable, then a small disturbance may cause the lung to collapse.

The principle of stability analysis is embodied in the four equations given above. The steps to be taken for a quantitative evaluation of lung stability are then very clear: One must evaluate the potential energy, i.e., the sum of strain energy, surface energy, and the potential of external load, as a function of arbitrary deformation of the lung.

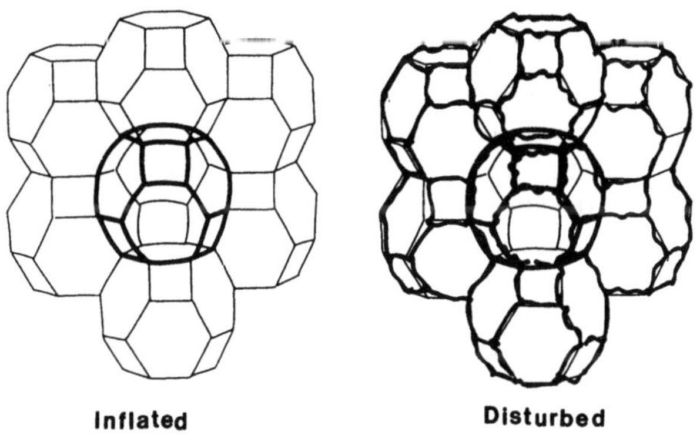

Fig. 2. A general and arbitrary deformation is considered in the stability study. *Left*, A mathematical model of a basic unit of pulmonary alveolar duct; *right*, a perturbation

How to Evaluate the Potential Energy Function

The study of atelectasis is, therefore, a study of the potential energy as a function of the strains in the lung. The lung is, however, made of many parts. The strains in different parts are not necessarily the same. The following should be distinguished:

1. The macroscopic strain of lung parenchyma, E_{ij}, which is averaged over a scale of millimeters and measured relative to a reference state, e.g., the functional residual state
2. The strains in collagen and elastin fiber bundles in the alveolar walls and mouths, measured relative to each fiber's zero-stress state
3. The strains in interalveolar septa and alveolar mouths relative to their respective zero-stress states

Technically, the calculation of the possible differences in the strains in the fibers, walls, and mouths from the macroscopic strains of the lung parenchyma is the most difficult step, requiring a large amount of anatomical and rheological data and sophisticated calculations. The procedure requires the following:

1. Collect data on all materials of construction of the lung
2. Determine the rheological properties of each material component.
3. Establish a model of the lung parenchyma, i.e., the alveolar ducts and alveoli
4. Determine surface tension as a function of the strains in the alveolar wall
5. Use the principles of continuum mechanics and calculate the strains in every structural component for any specified macroscopic strains of the parenchyma, E_{ij}
6. Calculate the potential energy of every structural component and sum them up

The status of the art is reviewed briefly below.

Structure of the Alveolar Walls

Structurally, the interalveolar septa (alveolar walls) are composed of collagen fibers, elastin fibers, ground substances (embedding matrix), cells, and capillary blood vessels. Collagen and elastin fibers can be stained and photographed. Many photographs and data on the fiber width and curvature are given in Sobin et al. (1988). Both collagen and elastin fibers are curved, and their average curvatures are of the same order of magnitude, although the elastin fibers are straighter. The elastic moduli of the ground substances and cells are much smaller than those of collagen and elastin.

Every alveolus must have a mouth opening to an alveolar duct for ventilation. The edge of the mouth is reinforced with thicker collagen and elastin fibers. Some statistical data on the fibers in the alveolar mouths of human lung have been obtained by Matsuda et al. (1987).

Model of the Alveoli and Alveolar Ducts

Miller (1947) reviewed the development of concepts related to the structure of the alveoli and alveolar ducts from Malpighi to Loeschcke. Orsos (1936), Weibel (1963), Hansen et al. (1975), Oldmixon and Hoppin (1987), Oldmixon et al. (1988), and Mercer et al. (1987) have added new results. Figure 3 shows a series of alveolar models published by various authors. The models in the upper row depict alveoli as bunches of grapes. Each alveolar wall has an "inside" and an "outside." On the inside, the alveolar gas pressure acts. On the outside, the pressure is presumably the pleural pressure. These models culminate in von Neergaard's model, shown in the first part figure in the lower row, which was taken from Clements' review (1965). This is the model that has asserted the importance of surface tension on the stability of the lung. One difficulty that this model leads to is shown in Fig. 4. If two soap bubbles are blown at the ends of two tubes and these two tubes are connected and open to each other, then at equilibrium the smaller bubble would collapse. Similarly, if a human lung were considered as 300 million bubbles connected in parallel to an airway, then one would conclude that at equilibrium all but one alveolus will be collapsed, unless the surface tension is zero or elastic force overwhelms the surface force. This is obviously not the case. The fault of this model is that it ignores the fact that an alveolar wall is an interalveolar septum. The inside of one alveolus is the outside of another alveolus. The pressure difference across each septum is negligibly small. A septum must be a minimal surface. Any calculation of septal deformation based on a pressure difference between airway and pleura would be wrong.

Other drawings in Fig. 3 show models of the alveolar duct as described by Weibel (1963), Hoppin and Hildebrandt (1977), who did not describe how these units are organized into an airway tree that fills the entire space of the lung.

To meet the space filling requirement, the author (Fung 1988) proposed a model based on the assumptions that: (1) all alveoli are equal and space filling before they are ventilated, (2) they are ventilated to ducts as uniformly as possible, and (3) the alveoli are reinforced at the edges of the alveolar mouths for structural integrity and distorted by lung weight and inflation according to the theory of elasticity.

It is well known that there exist only five regular convex polyhedra in three-dimensional space: the tetrahedron, cube, octahedron, pentagonal dodecahedron, and icosahedron. However, the last two are not space filling. On the other hand, the cube, the nonregular octahedron (every face a triangle), the rhombic dodecahedron (every face a rhombus), and the tetrakaidecahedron *(14-hedron)* are space filling. Photographs of the microstructure of the lung show that the alveolar walls are not all triangles, squares, rhombuses, or pentagons. Thus, a more acceptable choice is the tetrakaidecahedron. Now, a 14-hedron surrounded by 14 identical polyhedra contacting and matching each of its faces will form a solid unit in space which may be called a *14-hedron of order 2*. If all the walls of the central 14-hedron are removed, than all the alveoli

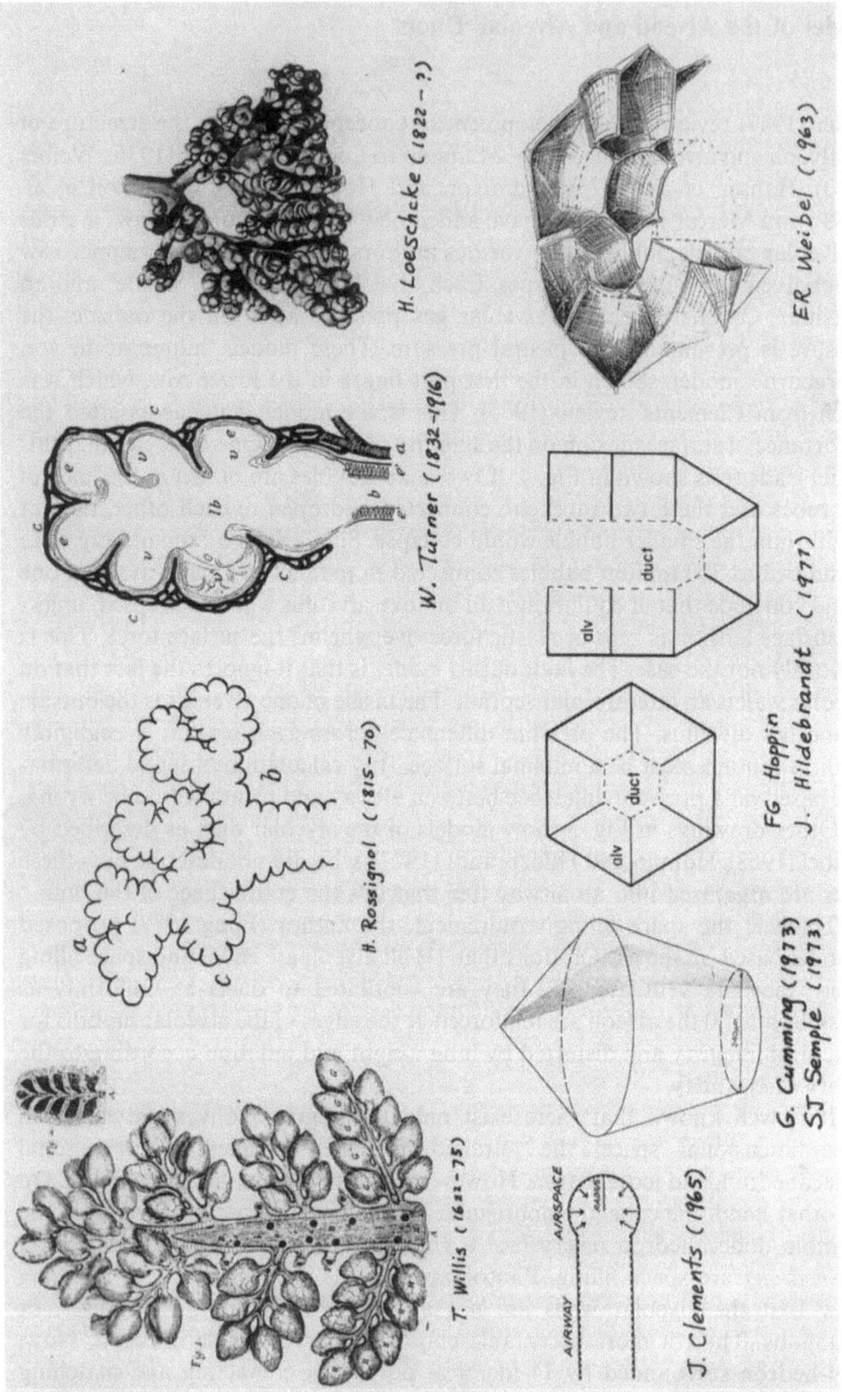

Fig. 3. A series of well-known alveolar models taken from the literature

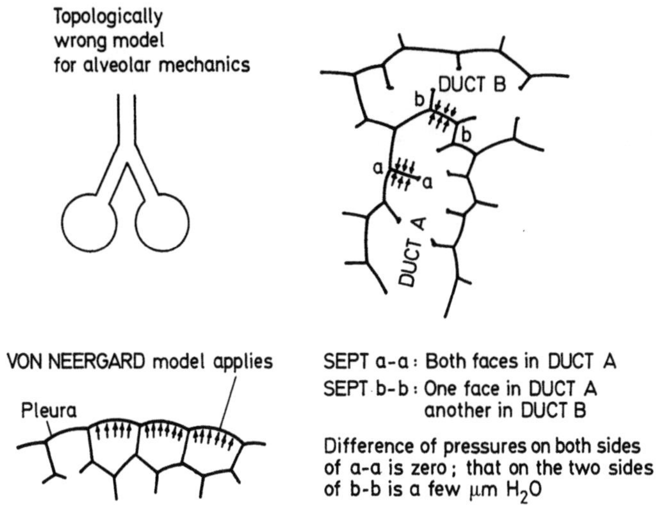

Fig. 4. Topological structure of pulmonary alveoli. *Top left*, Topologically wrong model for alveolar mechanics; *top right*, the typical topological arrangement of interalveolar septa. *Septum a–a*, Both sides are in the same alveolar duct; the net pressure difference between the two sides is zero. *Septum b–b*, One side is in duct *A*, and the other side is in duct *B*; the difference in the pressures acting on the two sides is on the order of a few μm H_2O. *Bottom left*, Equilibrium of pulmonary (visceral) pleura, to which von Neergaard's model applies. (From Fung 1975)

surrounding it are ventilated (Fig. 5). The edges at the center become the alveolar sacs. By proper reinforcement of the sacs, the integrity of the structure can be preserved.

In Fig. 5, it is shown how two or three order-2 14-hedra can be joined together, by removing one or more septa, to form a longer unit. A tree can be formed with these units. Comparison with Hansen et al.'s (1975) data suggests that human pulmonary ductal branches of generations 1–7 can be identified with these units. The order-2 14-polyhedra are not space filling by themselves, but a combination of order-1 and order-2 polyhedra is. The order-1 polyhedra can be ventilated to form a duct of order 8. This system matches the data of Hansen et al. (1975) quite well (see Fung 1988).

The alveolar shape will be changed if additional walls are perforated. Comparison with Hansen et al.'s (1975) data yields an estimate of the number of additional perforated walls (Fung 1988).

The Zero-Stress State

The need to know the zero-stress state has been mentioned above. As an example, consider the pulmonary artery. If we cut a short segment, we obtain a ring. If we cut the ring by a radial section, it will open up into a sector. A rough characterization can be obtained by the *opening angle*, defined as the angle

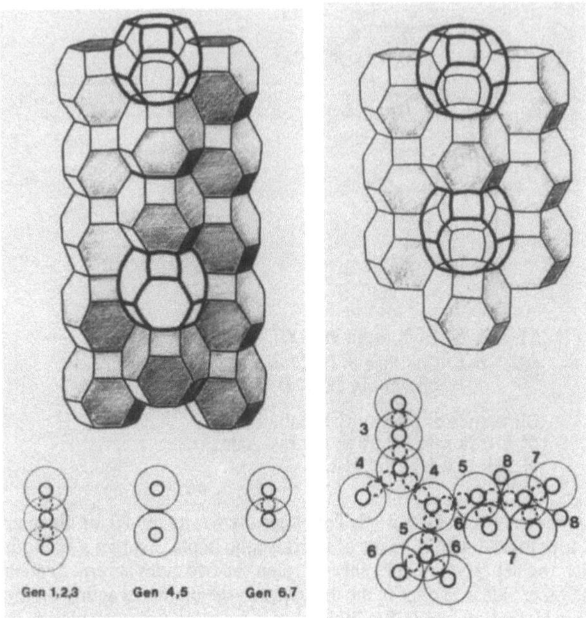

Fig. 5. A model of alveolar ducts. (From Fung 1988)

subtended between two radii joining the midpoint of the inner wall to the outer tips of the ends (see Liu and Fung 1989; Fung and Liu 1989). For a pulmonary artery of the rat, the opening angle from the junction with the heart to small branches of diameter about 100 μm is plotted in Fig. 6 (Fung and Liu, 1991). Note how large the opening angles of the main pulmonary arteries are! They are greater than 360° in the main trunk. The vessel will turn itself inside out when residual strains are removed!

The large opening angle will affect the strain energy in the vessel. Hence it is necessary to know the zero-stress state of the lung tissue. At the present time, a lack of information about the zero-stress state of lung tissue is the most serious problem in lung research.

The Surface Tension

The surface energy is revealed by the surface tension, which is equal to energy per unit area. Surface tension multiplied by the area of the interface yields total surface energy. Surface tension on the pulmonary alveolar wall has been investigated extensively. Comprehensive reviews and bibliographies have been written by Clements and Tierney (1965) and Goerke and Clements (1986). Recent contributions by Wilson and Bachofen (1982), Smith and Stamenovic (1986), are especially important.

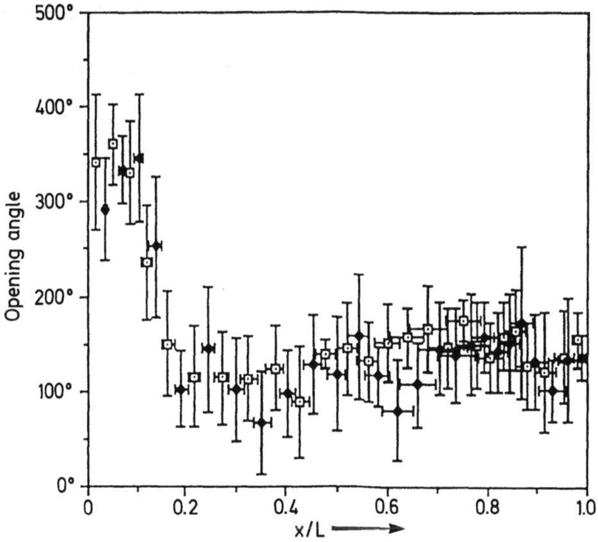

Fig. 6. The definition of the *opening angle* of the zero-stress state of a blood vessel, and the opening angle of the sections of a pulmonary artery of the rat. *L*, Length of the artery from the pulmonic valve to vessels of diameter about 100 μm; *x*, distance from the pulmonic valve. *Open squares*, In saline solution; *filled diamonds*, in Krebs solution

Potential Energy Function of the Lung

The potential energy function of the lung can be derived with the basic information mentioned in the preceding sections plus the rheological properties of every structural component.

Since the order-2 14-hedra model of the lung parenchyma is macroscopically isotropic, the strain energy function is a function of the three principal strains, or, equivalently, the three principal stretches, which may be denoted by λ_1, λ_2, λ_3. Hence we can write $\rho_0 W(\lambda_1, \lambda_2, \lambda_3)$.

In Fung (1975a), an explicit simplified example is given. A full expression for the refined model is not yet available.

The Stability Criterion

According to the ideas discussed earlier, arbitrary small perturbations of an inflated lung are considered. Let the stretch ratios at equilibrium be λ_{10}, λ_{20}, and λ_{30}. Let the stretch ratios of the perturbed lung be $\lambda_1 = \lambda_{10} + \delta\lambda_2$, and $\lambda_3 = \lambda_{30} + \delta\lambda_3$. The $\delta\lambda$ values are arbitrary, but infinitesimal. The strain energy $\rho_0 W$ is changed to $\rho_0 W + \delta(\rho_0 W)$. The stability is determined by the second variation of the strain energy, $\delta^2(\rho_0 W)$. The system is stable if $\delta^2(\rho_0 W) \geq 0$; otherwise it is unstable.

Substituting $\lambda_i = \lambda_{i0} + \delta\lambda_i$ into $\rho_0 W$ and retaining only the second-order terms results in:

$$\delta^2(\rho_0 W) = \sum_{i,\, j=1}^{3} k_{ij}\,\delta\lambda_i\,\delta\lambda_j, \tag{5}$$

where k_{ij} are the values of the second derivatives evaluated at $\lambda_i = \lambda_{i0}$:

$$k_{ij} = \frac{\partial^2 \rho_0 W}{\partial\lambda_i\,\partial\lambda_j}. \qquad (i, j = 1, 2, 3) \tag{6}$$

The right side of Eq. 5 is a quadratic form. If the equilibrium is to be stable, the quadratic form must be positive definite, i.e., > 0 for all values of $\delta\lambda_i$ and $\delta\lambda_j$, and 0 only when $\delta\lambda_i = \delta\lambda_j = 0$. The conditions for the positive definiteness are (see Fung 1965 pp. 29–30):

$$k_{11} + k_{22} + k_{33} > 0 \tag{7}$$

$$\begin{vmatrix} k_{11} & k_{12} \\ k_{21} & k_{22} \end{vmatrix} + \begin{vmatrix} k_{22} & k_{23} \\ k_{32} & k_{33} \end{vmatrix} + \begin{vmatrix} k_{33} & k_{31} \\ k_{13} & k_{11} \end{vmatrix} > 0 \tag{8}$$

$$\begin{vmatrix} k_{11} & k_{12} & k_{13} \\ k_{21} & k_{22} & k_{23} \\ k_{31} & k_{32} & k_{33} \end{vmatrix} > 0 \tag{9}$$

The quantities in Eqs. 8 and 9 are determinants. Thus, the problem of stability is reduced to the checking of the three equations 7, 8, and 9.

The simplest and most important case to check is the uniformly inflated state. Detailed examination shows (Fung 1975a) that the inflated state is stable above a critical pressure. On the other hand, an unstable state is obtained if the surface tension is a constant independent of area and the elastic stress is zero (in which case $k_{11} = 0$).

Three Types of Collapsed Lung

When the critical condition for instability is met, the lung will have a tendency toward collapse. The following three types of collapsed lung are of special interest: (1) atelectasis of the *focal type*, in which the alveoli collapse toward a central focus; (2) atelectasis of the *axial type*, in which the alveoli collapse toward a line; and (3) atelectasis of the *planar type*, in which the alveoli collapse toward a plane. These are illustrated in Fig. 7.

In each case it is assumed that, at the core, a number of the interalveolar septa are coalesced. When two interalveolar septa touch each other, their liquid

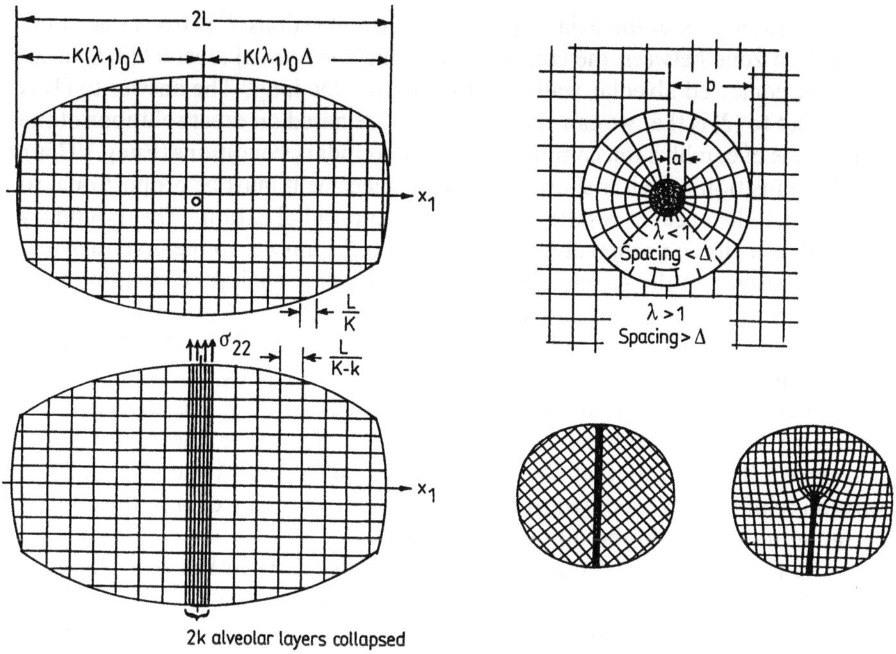

Fig. 7. Conceptual descriptions of three types of atelectasis. *Left panel, planar* atelectasis. $2k$ layers of alveoli are collapsed into a plaque. *Upper right*, an axial or a focal atelectasis. The alveoli in the central region are collapsed. A transition zone between circles of radius a and radius b is assumed. Beyond radius b is the normally inflated zone. A rigorous mathematical analysis shows that $b = a$, i.e., the transition zone does not exist. *Lower right*, Illustration that (1) the direction of the idealized alveoli is immaterial in the stability argument and (2) the edge of a planar atelectatic plaque provides a region in which the interalveolar septa can be pulled out to reinflate the alveoli

coverings will fuse, thus eliminating surface tension. Pressure, tension, and shear stress can be transmitted through the coalesced alveolar septa. Immediately next to these coalesced septa are the open alveoli, whose walls are moist and on which surface tension acts. The dimensions of the alveoli next to the coalesced region may conceivably be reduced because of the necessary continuity of the membranes (septa). Farther away from the atelectatic core, the alveoli are less and less influenced by the localized perturbation; they become those of the normally inflated lung.

There are, however, considerable differences in the behavior of the lung with the three types of atelectasis. In a lung with a planar atelectasis, the transition from the coalesced region to that of the normally inflated alveoli can be sharp. Hence, once created, a planar atelectasis can exist in an inflated lung. Since an inflated lung is stable with respect to all infinitesimal disturbances, an atelectic plaque can be introduced only by a large disturbance, such as obstruction of the airway, compression by a tumor, pressure by a surgeon's finger, or transient local reduction of stress to a level below the critical stress of instability. Since planar atelectasis is stable, it can be very persistent.

For atelectasis of the axial type, we ask two questions: (1) How large is the transition zone between the coalesced core and the normal alveoli? (2) Can we pull the coalesced alveolar walls out by inflating the lung? The answer to (1) is zero; that to (2) is that we can. These answers are based on exact solutions of the equations of equilibrium, compatibility, and boundary conditions (Fung 1975a). In the transition zone it is shown that the displacement must be proportional to the radial distance r, resulting in a constant radial strain. The boundary condition with the normal alveoli then leads to the answer to the first question. For the answer to the second question, we consider a small perturbation of the uniformly inflated region of the lung surrounding the core. For small perturbations a linearized theory suffices. An exact linear solution is that the radial displacement is inversely proportional to r. Consequently, the radial strain decreases with r, the circumferential strain increases with r, the areal strain is zero, i.e., the cross-sectional area of any small element in the r, θ plane is preserved. This means that the tissue can be pulled out of the core and the alveoli reinflated by an outward radial movement or coalesced into the core by a radial movement in the opposite direction.

The focal type of atelectasis behaves similarly. A transition zone does not exist. Small centripetal radial displacement may push the parenchyma into the core; outward radial displacement may pull the alveoli coalesced in the core out into the inflated lung.

Reinflation of the Atelectatic Lung

We have explained above that, from a mechanical point of view, focal and axial atelectases can be pulled out by reinflating the lung to a larger size; but how can a planar atelectasis be pulled out? It is not effective to pull the planar coalesced region which can transmit tensile stress; but the edges of a plaque of planar atelectasis must behave somewhat like half of an axial atelectatic core. Since there is no axial symmetry, the condition there is quite complex. It is clear that to remove a planar atelectasis one should work on the edges of the plaque. Overinflation will pull out the alveolar septa at the edges. One needs to overcome, in this process, not only the surface tension of the newly created interfaces, but also the viscous friction between the septa because of their relative motion. Therefore, the duration of overinflation should not be too brief. Excessive positive airway pressure, however, compresses the alveolar capillaries and decreases the blood flow; hence, the duration of overinflation should not be too long. Intermittently applied positive pressure breathing at a suitable frequency or negative pressure applied to the chest or abdomen are logical procedures. When a surgeon massages a lung after an operation to remove signs of atelectasis, he is applying this principle. The same principle explains why it is difficult to open an atelectatic plaque which borders on a pleura where the peeling action is ineffective.

Fleischner (1936) first described plate-like atelectasis in roentgenograms of the lung. The linear shadows in the lung, variously called Fleischner's lines, platter atelectasis, or discoid atelectasis, have been discussed in detail by Fraser and Paré (1970 p. 301). These lines are undoubtedly shadows of planar atelectasis. Fraser and Paré (pp. 196–239) presented detailed patterns of lobar and total pulmonary collapse. They showed that when atelectasis is approached a collapsed lobe or segment tends to look like a curved plate whose edges tend not to retract from the chest wall and the mediastinum. Thus, an atelectatic lobe is also planar.

Baby's First Breaths

The first breath, like all breaths afterwards, must be driven by the chest wall muscles and diaphragm. Prenatally, the lung is liquid-filled. At the first breath, air is sucked into the mouth. The questions are: What forces operate in the process? What role do surfactants play? What difficulties can one anticipate?

When air enters a liquid-filled trachea, the condition of the interface is indeed similar to what Laplace (1749–1827) investigated in his celestial mechanics. Von Neergaard (1929) applied Laplace's equation to the lung. To balance the surface tension, a pressure differential must exist across the two sides of the interface. In the trachea and bronchi, on one side of the interface, the air acts at atmospheric pressure, on the other side is the liquid, which must have a negative pressure of sufficient magnitude in order to suck the air into the lung. Where does the negative pressure come from?

The negative pressure in the liquid comes from the chest muscles which pull on the lung filled with an incompressible fluid. On the pleura a negative pleural pressure is produced by the muscle. In the airway, a far greater negative pressure comes from the motion of the liquid. The generalized Bernoulli's equation of a nonstationary flow of an incompressible fluid is (see e.g., Fung 1984 p. 48), for each streamline:

$$p + \frac{1}{2}\rho v^2 + \frac{\partial \phi}{\partial t} = \text{constant} \tag{10}$$

where p is pressure, ρ is fluid density, v is fluid velocity, ϕ is the velocity potential, t is time, and constant is an integration constant. Now in the first breath the movement of the liquid may be simulated by a source flow, for which the velocity potential is:

$$\phi = \frac{C(t)}{R}, \qquad v = \frac{\partial \phi}{\partial R} = -\frac{C(t)}{R^2} \tag{11}$$

$C(t)$ being a function of time and R being the radial distance from the source (it is a good approximation to take the origin at the air-liquid interface). The constant and $C(t)$ can be determined at the pleura where p is the pleural pressure and v is the velocity of the chest wall. From these equations it is seen that v^2 and $\partial\phi/\partial t$ tend to be large when R is small, implying a large negative pressure in the liquid at the source. This is the negative pressure that pulls the air-liquid interface into the lung.

In successive breaths, as the air-liquid interface moves further toward the periphery, the source flow approximation becomes less accurate. After a few breaths, most alveoli are inflated and the usual pressure-volume curves are seen.

At the end of the first breath, and for every successive breath, the breathing muscles relax and the negative fluid pressure is reduced. There is a possibility that the fluid will rush back into the small airways because of too high a surface tension, and there is also the possibility that the small airways in the partially inflated lung become collapsed because of the subatmospheric fluid pressure. These matters have been discussed extensively in the literature, but should be investigated more carefully in the future.

Perspectives on the Future

To improve the accuracy of prediction of the critical conditions of stability, it is necessary to improve our fundamental understanding of the zero-stress state of the alveolar walls and mouths, the fibrous structure of the lung parenchyma, the rheology of these fibers, and the spatial structure of the alveoli, ducts, airways, and blood vessels. With improved anatomical and rheological knowledge, we must improve the theoretical method of analysis of the stress and strain in the lung.

The basic principles and essential steps of stability analysis are outlined above. The analytical results, however, are as sketchy as the data that are available. I have outlined the type of data known today; but more extensive collections are needed and more thorough validation must be done.

When the equilibrium conditions are not satisfied, motion ensues. The investigation of the dynamics of atelectasis is an interesting research topic for the future.

The possible collapse of bronchi, bronchioles, and blood vessels is another important topic of research for the future. Alveoli in the neighborhood of such collapsed vessels may become atelectatic also. Perhaps focal and axial atelectasis are associated with these events. The physical principles governing the collapse of these vessels are the same as those outlined above.

References

Clements JA, Tierney DF (1965) Alveolar instability associated with altered surface tension. In: Fenn WO, Rahn H (eds) Respiration. American Physiological Society, Bethesda, pp 1565–1583 (Handbook of physiology, sect 3, vol II, chap 69)

Fleischner FG (1936) Über das Wesen der basalen horizontalen Schattenstreifen im Lungenfeld. Wien Arch Inn Med 28:461–480
Frasher RG, Paré JAP (1970) Diagnosis of diseases of the chest. Saunders, Philadelphia
Fung YC (1965) Foundations of solid mechanics. Prentice-Hall, New Jersey
Fung YC (1975a) Stress, deformation, and atelectasis of the lung. Circ Res 37:481–496
Fung YC (1975b) Does the surface tension make the lung inherently unstable? Circ Res 37:497–502
Fung YC (1984) Biodynamics: circulation. Springer, Berlin Heidelberg New York
Fung YC (1988) A model of the lung structure and its validation. J Appl Physiol 64:2132–2141
Fung YC, Liu SQ (1989) Change of residual strain in arteries due to hypertrophy caused by aortic constriction. Circ Res 65:1340–1349
Fung YC, Liu SQ (1991) Changes of zero-stress state of rat pulmonary arteries in hypoxic hypertension. J Appl Physiol 70:2455–2470
Goerke J, Clements JA (1986) Alveolar surface tension and lung surfactant. In: Fishman AP, Macklem PT, Mead J (eds) Mechanics of breathing, part 1. American Physiological Society, Bethesda, pp 247–261 (Handbook of physiology, sect 3. The respiratory system, vol III)
Hansen JE, Ampaya EP (1975) Human air space shapes, sizes, areas, and volumes. J Appl Physiol 38:990–995
Hansen JE, Ampaya EP, Bryant GH, Navin JJ (1975) The branching pattern of airways and air spaces of a single human terminal bronchiole. J Appl Physiol 38:983–989
Hoppin FG, Hildebrandt J (1977) Mechanical properties of the lung. In: West JB (ed) Bioengineering aspects of the lung. Dekker, New York
Liu SQ, Fung YC (1989) Relationship between hypertension, hypertrophy, and opening angle of zero-stress state of arteries following aortic constriction. J Biomech Eng 111:325–335
Matsuda M, Fung YC, Sobin SS (1987) Collagen and elastin fibers in human pulmonary alveolar mouths and ducts. J Appl Physiol 63:1185–1194
Mercer RR, Crapo JD (1987) Three-dimensional reconstruction of the rat acinus. J Appl Physiol 63: 785–794
Miller WS (1947) The lung, 2nd edn. Thomas, Springfield
Oldmixon EH, Hoppin FG (1987) Lengths and topology of septal borders (abstract). Fed Proc 46:820
Oldmixon EH, Butler JP, Hoppin FG Jr (1988) Dihedral angles between alveolar septa. J Appl Physiol 64:299–307
Orsos F (1936) Die Gerüstsysteme der Lunge und deren physiologische und pathologische Bedeutung. Beitr Klin Tuberk Spezifischen Tuberk Forsch 87:568–609
Smith JC, Stamenovic D (1986) Surface forces in lungs. I. Surface tension-lung volume relationships. J Physiol 60:1341–1350
Stamenovic D (1986) The mixture of phases and elastic stability of lungs with constant surface forces. Math Modeling 7:1071–1082
Sobin SS, Fung YC, Tremer HM (1988) Collagen and elastin fibers in human pulmonary alveolar walls. J Appl Physiol 64:1659–1675
Von Neergaard K (1929) Neue Auffassuxgen über einen Grundbegriff der Atemmechanik: die Retraktionskraft der Lunge, abhängig von der Oberflächenspannung in den Alveolen. Z Gesamte Exp Med 66:373–394
Weibel EG (1963) Morphometry of the human lung. Academic, New York
Wilson TA (1982) Surface tension – surface area curves calculated from pressure-volume loops. J Appl Physiol 53:1512–1520
Wilson TA, Bachofen H (1982) A model for mechanical structure of the alveolar duct. J Appl Physiol 56:1064–1070

Oscillation Mechanics in Respiratory Monitoring

H. Mang and A. Jaegers

Introduction

Recent advances in biomedical engineering and computer technology have considerably improved the capability for monitoring almost all organ systems. Continuous monitoring of respiratory function may enable us to predict catastrophes and may provide an opportunity for the timely institution of livesaving measures. Unfortunately, such monitoring has experienced slow advancement, frequently being limited to the intermittent measurement of arterial blood gases. There is a general lack of sophistication in the field of respiratory monitoring, in contrast to those methods and devices used for the control of other organ systems, especially the cardiovascular system (Wilson 1976). Assessment of pulmonary function largely differs in the ambulatory and critically ill patient. In the pulmonary function testing (PFT) laboratory, detailed information can be obtained on lung volumes, flow rates, airway resistance, and diffusing capacity, whereas in the intensive care unit only limited information can be obtained on lung volumes and there is greater emphasis on breathing pattern and inspiratory pressure monitoring (Tobin 1988). In addition, patients who are being mechanically ventilated cannot be asked to participate in pulmonary function testing. Therefore, a test must be employed which would not require subject cooperation and could be performed without disconnection from the ventilator.

Sinusoidal Forcing and Complex Impedance

One method of collecting pulmonary data on subjects unable to cooperate is the forced oscillation technique of DuBois (1956). This technique utilizes a loudspeaker to produce small amplitude flow oscillations which are transmitted to the subject via a mouthpiece or endotracheal tube. This results in a reflected alternating pressure which is picked up by a pressure transducer and, after filtering, demodulation, and smoothing, is digitized by a computer. The imposed flows and the resulting pressure signals are used to calculate impedance. Using linear regression, these data can be fitted to three or more parameter models to yield estimates not only of resistance, but also of reactance (Fig. 1). We applied a three parameter model in which energy dissipation is represented by viscous resistance and energy storage is represented by both a capacitive component

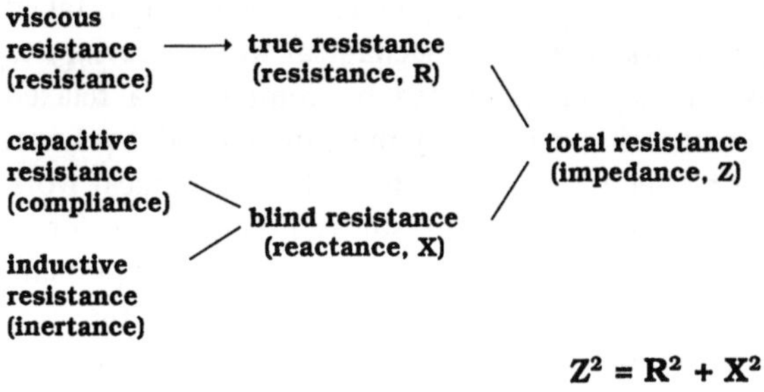

Fig. 1 Components of complex resistance (impedance)

(compliance) and an inductive component (inertance). Simultaneous registration of resistance and reactance and the calculation of impedance meets the power demand of respiration more exactly than the measurement of airway resistance in a whole-body plethysmograph or of the work of breathing with the esophageal balloon method because impedance of the chest wall is taken into consideration. For a sinusoidal breathing pattern the total power of breathing is calculated, analogous to the effective power of alternating current, from the flow amplitude and impedance according to the following equations (Jung 1990) (complex quantities in bold face):

$$\mathbf{Z}^2 = \mathbf{R}^2 + \mathbf{X}^2$$

$$\dot{W}^2_{\mathrm{eff}} = \dot{W}^2_{\mathrm{irr}} + \dot{W}^2_{\mathrm{rev}}$$

$$\dot{\mathbf{W}} = \mathbf{P}\cdot\dot{\mathbf{V}} \quad \text{and} \quad \mathbf{P} = \mathbf{Z}\cdot\dot{\mathbf{V}}$$

$$\dot{\mathbf{W}} = \mathbf{Z}\cdot\dot{\mathbf{V}}^2 \quad \text{or} \quad \dot{W}_{\mathrm{eff}} = \mathbf{Z}\cdot\dot{V}^2_{\mathrm{eff}}$$

$$\dot{V}^2_{\mathrm{eff}} = 1/2\cdot\dot{V}^2_0$$

$$\dot{\mathbf{W}} = 1/2\cdot Z\cdot\dot{V}^2_0$$

Impedance and the Power of Breathing

The respiratory muscles work against three main types of forces: (1) flow-resistive forces offered by the airways and by the nonelastic deformation of tissue, (2) elastic forces that develop in the tissues of the lung and chest when a change in volume occurs, and (3) inertial forces that depend on the mass of the tissues and gases. Inertial forces are not usually considered because they seem negligible (Sharp et al. 1964). Flow-resistive forces offered by the airways alone can be determined by measuring alveolar pressure with a body plethysmograph. The esophageal balloon is the most common method for measuring the elastic forces that develop in the tissues of the lung and the flow-resistive forces offered by the airways. However, with this technique it is not possible to measure flow-resistive work done to the thorax, which can account for one-third of the total mechanical work of breathing. Similarly, it is not possible to estimate the elastic work done on the chest wall unless the compliance of the thorax is taken into account, which is a difficult task. The total mechanical work necessary to ventilate the respiratory system may be estimated by ventilating a relaxed subject with a respirator and measuring inspiratory pressure and tidal volume. There has been no method for directly measuring the total mechanical work performed during spontaneous breathing. In our study, flow-resistive forces offered by the airways alone were determined by measuring alveolar pressure with a body plethysmograph. Airway work was calculated from the area enclosed by the alveolar pressure tidal volume loop. We used the esophageal balloon technique to measure the elastic forces that develop in the lung tissues and the flow-resistive forces caused by the airways. Thus, lung work was computed from the area enclosed by the esophageal pressure tidal volume loop.

The basic principle of our method to measure the flow-resistive, elastic, and inertial forces offered by airways, lung, and chest wall is derived from a variant of the forced oscillation technique described by Franetzki et al. (1979). The alternating airflow first follows the airways: mouth, trachea, bronchi, bronchioli, and alveoli. The pressure fluctuations in the alveoli are then transmitted to the alveolar walls, which, being elastic, react accordingly. The elastic "deformation" is transmitted via the parenchyma of the lung to the pleura and hence to the chest wall. Finally they appear as minute, though not noticeable, vibrations at the surface of the body. The oscillating flow must overcome the same types of forces against which the respiratory muscles work during spontaneous breathing or a ventilator in case of artificial ventilation: (a) flow-resistive forces by the airways and friction in the tissues (resistance), (b) elastic forces due to the elasticity of tissues and the compressibility of intrathoracic gases (compliance), and (c) inertial forces that depend on the mass of tissues and gases (inertance). The sum of inertance and compliance is reactance. If we account for reactance which geometrically adds to resistance we obtain impedance. Impedance is an index of the impediment the respiratory system presents to alternating flow. Therefore, in contrast to other techniques, the forced oscillation method studies the respiratory resistance as a complex parameter. The mathematical connection between impedance and total power of breathing is given in Eqs. 1–6.

It was the purpose of our study to examine the relationships between airway, lung, and total work of breathing in normal subjects. We were especially interested in the question whether the forced oscillation method provides results comparable to the established methods for measuring work of breathing. We studied 23 male and 3 female healthy volunteers between 20 and 30 years of age. Airway work per breath was measured with a Jaeger Bodytest plethysmograph and lung work per breath with the esophageal balloon technique. Work per breath was multiplied by the breathing frequency to obtain work per minute, i.e., power of breathing. We determined impedance at 10 Hz with a Siemens Siregnost FD 5 and measured peak inspiratory flow ("flow amplitude") with a variable orifice flow sensor. Descriptive statistics were used to characterize data and linear regression to test coherence of airway, lung, and total power of breathing (Table 1). Even in this homogeneous group of young and healthy volunteers there was a wide range of values for power of breathing. Airway and lung work are in accordance with values reported in the literature (Kacmarek 1988).

As we anticipated, the impedance method constantly provided higher estimates for the total power of breathing than the standard methods, which measure work done on the airways or lung (Fig. 2). Correlations were poor, in particular in the established methods, but highly significant due to a large sample size. The variability of values for the power of breathing may be attributed either to true physiological differences between subjects, the variability of resting respiratory drive and timing (Tobin et al. 1983), or to a change in breathing pattern induced by instrumentation (Gilbert et al. 1972).

The main short-coming of our evaluation is the fact that we could not apply the three methods simultaneously but had to perform the measurements successively in a random order. With regard to the variability of breathing patterns this could also account for the scattering of our values. The determination of the total power of breathing with the impedance method is based on the assumption that the inspiratory airflow wave is a sine function of time. Several studies have pointed out that a rectangular airflow wave might be preferred for economical

Table 1. Values for airway, lung, and total power of breathing in 26 healthy volunteers

$n = 26$	Airway	Lung	Total	Power
Mean	3.0	3.2	6.3	J/min
S.D.	1.3	1.2	3.3	J/min
Median	2.9	3.1	5.8	J/min
Minimum	1.2	1.4	2.5	J/min
Maximum	6.0	6.0	16.2	J/min
Span	4.8	4.6	13.7	J/min
Correlation	$r = 0.46$*	$r = 0.56$*		
	$r = 0.56$**			

*$p < 0.001$
**$p < 0.0001$

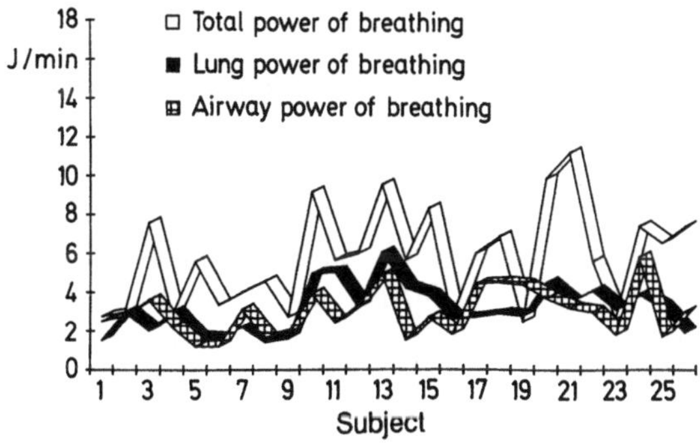

Fig. 2. Different measures of breathing power

reasons during exercise. Furthermore, all methods described here imply a linear relationship between pressure and flow. This assumption only can be accepted for quiet breathing through natural airways.

In contrast to body plethysmography and the esophageal balloon technique, the impedance method takes into consideration the flow-resistive and elastic work of the chest wall and the inertia of the whole respiratory system. Thus, according to our model, direct measurement of the total mechanical work or power performed during spontaneous breathing has become possible.

Other Physiological Implications of Oscillation Mechanics

In a few studies, lung and chest wall properties were partitioned by measuring intrathoracic pressure with an esophageal balloon. In Nagel's study (Nagel et al. 1980) of 15 healthy, seated, and spontaneously breathing subjects the chest wall represented 20%–30% of total respiratory resistance at frequencies between 2 and 32 Hz. In anesthetized, tracheostomized, and paralyzed dogs in the supine position Jackson et al. (1984) analyzed impedance data between 4 and 32 Hz and found that, at FRC, 41% of the respiratory system resistance was due to the lung and 59% was associated with the chest wall; 98% of the respiratory inertance was contributed by the lung and only 2% by the chest wall. Quiet breathing takes place at frequencies between 0.2 and 0.3 Hz (12–18 breaths per minute). Over this range of frequencies chest wall impedance is markedly higher and the work of breathing is accordingly larger than formerly thought (Barnas et al. 1987); however, the energy cost would still be a small fraction of the total resting energy expenditure. During exercise breathing frequency increases up to 1 Hz, where the real part of chest wall impedance is substantially lower and the imaginary part only moderately increased. Total work of breathing in this case would not be considerably different from previous estimates.

Barnas et al. (1989) also found that during respiratory muscle contraction chest wall impedance increases. Changes in regional chest wall impedances can be somewhat independent, depending on which muscles contract, and increases in chest wall impedance are due, at least in part, to changes in the passive properties of the muscles themselves. During many nonrespiratory tasks some of the respiratory muscles must be maintained in a state of contraction.

These results imply that chest wall impedance is greatly increased, depending on which muscles are contracting and the degree of effort. Somehow activation of the respiratory muscles must be coordinated to facilitate breathing despite these increases. When inspiratory muscle fatigue is impending, respiratory muscle discoordination frequently occurs and spontaneous breathing may become insufficient. After laparotomy, in case of increased intra-abdominal pressure, chest wall impedance may increase and further impair natural breathing. Timely initiation of respiratory care or artificial ventilation will depend on the awareness of these relationships and meticulous monitoring of breathing mechanics.

The airways have been shown to be responsible for most lung resistance and inertance. Combining sinusoidal forcing at the mouth and body plethysmography, Finucane et al. (1975) described a method to estimate alveolar pressure swings during forced oscillation measurement. Fredberg and Mead (1979) used a model of the lung in which the following factors could be controlled: gas compressibility within the airways, distortion of velocity profile in relation to gas inertia, parallel inhomogeneity, and airway wall impedance. The frequency dependence of resistance could be explained mainly by parallel inhomogeneities (47%), distortion of velocity profiles (35%), and to a smaller extent by gas compliance (11%) and airway wall distensibility (7%). Subsequently, Fredberg et al. (1984) demonstrated that alveolar pressure swings can exceed airway opening pressure swings when small amplitude high frequency oscillation is applied at the airway opening. Alveolar pressure swings at resonance were larger than those at the airway opening by approximately 200% near 50% vital capacity and 500% near 100% vital capacity. This increase in the resonant amplification of alveolar pressure with increasing lung volume is due to an increase in lung stiffness. Thus, there may be some advantage in applying high frequency ventilation at frequencies higher than lung resonant frequency.

Clinical Application of Oscillation Mechanics

The forced oscillation technique is, although not widely used method for monitoring an established method for investigating, the respiratory system. In most clinical studies measurements have been made at a single frequency, the method being used little more than a convenient tool to estimate total respiratory resistance. The rapid, noninvasive, and relatively effortless nature of this approach makes it especially useful for epidemiological studies (i.e., in smokers and miners) and for studies involving noncooperative subjects (i.e., young children and ICU patients). In this paper we want to focus on the application of the forced oscillation technique in anesthesia and critical care medicine.

Lehane et al. (1980) developed a method for the measurement of respiratory system resistance (impedance) and specific airways conductance using the forced oscillation method. He used it to study the effects of halothane and enflurane on airway mechanics in anesthetized patients. Impedance was determined over a range of lung volumes, and specific airways conductance was obtained by computer aided analysis of the hyperbolic relationship between impedance and lung volume. There was a significant reduction in impedance with halothane and enflurane. Expiratory reserve volume (ERV) was found to be small and contributed to the high impedances observed: mean impedance was 0.59 kPa/l/s, range 0.15–1.71. Small changes in ERV were also shown to produce changes in impedance independent of changes in bronchomotor tone. Neither halothane nor enflurane produced significant mean changes in ERV.

In another study, Jones et al. (1987) compared the effect of salbutamol (200 μg, aerosol), high-dose aminophyllin (i.v., 670 mg), or placebo (aerosol and infusion) on bronchomotor tone in normal volunteers before and after bronchial provocation with histamine (aerosol, 500 μg). Specific airways, conductance of the lower airways was measured using a forced airflow oscillation technique. All subjects receiving aminophyllin had tremor and irritability, whereas after salbutamol there were no noticeable systemic or psychological effects. Before the administration of histamine, salbutamol caused significant bronchodilatation compared with control: aminophyllin did not induce a significant change in airway conductance. The effect of histamine administration on specific airways conductance was only partially blocked by the high dose of aminophyllin but was completely blocked by salbutamol. These results suggest that salbutamol, given prophylactically, is more efficient in blocking the effects of histamine in the airways than is aminophyllin. Therefore, consideration should be given to the prophylactic administration of this drug in patients with a history of histamine-like reactions during anesthesia.

Finally, a few studies have been performed in subjects with various acute respiratory or cardiac conditions. Impedance was found to be initially increased, abnormally frequency-dependent, and to come back to normal values within a few weeks. Interiano et al. (1973) evaluated pulmonary mechanics in 30 patients with acute myocardial infarction by measuring impedance with forced oscillations from 3 to 9 Hz. Initially, impedance was 52% greater than predicted, but was only 4% greater 10 or more weeks later. At that time, frequency-dependence of impedance had disappeared. Impedance showed a highly significant correlation with elevation of both the pulmonary artery pressure and the pulmonary capillary wedge pressure. Vascular engorgement and interstitial edema from elevated vascular pressures causing narrowing of the peripheral airways and closure of collateral airways could account for increased impedance.

To further investigate the relationship between alterations in lung mechanics and acute pulmonary vascular congestion, Depeursinge et al. (1986) performed repeated measurements of respiratory system impedance in 11 patients with and in 7 without acute left ventricular failure. Indices of impedance were obtained by calculating the average and slope of the resistance and reactance in low (10–20 Hz) and high (20–50 Hz) frequency intervals. Impedance indices in patients with ventricular failure differed significantly from those in patients without failure. Pulmonary vascular congestion was regularly associated with an abnormal frequency-dependence of resistance at low frequencies and with an increased resonant frequency. Impedance differences between patients with and without left ventricular failure were consistent with the presence of a small airways obstruction even in patients with mild left ventricular failure. Furthermore, impedance indices were able to distinguish between moderate and severe pulmonary vascular congestion, probably because of significant narrowing of the large airways during severe and acute left ventricular failure. The specificity of the frequency-dependence of impedance for lung mechanical alterations induced by vascular congestion vs those induced by obstructive lung disease must be further investigated. This might be of clinical value in patients with

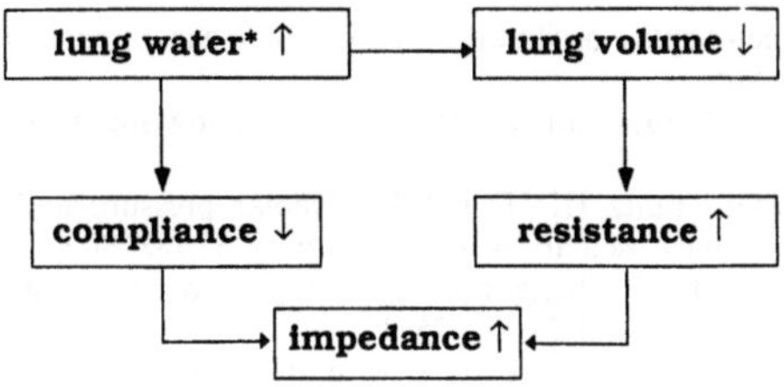

* e.g.: ARDS (EVLW ↑) and CHF (PCWP ↑)

Fig. 3. Lung water content and impedance

obstructive lung disease who also suffer from congestive heart failure. In the adult respiratory distress syndrome it is probably impossible to analyze the contributions of atelectasis, pulmonary edema, pulmonary vascular congestion, increased tissue resistance to inflation, and increased resistance to airflow to the altered lung mechanics (Fig. 3).

For patients requiring PEEP during ventilation, performing traditional tests of lung function is a complicated problem. The pulmonary mechanics of these patients can change rapidly with potential for a negative impact on oxygenation. In an effort to address this problem, Fouke and Wolin (1989) designed a system with a three-way valve that permits the patient to be switched from the ventilator to the forced oscillations system for data collection. A unique feature of the valved system is that it serves to maintain positive airway pressure during the short periods required for data collection (20–30 s), which do not interfere with patient care and are well within the limits of safety.

It is tempting to imagine an automatically recurring oscillometric measurement of respiratory system impedance integrated within advanced ICU ventilators. In contrast to resistance and compliance, impedance would not be a calculated but a measured quantity which reflects the energy cost of breathing, and is suitable to follow the course of a patient's rapidly changing disease state.

References

Barnas GM, Yoshino K, Loring SH (1987) Impedance and relative displacements of relaxed chest wall up to 4 Hz. J Appl Physiol 62:71–81

Barnas GM, Heglund NC, Yager D, Yoshino K, Loring SH, Mead J (1989) Impedance of the chest wall during sustained respiratory muscle contraction. J Appl Physiol 66:360–369

Depeursinge FB, Depeursinge CD, Boutaleb AK, Feihl F, Perret CH (1986) Respiratory system impedance in patients with acute left ventricular failure: pathophysiology and clinical interest. Circulation 73:386–395

DuBois AB, Brody AW, Lewis DH, Burgess BF (1956) Oscillation mechanics of lungs and chest in man. J Appl Physiol 8:587–594

Finucane KE, Dawson SV, Phelan PD, Mead J (1975) Resistance of intrathoracic airways of healthy subjects during periodic flow. J Appl Physiol 38:517–530

Fouke JM, Wolin AD (1989) Instrumentation for estimating pulmonary function in patients on positive end-expiratory pressure. Crit Care Med 17:265–268

Franetzki M, Prestele K, Korn V (1979) A direct-display oscillation method for measurement of repiratory impedance. J Appl Physiol 46:956–965
Fredberg JJ, Mead J (1979) Impedance of intrathoracic airway models during low-frequency periodic flow. J Appl Physiol 47:347–351
Fredberg JJ, Keefe DH, Glass GM, Castile RG, Frantz III ID (1984) Alveolar pressure non-homogeneity during small-amplitude high-frequency oscillation. J Appl Physiol 57:788–800
Gilbert R, Auchincloss Jr JH, Brodsky J, Boden W (1972) Changes in tidal volume, frequency, and ventilation induced by their measurement. J Appl Physiol 33:252–254
Interiano B, Hyde RW, Hodges M, Yu PN (1973) Interrelation between alterations in pulmonary mechanics and hemodynamics in acute myocardial infarction. J Clin Invest 52:1994–2006
Jackson AC, Watson JW, Kotlikoff MI (1984) Respiratory system, lung, and chest wall impedances in anesthetized dogs. J Appl Physiol 57:34–39
Jones JG, Jordan C, Slavin B, Lehane JR (1987) Prophylactic effects of aminophyllin and salbutamol on histamine-induced bronchoconstriction. Br J Anaesth 59:498–502
Jung R (1990) Atemarbeit und Atemleistung als komplexe Parameter der Atemmechanik. Thesis, University of Erlangen
Kacmarek RM (1988) The role of pressure support ventilation in reducing work of breathing. Respir Care 33:99–120
Lehane JR, Jordan C, Jones JG (1980) Influence of halothane and enflurane on respiratory airflow resistance and specific conductance in anaesthetized man. Br J Anaesth 52:773–781
Nagels J, Landser FJ, Van der Linden L, Clement J, Van de Woestijne KP (1980) Mechanical properties of lungs and chest wall during spontaneous breathing. J Appl Physiol 49:408–416
Sharp JT, Henry JP, Sweany SK, Meadows WR, Pietras RJ (1964) Total respiratory inertance and its gas and tissue components in normal and obese men. J Clin Invest 43:503–509
Tobin MJ (1988) Respiratory monitoring in the intensive care unit. Am Rev Respir Dis 138:1625–1642
Tobin MJ, Chadha TS, Jenouri G, Birch SJ, Gazeroglu HB, Sackner MA (1983) Breathing patterns. 1. Normal subjects. Chest 84:202–205
Wilson RS (1976) Monitoring the lung: mechanics and volume. Anesthesiology 45:135–145

The Pulmonary Surfactant System: Its Contribution to Lung Alveolar Stability, Alteration in Acute Respiratory Failure, and Replacement as a Therapeutical Concept*

U. Pison and S. Hawgood

Introduction

Sufficient amounts of biologically active pulmonary surfactant, a lipoprotein complex that lines air sacs in all mammalian lungs, are crucial for normal lung function [10]. Deficient pulmonary surfactant is the primary cause of the respiratory distress syndrome so common in premature infants [14] and alterations have also been found in adult patients with acute respiratory failure [21, 47, 48]. Therefore, replacement of deficient or inactive surfactant for the prevention and treatment of respiratory distress syndrome of various etiologies might become an important pharmacological approach. Clinical studies in new born infants have reported consistent short-term effects on lung function following tracheal instillation of both natural surfactant, derived from animal lung tissue or human amniotic fluid, and synthetic preparations [11, 25, 29]. Comparable effects have been reported for surfactant replacement in adult patients with severe respiratory failure [38].

This paper is not meant to be an exhaustive review, but summarizes some of our basic knowledge on the pulmonary surfactant system, demonstrates that surfactant is altered in adults with acute respiratory failure, explains how it might be altered, and points out criteria and questions to be answered in clinical trials involving adults using exogenous surfactant as a replacement. For details and primary references, the reader is referred to several recent reviews addressing the biochemical and biosynthetic aspects [44, 53, 60], molecular aspects [22, 51], metabolism [71, 72], ontogeny [52], and morphological aspects [4, 19, 58, 68, 69] of surfactant.

Physiological Relevance of Pulmonary Surfactant

The importance of the lung air-liquid interfacial film for lung mechanics has been known since von Neergard, in 1929, attributed the differences in recoil forces between fluid- and air-filled lungs to surface tension [42]. When gas-free normal lungs are inflated stepwise with air or with fluid (Fig. 1), the pressure

* This study was supported by Deutsche Forchungsgemeinschaft

required to maintain any given volume in a fluid-filled lung under static conditions is less than half that required to maintain the same volume in an air-filled lung. A second difference is that, using a fluid, the filling and emptying pressures in the lung are nearly equal at given volumes. In contrast, the pressures are different during filling and emptying of the lung using air, forming the so-called hysteresis area in the pressure-volume diagram. Such differences in the pressure-volume curves can be explained if one considers that the retractive force is due to elasticity of the tissue and surface tension in the air spaces.

Pattle [45] and Clements [8] first demonstrated that a substance providing very low surface tension is present in pulmonary edema fluid and lung tissue. Treating the lung as an aggregation of individual units, Clements suggested that each unit is represented by a model consisting of an elastic balloon, with a moist inner surface, at the end of a collapsible tube [10]. Applying Laplace's law (pressure × radius = twice the total tension) to such a lung unit, total tension should be the sum of tissue and surface tension. Since the lung consists of hundreds of millions of alveoli of varying sizes, surface tension has to change as surface area changes, otherwise the lung would empty its smaller air spaces into larger ones and would then consist only of collapsed alveoli and hyperinflated alveolar ducts (Fig. 2). Surface tension of extracted lung lavage material, but not of water or detergent, decreases markedly during compression of the surface film in a Wilhelmy balance, an apparatus measuring surface tension. Compression of the film is consistent with reduction of surface area; therefore, this in vitro process might simulate in vivo expiration in which the radii of alveoli become smaller. Assuming that surface-active material acts in the same way at the unit surface in the lung as it does when extracted and studied in the Wilhelmy balance, the alveolar lining layer indeed is sufficient to insure the stability and prevent the collapse of small alveoli during expiration and to lead to a stable balance between small and large alveoli [10, 44]. Direct measurements of

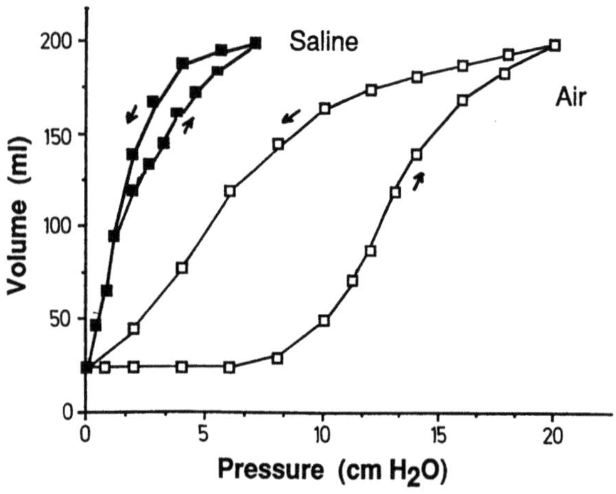

Fig. 1. Pressure-volume relationship of excised canine lungs

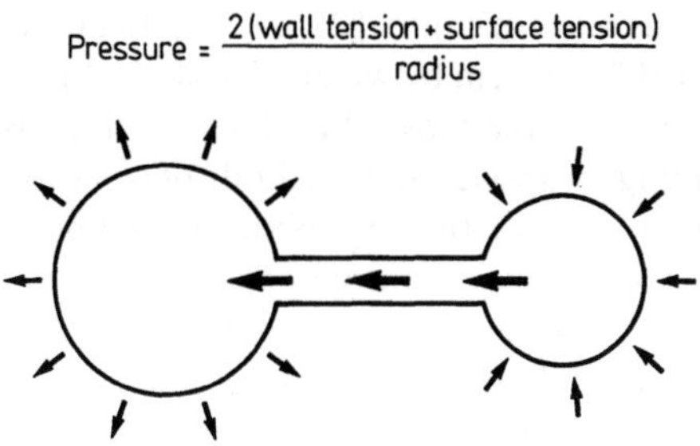

Fig. 2. Balloons are blown up to different volumes and connected to each other. The smaller balloon empties into the larger, fulfilling Laplace's law

surface tension in intact lungs of living animals [55] and energy analyses based on well defined structure-function relationships of isolated, air-filled and perfused lungs have been carried out [70]. These studies have provided striking evidence that the surface tension within alveoli indeed is very low at lung volume levels of normal breathing and changes with alveolar size.

In addition to the mechanisms by which surfactant provides and maintains low surface tension, which are obviously of critical importance to normal lung funtion, other properties of surfactant have been noted. One is surfactant's hypothetical involvement in lung fluid balance [9, 20, 46]; another is its contribution to alveolar transport and clearance mechanisms [31]. Surfactant functions that are apparently unrelated to lowering surface tension include interactions with alveolar macrophages [2, 30, 39, 62] and lymphocytes [57]. Surfactant components might thus regulate the immune response [3] and be involved in endogenous host defenses [12, 28] in the alveolar space of the lungs.

Components of Pulmonary Surfactant

Since initial interest in the alveolar lining material focused on its intriguing ability to lower surface tension, methods of isolating this material were developed, using as the sole criterion whether the product could establish and maintain a very low surface tension in vitro. King and Clements used a preparation procedure that combined density gradients and differential centrifugation to isolate a material from lung lavage that met this criterion. This has become the conventional technique to prepare pulmonary surfactant [32]. The material is chemically heterogeneous [33], consisting of various lipids and proteins. It should be noted that surfactant prepared from whole lung tissue or lung lavage, employing techniques such as centrifugation in aqueous media and extraction using organic solvents, may not reflect the actual alveolar lining material. Various components might be lost, gained, or modified during the preparation procedure.

Although there are major concerns associated with the isolation of a homogeneous surfactant preparation from whole lung or lavage fluid, surfactant prepared from either source in many different species is surprisingly similar, varying only during development [36] or acute lung injury [21, 41, 47]. In adults it contains approximately 90% lipid and 10% protein by weight (Table 1). More than 80% of the lipid is phospholipid [34, 53], the most abundant of which is phosphatidylcholine (60%–80%, depending on species and methods of isolation and detection employed). Approximately 60% of the phosphatidylcholine is disaturated, with more than 90% of the acyl groups palmitoyl [7]. Dipalmitoylphosphatidylcholine is one of the surfactant components important for lowering surface tension [18, 43]. Although phosphatidylglycerol makes up 5%–10% of the phospholipid fraction, a very high proportion compared to other mammalian tissues, it is not required for surface tension reducing properties [6, 40].

The proteins associated with surfactant contain at least three different groups now called SP-A, SP-B, and SP-C [51]. For functional aspects of the proteins see Table 2.

SP-A, the most abundant surfactant-associated protein, has an apparent molecular weight under reduced conditions of 26000–36000. The heterogeneous molecular weight results from differences in post-translational modification, especially variable degrees of glycosylation [23, 66]. Under nonreduced conditions the molecular weight of SP-A has been estimated to be 700000 [35], suggesting that in its native state SP-A is highly oligomerized. The complete amino acid sequences of dog [5], human [15, 65], and rat SP-A [54] have been deduced from their respective cDNA sequences. The NH_2-terminus of the mature protein contains 7–10 amino acids depending on the species, followed by a collagen-like sequence characterized by a series of 24 repeats of the sequence glycine-X-Y where Y is frequently 4-hydroxyproline [22]. The collagen-like series of reiterated sequences is disrupted in triplet 13 by the insertion of an additional residue, which is also a feature of the complement protein Clq [61] and the mannose-binding proteins [13].

Table 1. Alveolar surfactant composition

Phospholipids		85
Staturated phosphatidylcholine	60	
Unsaturated phosphatidylcholine	20	
Phosphatidylglycerol	8	
Phosphatidylethanolamine	5	
Phosphatidylinositol	2	
Sphingomyelin	2	
Others	3	
Neutral lipids and cholesterol		5
Proteins		10
Contaminating serum proteins	80	
SP-A	10	
SP-B and SP-C	10	

Average values in percent of the total are given as determined in lung washings obtained from various mammalian species and processed by conventional techniques.

Table 2. Properties and functions of surfactant-associated proteins. (Modified from [71])

Protein	Molecular weight (10^{-3}) Reduced	Nonreduced	Characteristics	Proposed functions
SP-A	26–36	700	Glycoprotein, N-linked oligosacchaaride Stretch of collagen-like sequence Lectin Structure analogue of C1q and mannose-binding proteins	Binds to lipids Binds to carbohydrates Enhances lipid adsorption via SP-B/SP-C interaction Induces lipid aggregation Inhibits type II cell lipid secretion Enhances type II cell lipid uptake
SP-B	5–8	18	Hydrophobic	Enhances lipid absorption Enhances type II cell lipid uptake Inhibits type II cell lipid synthesis
SP-C	5–10	5–10	Hydrophobic	Enhances lipid adsorption

SP-B and SP-C are two very hydrophobic proteins with distinctive molecular weights under nonreduced conditions of 18000–20000 and 5000–6000, respectively. The nominal molecular weights for the proteins under reduced conditions, however, are very similar (between 5000 and 8000). The amino acid sequences for both proteins have been derived from cDNA [17, 24, 63], predicting a precursor with a molecular weight of approximately 42000 for SP-B and one of approximately 21000 for SP-C. It is not known whether or to what extent these precursor proteins are cleaved to their smaller forms intracellularly, extracellularly, or during the isolation procedure.

Alteration of Surfactant in Lung Disease

Much of surfactant research has been motivated by the finding of Avery and Mead, in 1959 [1], that a deficiency of pulmonary surfactant is the primary cause of the respiratory distress syndrome of premature infants. Evidence is now growing that surfactant is also altered in adult patients who have acute respiratory failure [21, 48].

In a prospective study, surfactant abnormalities were evaluated in severely injured patients during the course of post-traumatic pulmonary dysfunction [47]. Trauma patients were selected because of the homogeneity of the underlying disease and the consistency in time relationship between the insult and the development of respiratory failure in several of these patients. Serially obtained bronchoalveolar lavage fluids from noncontused lung areas were analyzed for alveolar phospholipid composition and surface tension characteristics in a Wilhelmy balance and compared with data determined in lung washings obtained from normal probands. Phospholipid composition is dramatically changed very early after the initial insult, but total phospholipid concentration is not. One of the most pronounced alterations was a decreased relative amount of phosphatidylcholine. This decrease was significantly correlated to both severity of respiratory failure in vivo ($r = 0.77$) and hysteresis area of the surface tension isotherm in vitro ($r = 0.62$).

In patients who developed septicemia during the course of post-traumatic respiratory failure, but not in patients who had uncomplicated courses, the relative amount of alveolar phosphatidylethanolamine (normally 4.8% of total phospholipids) and alveolar phosphatidylcholine (normally 62.8%) both approached the proportions found in the trachea (phosphatidylethanolamine 33.4%, phosphatidylcholine 35.6%). This suggests that the alveolar surfactant phospholipid pool size had progressively decreased [48].

Since various phospholipid ratios could serve as predictors for lung maturity [36], ratios between phosphatidylcholine and sphingomyelin (PC/SPH; normally 8.9) and phosphatidylinositol and phosphatidylglycerol (PI/PG; normally 0.8) were calculated for patients who had acute respiratory failure following multiple injury. In patients without any complications both ratios normalized during approximately 10–15 days after trauma (Fig. 3a). In patients who had complicating septicemia these ratios often did not change during the course of respiratory failure (Fig. 3).

Sensitive techniques to detect surfactant-associated proteins have become available recently; thus, SP-A, SP-B, and SP-C levels in lung lavage samples are under current investigation. Information about the concentration of

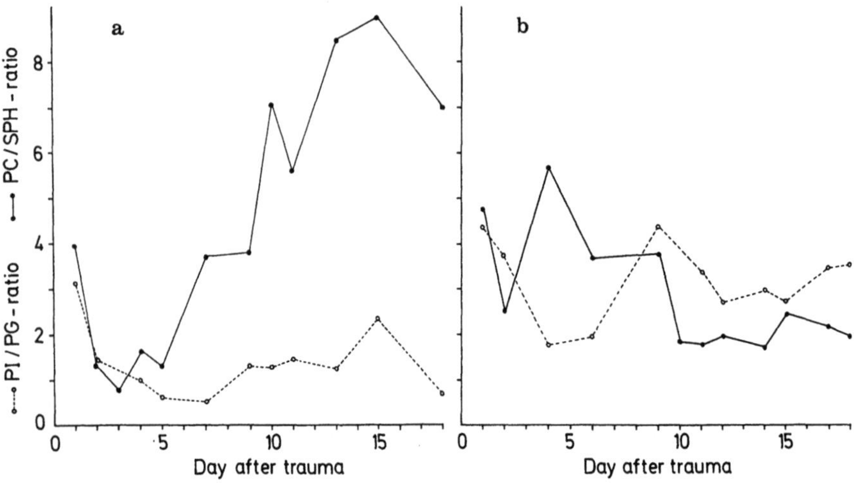

Fig. 3a,b. Phosphatidylcholine/sphingomyelin ratio (PC/SPH) and phosphatidylinositol/phosphatidylglycerol ratio (PI/PG) in lung washings obtained from a multiple traumatized patient **a** without any complication during the course of post-traumatic respiratory dysfunction and **b** with septicemia complicating the course of post-traumatic respiratory dysfunction. The normal ratio for PC/SPH is 8.9, for PI/PG 0.8.

surfactant-associated proteins will help us to understand complex metabolic events in the alveolar compartment of the lungs during various lung diseases.

Mechanisms of Surfactant Alteration

Lung surfactant dysfunction is the consequence of an altered pulmonary surfactant system and might be due to several mechanisms (Fig. 4). One mechanism is related to type II cell death or metabolic changes of this cell during lung injury. Both events could affect phospholipid and surfactant protein levels and composition. Another mechanism by which intra-alveolar surfactant could be altered is via surfactant inhibitors. A specific inhibitor has been described in premature infants who have respiratory distress [26] and numerous serum proteins, including albumin, have been found to inactivate pulmonary surfactant in vitro. The most pronounced inhibitory effect in this regard was found for fibrinogen [16, 56]. Since increased capillary permeability is a general feature of lung injury, it is likely that several surfactant inhibitors might be present in the alveoli of the lungs during acute respiratory failure. In addition, increased capillary permeability might change the alveolar phospholipid composition and protein/phospholipid ratios in the alveolar lung compartment. Such events might thus change surfactant reassembly at the air-liquid interface, the event leading to the biologically active form of surfactant [18]. Finally, lack or degradation of surfactant-associated proteins might be important mechanisms by which pulmonary surfactant could be inactivated. The former has been found in premature infants [37]; the latter has been demonstrated in vitro [49]. Neutrophil elastase degrades SP-A and probably SP-B thereby inactivating surfactant function in vitro.

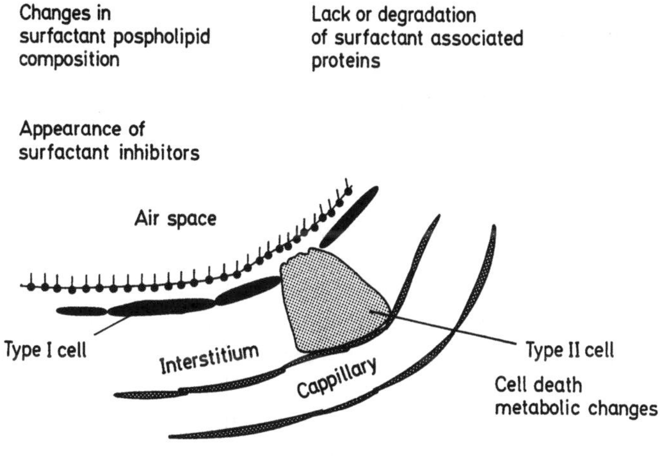

Fig. 4. Mechanisms of lung surfactant dysfunction

Surfactant Replacement

The therapeutical concept and results from clinical trials using exogenous surfactant for replacement in premature infants have been reviewed recently [29]. For our purpose, exogenous surfactant substitution should be discussed as a pharmacological approach in adults who have acute respiratory failure. Four major questions should be answered before testing the hypothesis that surfactant replacement is beneficial to adults who have acute respiratory failure: (1) In what group of adult patients should exogenous surfactant be replaced? (2) What kind of exogenous surfactant should be used? (3) How much should be replaced, in what time frame, and how should it be administered? (4) How should therapeutical effects be established.

In what group of adult patients should exogenous surfactant be replaced? It is obvious that a new experimental therapy, such as surfactant replacement in adults who have acute respiratory failure, should be tested in pilot studies in which the patient collective to be tested is highly selected. For prevention studies there are two approaches. One would be to select a homogeneous group in which the time relationship between the initial insult and the development of respiratory failure is known and consistent. Trauma patients and patients after esophagectomy both fulfill these criteria and would therefore be ideal groups to test the above stated hypothesis. Another approach might be to select for adult patients at risk of developing respiratory failure and test whether surfactant is present and active or not. However, at the moment there is no easy and specific test available and it might be better to select patients for prevention studies using the first approach. For rescue studies patients have to be selected by a defined respiratory failure scoring system, so that any effect could be measured by improvement in the degree of respiratory distress.

What kind of exogenous surfactant should be used? The report of the Mackinac Workshop on Exogenous Surfactant for Human Lung Disease, held in 1982, listed a number of tests that should be considered when choosing a surfactant for clinical use, including tests for biophysical activity, biochemical composition, efficacy in vivo, and stability, storage, and sterility characteristics [59]. Although natural surfactants are most effective, artificial surfactants are without the risk of contaminating infectious or other hazardous agents. The ideal exogenous surfactant for both prevention and rescue studies would be a material composed from synthetic phospholipids and genetically engineered surfactant-associated proteins A, B, and C in an appropriate ratio, since lipids and SP-A, B, and C all contribute to surface film formation [24, 50, 64, 67]. This material would be without the hazard of contaminating pathogens. The ideal exogenous surfactant is not available; thus, surfactant replacement therapy in adults might be tested using sources selected by availability.

How much surfactant should be replaced, in what time frame, and how should it be administered? The surface area of adult human lungs is 60–80 m^2. Assuming a limiting surface area of 42.5 $Å^2$ for dipalmitoyl phosphatidylcholine,

2.5–3.3 mg/kg are required to coat the alveolar surface with one monolayer of the phospholipid. However, there are various degrees of alveolar edema and, consequently, various amounts of surfactant inhibitor(s) in patients with acute respiratory failure. Furthermore, loss of exogenous material will probably occur during application. It is therefore reasonable to expect that several monolayer equivalents are required for an effective surfactant replacement therapy. Doses of from 25 to 200 mg surfactant lipid/kg body weight have been used in clinical trials in premature infants, mostly instilled as a single dose intratracheally [11, 25]. In ventilated preterm lambs the optimal dose was dependent on which end point was selected. Pressure-volume relationships of the lungs were maximally improved at doses at or above 53 mg/kg body weight; the minimal surface tensions and stability indices of the alveolar washes were optimized with doses at or above 64 mg/kg body weight [27]. The duration of effects of exogenous surfactant should follow the biological half-life of the material. The biological half-life of a given surfactant phospholipid as estimated in animal studies depended on the precursor used. It ranged from 17 to 20 h if palmitate was used, from 35 to 45 h if choline was the precursor, and from 61 to 90 h with [^{32}P]phosphate [72], but might be much shorter during lung injury. The dose and time frame to repeat any exogenous surfactant administration in adults has to be developed empirically, as it has been done in premature infants. The experiences from clinical trials in premature newborns and results obtained from animal studies on metabolism and turnover of pulmonary surfactant may help to design a pilot study in adults who have acute respiratory failure. One possible approach in this regard might be as follows: Initial administration of 100 mg surfactant lipid/kg body weight divided into five aliquots and instilled as a liquid bolus via a bronchoscope in each of the lung lobes. Since the biological half-life of the applied material and the amount of surfactant inhibitors cannot be predicted, further administration should follow the clinical course of gas exchange and lung mechanics in pretreated patients, repeating treatment when initial improvement decreases by 50% or when no effect can be demonstrated 2 h after initial administration.

How should therapeutical effects be established? Acute effects can be estimated using conventional arterial blood gas measurements and the ventilator pressures and oxygen fraction necessary to maintain normal gas exchange. Long-term effects after surfactant replacement therapy might be measured by duration of mechanical ventilator support required, survival time, and pulmonary function associated with survival.

Summary

Pulmonary surfactant is a unique material of specialized composition and structure. It includes different phospholipids and at least three associated proteins. The main function of pulmonary surfactant is to reduce the surface tension of the interface where air and liquid meet in the alveolar space of the lung. Surfactant thus provides mechanical stability of the alveolar units and prevents alveolar collapse and atelectasis at normal transpulmonary pressures. A deficiency of surfactant in premature newborns causes the respiratory distress syndrome and alterations of pulmonary surfactant have been demonstrated in adults who have acute respiratory failure. Mechanisms which lead to surfactant dysfunction might be: type II cell death/alteration leading to changes in surfactant metabolism and turnover; changes in surfactant phospholipid and protein composition; appearance of surfactant inhibitors due to capillary leakage; and lack or enzymatic degradation of surfactant-associated proteins. Replacement of deficient or inactive surfactant for the prevention and treatment of respiratory distress syndrome of various etiologies might become an important pharmacological approach.

References

1. Avery ME, Mead J (1959) Surface properties in relation to atelectasis and hyaline membrane disease. Am J Dis Child 97:517–523
2. Baughman RP, Mangels DJ, Strohofer S, Corser BC (1987) Enhancement of macrophage and monocyte cytotoxicity by the surface active material of lung lining fluid. J Lab Clin Med 109:692–697
3. Benson BJ, Dobbs LG, Ansfield MJ (1983) Immunopharmacology of lung surfactant. In: Newball HH (ed) Immunopharmacology of the lung. Dekker, New York, pp 209–241
4. Benson BJ, Williams MC, Sueishi K, Goerke J, Sargeant T (1984) Role of calcium ions in the structure and function of pulmonary surfactant. Biochim Biophys Acta 793:18–27
5. Benson BJ, Hawgood S, Schilling J, Clements JA, Damm D, Cordell B, White RT (1985) Structure of canine pulmonary surfactant apoprotein: cDNA and complete amino acid sequence. Proc Natl Acad Sci USA 82:6379–6383
6. Beppu OS, Clements JA, Goerke J (1983) Phosphatidylglycerol-deficient lung surfactant has normal properties. J Appl Physiol 55:496–502
7. Brown ES (1964) Isolation and assay of dipalmityl lecithin in lung extracts. Am J Physiol 207:402–406
8. Clements JA (1957) Surface tension of lung extracts. Proc Soc Exp Biol Med 95:170–172
9. Clements JA (1961) Pulmonary edema and permeability of alveolar membranes. Arch Environ Health 2:280–283
10. Clements JA, Tierney DF (1965) Alveolar instability associated with altered surface tension. In: Fenn WO, Rahn H (eds) Respiration. American Physiological Society, Washington, pp 1565–1583 (Handbook of physiology, Sect 3, vol 2)
11. Collaborative European Multicenter Study Group (1988) Surfactant replacement therapy for severe respiratory distress syndrome: an international randomized clinical trial. Pediatrics 82:683–691
12. Coonrod JD, Jarrells MC, Yoneda K (1986) Effect of rat surfactant lipids on complement and Fc receptors of macrophages. Infect Immun 54:371–378
13. Drickamer K, Dordal MS, Reynolds L (1986) Mannose-binding proteins isolated from rat liver contain carbohydrate-recognition domains linked to collagenous tails. J Biol Chem 161:6878–6887
14. Farrell PM, Avery ME (1975) Hyaline membrane disease. Am Rev Respir Dis 111:657–688
15. Floros J, Steinbrink R, Jacobs K, Phelbs D, Kriz R, Recny M, Sultzman L, Jones S, Taesch HW, Frank HA, Fritsch EF (1986) Isolation and characterization of cDNA clones for the 35-kDa pulmonary surfactant-associated protein. J Biol Chem 261:9029–9033
16. Fuchimukai T, Fujiwara T, Takahashi A, Enhorning G (1987) Artificial pulmonary surfactant inhibited by proteins. J Appl Physiol 62:429–437

17. Glasser SW, Korfhagen TR, Weaver T, Pilot-Matias T, Fox JL, Whitsett JA (1987) cDNA and deduced amino acid sequence of human pulmonary surfactant-associated proteolipid SPL(Phe). Proc Natl Acad Sci USA 84:4007–4011
18. Goerke J, Clements JA (1986) Alveolar surface tension and lung surfactant. In: Macklem PT, Mead J (eds) The respiratory system. American Physiological Society Washington, pp 247–261 (Handbook of physiology, vol 3)
19. Groniowski JA (1983) Fine structure basis of pulmonary surfactant. Int Rev Exp Pathol 25:183–238
20. Guyton AC, Moffatt DS (1981) Role of surface tension and surfactant in the transepithelial movement of pulmonary edema. Prog Respir Res 15:62–75
21. Hallman M, Spragg R, Harrell JH, Moser KM, Gluck L (1982) Evidence of lung surfactant abnormality in respiratory failure. J Clin Invest 70:673–683
22. Hawgood S, Benson BJ (1989) The molecular biology of surfactant apoproteins. In: Massaro D (ed) Lung cell biology. Dekker, New York, pp 701–734
23. Hawgood S, Efrati H, Schilling J, Benson BJ (1985) Chemical characterization of lung surfactant apoproteins: amino acid composition, N-terminal sequence and enzymic digestion. Biochem Soc Trans 13:1092–1096
24. Hawgood S, Benson BJ, Schilling J, Damm D, Clements JA, White RT (1987) Nucleotide and amino acid sequences of pulmonary surfactant protein SP 18 and evidence for cooperation between SP 18 and SP 28–36 in surfactant lipid adsorption. Proc Natl Acad Sci USA 84:66–70
25. Horbar JD, Soll RF, Sutherland JM, Kotagal U, Philip AGS, Kessler DL, Little GA, Edwards WH, Vidyasagar D, Raju TNK, Jobe AH, Ikegami M, Mullett MD, Myerberg DZ, McAuliffe TL, Lucey JF (1989) A multicenter randomized, placebo-controlled trial of surfactant therapy for respiratory distress syndrome. N Engl J Med 320:959–965
26. Ikegami M, Jobe A, Berry D (1986) A protein that inhibits surfactant in respiratory distress syndrome. Biol Neonate 50:121–129
27. Ikegami M, Adams FH, Towers B, Osher AB (1980) The quantity of natural surfactant necessary to prevent the respiratory distress syndrome in premature lambs. Pediatr Res 14:1082–1085
28. Jarstrand C (1984) Role of surfactant in the pulmonary defense system. In: Robertson B, van Golde LMG, Batenburg JJ (eds) Pulmonary surfactant. Elsevier, Amsterdam, pp 187–201
29. Jobe A, Ikegami M (1987) Surfactant for the treatment of respiratory distress syndrome. Am Rev Respir Dis 136:1256–1275
30. Juers JA, Rogers RM, McCurdy JB, Cook WW (1976) Enhancement of bactericidal capacity of alveolar macrophages by human alveolar lining material. J Clin Invest 58:271–275
31. Kilburn KH (1968) A hypothesis for pulmonary clearance and its implication. Am Rev Respir Dis 98:449–463
32. King RJ, Clements JA (1972) Surface active materials from dog lung. I. Methods of isolation. Am J Physiol 223:707–714
33. King RJ, Clements JA (1972) Surface active materials from dog lung. II. Composition and physiological correlations. Am J Physiol 223:715–726
34. King RJ, Clements JA (1985) Lipid synthesis and surfactant turnover in the lungs. In: Fishman AP, Fisher AB (eds) Circulation and nonrespiratory functions. American Physiological Society, Washington, pp 309–336 (Handbook of physiology, sect 3, vol 1)
35. King RJ, Simon D, Horowitz PM (1989) Aspects of secondary and quarternary structure of surfactant protein A from canine lung. Biochim Biophys Acta 1001:294–301
36. Kulovich MV, Hallman M, Gluck L (1979) The lung profile: normal pregnancy. Am J Obstet Gynecol 135:57–63
37. Kuroki Y, Takahashi H, Fukada Y, Mikawa M, Inagawa A, Fujemoto S, Akino T (1985) Two site "simultaneous" immunoassay with monoclonal antibodies for the determination of surfactant apoproteins in human amniotic fluid. Pediatr Res 19:1017–1020
38. Lachmann B (1987) The role of pulmonary surfactant in the pathogenesis and therapy of ARDS. In: Vincent JL (ed) Update in intensive care and emergency medicine. Springer, Berlin Heidelberg New York, pp 123–134
39. LaForce FM, Kelly WJ, Huber GL (1973) Inactivation of Staphylococci by alveolar macrophages with preliminary observations on the importance of alveolar lining material. Am Rev Respir Dis 108:784–790
40. Liau DF, Barrett CR, Bell ALL, Cermansky G, Ryan SF (1984) diphsophatidylglycerol in experimental acute alveolar injury in the dog. J Lipid Res 25:678–683

41. Liau DF, Barrett CR, Bell ALL, Ryan SF (1987) Functional abnormalities of lung surfactant in experimental acute alveolar injury in the dog. Am Rev Respir Dis 136:395–401
42. Neergaard K von (1929) Neue Auffassungen über einen Grundbegriff der Atemmechanik. Die Retraktionskraft der Lunge, abhängig von der Oberflächenspannung in den Alveolen. Z Gesamte Exp Med 66:373–394
43. Notter RH (1984) Surface chemistry of pulmonary surfactant: the role of individual components. In: Robertson B, van Golde LMG, Batenburg JJ (eds) Pulmonary surfactant. Elsevier, Amsterdam, pp 17–65
44. Notter RH, Finkelstein JN (1984) Pulmonary surfactant: an interdisciplinary approach. J Appl Physiol 57:1613–1624
45. Pattle RE (1955) Properties, function and origin of the alveolar lining layer. Nature 175:1125–1126
46. Pattle RE (1965) Surface lining of lung alveoli. Physiol Rev 45:48–79
47. Pison U, Seeger W, Buchhorn R, Brand M, Joka T, Obertacke U, Schmit-Neuerburg KP, Neuhof H (1989) Surfactant abnormalities in patients with respiratory failure following multiple trauma. Am Rev Respir Dis 140:1033–1039
48. Pison U, Obertacke U, Brand M, Seeger W, Joka T, Bruch J, Schmit-Neuerburg KP (1990) Altered pulmonary surfactant in uncomplicated and septicemia-complicated courses of acute respiratory failure. J Trauma 30:19–26
49. Pison U, Tam EK, Caughey GH, Hawgood S (1989) Proteolytic inactivation of dog lung surfactant-associated proteins by neutrophil elastase. Biochim Biophys Acta 992: 251–7
50. Pison U, Shiffer K, Hawgood S, Goerke J (1989) Effects of the surfactant-associated proteins, SP-A, SP-B and SP-C, on phospholipid surface film formation. Prog Respir Res 25: 1–3
51. Possmayer F (1988) Perspective: A proposed nomenclature for pulmonary surfactant-associated proteins. Am Rev Respir Dis 138:990–998
52. Post M, van Golde LMG (1988) Metabolic and developmental aspects of the pulmonary surfactant system. Biochim Biophys Acta 947:249–286
53. Rooney SA (1985) The surfactant system and lung phospholipid biochemistry. Am Rev Respir Dis 131:439–460
54. Sano K, Fisher J, Mason RJ, Kuroki Y, Schilling J, Benson B, Voelker D (1987) Isolation and sequence of a cDNA clone for the rat pulmonary surfactant-associated protein (PSP-A). Biochem Biophys Res Commun 144:367–374
55. Schürch S, Goerke J, Clements JA (1976) Direct determination of surface tension in the lung. Proc Natl Acad Sci USA 75:3417–3421
56. Seeger W, Stohr G, Wolf HRD, Neuhof H (1985) Alteration of surfactant due to protein leakage: special interaction with fibrin monomer. J Appl Physiol 58:326–338
57. Sitrin RG, Ansfield MJ, Kaltreider HB (1985) The effect of pulmonary surface-active material on the generation and expression of murine B and T-lymphocyte effector functions in vitro. Exp Lung Res 9:85–97
58. Suzuki Y, Fujita Y, Kogishi K (1989) Reconstitution of tubular myelin from synthetic lipids and proteins associated with pig pulmonary surfactant. Am Rev Respir Dis 140:75–81
59. Taeusch HW, Clements JA, Benson B (1983) Exogenous surfactant for human lung disease. Am Rev Respir Dis 128:791–793
60. Van Golde LMG, Batenburg JJ, Robertson B (1988) Metabolism of phospholipids in the lung. Physiol Rev 68:374–455
61. Voss T, Eistetter H, Schäfer KP, Engel J (1988) Macromolecular organization of natural and recombinant lung surfactant protein SP 28–36. Structural homology with the complement factor Clq. J Mol Biol 201:219–227
62. Walker SR, Williams MC, Benson BJ (1986) Immunocytochemical localization of the major surfactant apoproteins in type II cells, Clara cells, and alveolar macrophages of rat lung. J Histochem Cytochem 34:1137–1148
63. Warr RG, Hawgood S, Buckley DI, Crisp TM, Schilling J, Benson BJ, Clements JA, White RT (1987) Low molecular weight human surfactant protein (SP 5): isolation, characteristics and cDNA and amino acid sequences. Proc Natl Acad Sci USA 84:7915–7919
64. White RT, Damm D, Buckley D, Hawgood S, Spratt K, Schilling J, Benson B (1987) Expression, characterization and in vitro activity of recombinant surfactant protein SP 28–36. Pediatr Res 21:469a

65. White RT, Damm D, Miller J, Spratt K, Schilling J, Hawgood S, Benson B, Cordell B (1985) Isolation and characterization of the human pulmonary surfactant apoprotein gene. Nature 317:361–363
66. Whitsett JA, Weaver T, Hull W, Ross G, Dion C (1985) Synthesis of surfactant-associated glycoprotein A by rat type II epithelial cells. Primary translation products and post-translational modification. Biochim Biophys Acta 828:162–171
67. Whitsett JA, Ohning BL, Ross G, Meuth J, Weaver T, Holm BA, Shapiro DL, Notter RH (1986) Hydrophobic surfactant-associated protein in whole lung surfactant and its importance for biophysical activity in lung surfactant extracts used for replacement therapy. Pediatr Res 20:460–467
68. Williams MC (1977) Conversion of lamellar body membranes into tubular myelin in alveoli of fetal rat lungs. J Cell Biol 72:260–277
69. Williams MC (1987) Vesicles within vesicles: what role do multivesicular bodies play in alveolar type II cells? Am Rev Respir Dis 135:744–746
70. Wilson TA, Bachofen H (1982) A Model for the mechanical structure of the alveolar duct. J Appl Physiol 52:1064–1070
71. Wright JR, Clements JA (1989) Lung surfactant turnovers and factors that affect turnover. In: Massaro D (ed) Lung cell biology. Dekker, New York, pp 655–699
72. Wright JR, Clements JA (1987) Metabolism and turnover of lung surfactant. Am Rev Respir Dis 135:426–444

Effects of Artificial Ventilation on Surfactant Function*

J.A.H. Bos and B. Lachmann

Introduction

Since its introduction for clinical routine use more than 40 years ago, artificial ventilation has proven to be a life-saving method or therapy in intensive care. It has also remained a topic of much discussion and controversy because artificial ventilation involves a disturbance of normal cardiovascular and respiratory function (Price et al. 1954). That artificial ventilation can lead to decreased lung compliance and a dysfunction of gas exchange is well-known. Even more important is that ventilation by itself can lead to formation of atelectasis, pulmonary edema, pneumonitis, and fibrosis (for review see Tables 1 and 2). To date, no adequate explanation of the pathophysiological basis of all the changes due to artificial ventilation has been documented. However, there is evidence that some of them are induced by alterations to the surfactant system. These findings have stimulated ongoing extensive research in this area in an attempt to explain the side effects of artificial ventilation and to find improved methods of artificial ventilation in which these effects are minimized.

This paper focuses on investigations in which surfactant or surfactant-dependent functions have been studied in combination with artificial ventilation and what the immediate effects are of the ventilator setting used. First, the normal surfactant functions and the methods used for in vivo and in vitro characterization of the surfactant system will be briefly described; second, the influence of artificial ventilation on these functions will be discussed.

Surfactant Functions

Mechanical Stabilization of Lung Alveoli

The integrity of the surfactant system of the lung is a prerequisite for normal breathing with the least possible effort. Surfactant produces this effect by decreasing the surface tension of the interface between the alveoli and air. This provides an explanation for why we have to generate a pressure of only 4–8 cm H_2O during each inspiration, while at the air-liquid interface only the surface

* Thanks are due to the Dutch Foundation for Medical Research (SFMO) for financially supporting this work.

Table 1. Overview of effects of artificial ventilation on lung mechanics and the surfactant system: Conventional mechanical ventilation

Author(s)	Year	Form of ventilation	Method of investigation	Findings
Mead and Collier	1959	Ventilation of dogs in normal range (12 ml/kg) followed by inflations (40 cm H_2O) or suction (− 70 cm H_2O).	PV	Ventilation reduced lung compliance; suction reduced compliance even further; inflation restored lung compliance.
Greenfield et al.	1964	Normoventilation (P_{PAW}) = 10 cm H_2O) and hyperventilation (P_{PAW} = 28 cm H_2O) in dogs for 6 h.	ST, MS	Overinflation of the lung resulted in a decrease of surface activity and severe atelectasis. Ventilation at normal pressure and volume did not alter surfactant and did not result in atelectasis of the lung.
Faridy et al.	1966	Ventilation of excised dog lungs; parameters studied: (1) V_T, (2) duration, (3) end-expiratory pressure	PV, ST	Ventilation in vitro decreased compliance and surface activity. These effects are directly related to the tidal volume and duration of ventilation and inversely related to the end-expiratory pressure PEEP (e.g., PEEP > 4 cm H_2O prevented the negative effects of ventilation).
McClenahan and Urtnowski	1967	Ventilation of excised rat and dog lungs with a V_T of 66% of TLC at a rate varied from 10–40/min for 15–30 min.	PV, ST	Greater than tidal volume ventilation rapidly caused decreased distensibility and decreased surface activity in these lungs. The higher the ventilatory rate the greater the changes.
Benzer	1969	Pressure controlled ventilation (30 cm H_2O) of dead, or living rabbits, respectively, with an open or closed chest at different PEEP levels (0 and 5 cm H_2O) over 75 min	PV, ST	Ventilation of dead animals without PEEP resulted in a large decrease in compliance and surfce activity. When alive animals were ventilated the damage was less and the application of PEEP could entirely prevent any damaging effect of ventilation.
Forrest	1972	Ventilation of anesthetized guinea pigs; parameters studied: V_T changes (15 and 75% of predicted VC) over time	PV, ST	Hyperventilation reduced lung compliance, total lung volume, and surface activity to a degree which was related to the duration of hyperventilation. Opening pressure of lungs and pressure needed to maximally inflate lungs increased following hyperventilation.
Wauer and Lachmann	1972	Ventilation of anesthetized guinea pigs either with PEEP of 3 cm H_2O or with NEEP of 12 cm H_2O for 30 min followed by inflation with pressure of 40 cm H_2O	PV	NEEP reduced lung compliance within 30 min to 50% of the initial value. Inflation after NEEP did not fully restore lung compliance. Ventilation with a PEEP kept compliance unchanged.

Table 1. (Continued)

Author(s)	Year	Form of ventilation	Method of investigation	Findings
Webb and Tierney	1974	Ventilation anesthetized rats; parameters studied: HIPPV of 30/0 and 45/0 cm H_2O and HIPPV of 30 and 45 cm H_2O combined with a PEEP of 10 cm H_2O	LM, BG, MS	HIPPV (30/0 and 30/10) resulted in perivascular edema but no alveolar edema. HIPPV 45/0 animals had alveolar and perivascular edema, severe hypoxemia, and decreased compliance, and died within 1 h. HIPPV 45/10 animals had no alveolar edema and survived.
Wyszogrodski et al.	1975	Hyperventilation in open-chested anesthetized cats; parameters studied: V_T of 65% of TLC and no PEEP; V_T of 65% of TLC and PEEP of 2.5 cm H_2O; V_T of 45% of TLC and PEEP of 2.5 cm H_2O	PV, BC, ST	Hyperventilation without PEEP increased elastic recoil and decreased surface activity of lung extracts. Hyperventilation promoted release of surfactant from tissue to alveolus, but released material was inactivated. PEEP prevented adverse effects of hyperventilaion.
Faridy	1976a	Ventilation of rat lung for studying movement of surfactant from alveoli to the airways; parameters studied: lungs were kept at 0 cm H_2O or were inflated at 30 cm H_2O or were ventilated with air, O_2, or N_2. In the latter, V_T was varied between 15% and 60% of TLV. PEEP varied between 0 and 3 cm H_2O, frequency was also altered between 30–150/min. EPA were investigated	ST, BC	Surface tension and lecithin content of EPA did not change if the lungs were kept at minimal lung volume or at constant inflation but increased following ventilation. This increase was directly related to duration of ventilation and to V_T and was inversely related to PEEP. Different O_2 and N_2 concentration of the gas used for ventilation had no influence.
Faridy	1976b	Excised lung lobes from dogs were surfactant depleted and kept for 3 h either at FRC level or inflated from 5–30 cm H_2O at static pressures. For inflation either air, pure N_2, or O_2 were used.	ST, BC	Increase in surface activity was directly related to inflating pressure. The release of surfactant is a metabolically active process: 100% O_2 and N_2 inhibit this process.
Oyarzun and Clements	1977	Normo- and hyperventilation in spontaneous breathing rabbits; parameters studied: alveolar surfactant phospholipid.	BC	Hyperventilation during spontaneous breathing significantly increased the alveolar phospholipid content. Administration of atropine prevented the increase in alveolar phospholipids by hyperventilation.
Nilsson et al.	1978	Ventilation of surfactant deficient premature newborn rabbits with a V_t of 10 ml/kg; parameters studied: influence of surfactant instillation on lung mechanics and morphology.	PV, MS	Widespread necrosis and desquamation of bronchiolar epithelium in controls, whereas such lesions were scarce or absent in surfactant treated animals. Lung compliance in the surfactant treated group was increased compared with controls.

Table 1. (Continued)

Author(s)	Year	Form of ventilation	Method of investigation	Findings
Thet et al.	1979	Ventilation of excised rat lungs; parameters studied: CTV combined either with large inflations (CTVI) (+ 40 cm H_2O) or with a PEEP of 10 cm H_2O (CTVP).	PV, BC, MS	Opening pressure and recoil pressure was significantly higher in CTV group than in CTVI and CTVP groups. CTV animals also had areas of atelectasis which could be reversed by large inflation or the application of PEEP. CTV led to increases of inactivated surfactant in the alveolar space.
Oyarzun et al.	1980	Ventilation of anesthetized rabbits; parameters studied: DPPC clearance in dependence of either normo- or hyperventilation.	BC	Increased ventilation increased alveolar clearance of radiolabeled DPPC.
Hildebran et al.	1981	After initial surfactant depletion, over-distension of excised rat lungs to TLC with air.	PV, BC, ST	Air inflation to TLC leads to release of surfactant into the alveolar space.
Lachmann et al.	1981	Ventilation of immature surfactant deficient rabbits; ventilation modes studied: different I/E ratios.	LM, MS	Inspiration time which covered 80% of ventilator cycle led to greater compliance and less morphological damage than short inspiration times.
Lachmann et al.	1982	Ventilation of surfactant depleted adult rabbits; ventilation modes studied: volume controlled vs pressure controlled ventilation; inversed I/E ratio ventilation.	PV, BG, MS	Reduced recoil pressure, increased blood gases, less morphological damage in pressure-controlled inversed ratio ventilation than with volume-controlled ventilation.
Thet and Alvarez	1982	Hyperventilation of excised rats with or without a prior period of starvation.	PV, BC	Starvation did not change recoil but decreased alveolar pool of surfactant. Hyperventilation increased surface recoil. Hyperventilation induced dysfunction of surfactant was greater when the alveolar pool of surfactant was reduced by starvation.
Massaro and Massaro	1983	Ventilation of anesthetized rats; parameters studied: volume density of lamellar body in type II cells in dependency of inflation during ventilation (Periodic inflation: $4 \times V_T$ every 5 min for 1 h).	MS	Periodic large sighs reduced density and volume of lamellar bodies in type II cells within 60 min to 2/3 of the initial value.
Ennema et al.	1984a	Ventilation of anesthetized rabbits. One group breathed spontaneously, another group was ventilated mechanically with a PEEP of 5 cm H_2O for 6h; parameters studied: lung mechanics and surfactant metabolism.	PV, BC	Despite a PEEP of 5 cm H_2O, dynamic lung compliance decreased during ventilation. Static compliance and amount and composition of surfactant phospholipids remained unaltered. Incorporation of labeled palmitate into SPC of the

Table 1. (Continued)

Author(s)	Year	Form of ventilation	Method of investigation	Findings
				lamellar body fraction increased in the ventilated group. The clearance of radioactivity from the lamellar bodies into the alveolar lumen was greatly enhanced in the ventilated group.
Lachmann	1985	Ventilation of guinea pigs combined with tracheal saline instillation (3 ml/kg). Control animals either ventilated without saline or breathing spontaneously with 3 ml/kg saline instillation.	BG, PV	Combination of artificial ventilation with saline instillation led to deterioration of blood gases and increase of opening pressure and animals died without additional PEEP. Surfactant replacement did restore these effects. Saline instillation in spontaneous breathing animals or only artificial ventilation had no effect on any mentioned parameters.
Evander et al.	1990	Ventilation of anesthetized rabbits; ventilation modes studied: deep slow ventilation ($V_T = 30 \pm 4$ ml/kg, f = 20 min) and rapid shallow ventilation ($V_T = 11 \pm 2$ ml/kg^{-1}, f = 80 min^{-1}).	^{99m}Tc-DTPA	Clearance of ^{99m}Tc-DTPA from the lung was significantly faster during deep slow ventilation with large tidal volumes than during rapid shallow ventilation. There was no dependency on lung volume

Abbreviations: ^{99m}Tc-DTPA, ^{99m}Tc-DTPA clearance measurement; BC, biochemical measurement; BG, blood gases; CMV, conventional mode of ventilation; CTV, constant tidal volume ventilation; DPPC, dipalmitoyl phosphatidylcholine; EPA, extra pulmonary airways; HFJV, high frequency jet ventilation; HFO, high frequency oscillation; HFOV, high frequency oscillatory ventilation; HIPPV, high inflation positive pressure ventilation; IMV, intermittent mandatory ventilation; IPPV, intermittent positive pressure ventilation; LM, lung mechanics; MAP, mean airway pressure; Mortality, mortality rate; MS, morphology study; NEEP, negative end-expiratory pressure; PEEP, positive end-expiratory pressure; P_{PAW}, peak inspiratory pressure; PV, pressure-volume diagram; ST, surface tension; TLC, total lung capacity; TLV, total lung volume; VC, vital capacity; V_T, tidal volume

Table 2. Overview of effects of artificial ventilation on lung mechanics and the surfactant system: High frequency ventilation

Author(s)	Year	Form of ventilation	Method of investigation	Findings
Frantz III et al.	1982	Adult anesthetized cats were ventilated with the following modes for 4 h: (1) HFJV at 12 Hz and (2) CMV. In the ventilated groups PEEP was maintained. The control group was not ventilated.	BG, PV, BC, MS, ST	PV diagrams were identical in all groups. No effect was measured on pulmonary lavage surfactant (functionally or biochemically). Lung liquid and morphological aspects were not different.
Ennema et al.	1984b	Healthy adult anesthetized rabbits were ventilated with HFO at 5 Hz with a MAP of 5 cm H_2O. Control group was not ventilated.	PV, BC	Static compliance of the lungs; amount and composition of surfactant phospholipids of lamellar body and alveolar lavage fraction were comparable to values found for spontaneously breathing animals.
Solimano et al.	1985	Ventilation of surfactant deficient premature lambs with: (1) HFO at 15 Hz and (2) CMV; parameters studied: bidirectional protein leak and turnover of labeled natural surfactant.	BC, ST, MS, BG	No differences between CMV and HFOV regarding blood gases, large protein leaks and pathological findings typical for RDS lungs. HFO resulted in a decrease of secretion of surfactant and/or a stimulation of reuptake.
Man et al.	1987	Ventilation of dogs with the following modes: spontaneous breathing, IPPV ($V_T = 15$ ml/kg, $f = 10$–12 min^{-1}) with or without PEEP (2 cm H_2O), HFOV at 8 Hz, and HFOV at 16 Hz. Duration of ventilation: 4 h.	^{99m}Tc-DTPA	Spontaneous breathing and IPPV did not increase clearance rate. IPPV and PEEP as well as HFOV (8 and 16 Hz) increased clearance of ^{99m}Tc-DTPA.
Obara et al.	1987	HFOV with IMV was compared with CMV by matching the MAP in adult rabbits. Both groups had PEEP (5 cm H_2O). Controls were not ventilated.	MS	Volume and density of lamellar bodies in type II cells in the HFOV-IMV animals were significantly reduced compared with other groups suggesting enhancement of secretion of surfactant from alveolar type II cells by HFOV-IMV compared with CMV.
Delemos et al.	1987	Ventilation of premature baboons either with HFO at 10 Hz or with CMV combined with PEEP.	Mortality, MS, BG, LM	Improved blood gases, little evidence of barotrauma in HFO animals in comparison to CMV animals.

Table 2. (Continued)

Author(s)	Year	Form of ventilation	Method of investigation	Findings
McCulloch et al.	1988	Ventilation of surfactant deficient adult rabbits with the following mode: HFO or CMV over a period of 7 h at a high or low FRC.	MS, BG	PaO_2 and lung mechanics were excellent in HFO at high FRC, whereas there were large decreases at HFO and CMV at low FRC. In these animals there were also significantly more hyaline membranes present.
Bos et al.	1989	Surfactant deficient adult rabbits were ventilated by different modes: HFJV at 2 Hz and 15 Hz and volume-controlled ventilation with PEEP. Mean airway pressure was adjusted to get, at 100% oxygen, a PaO_2 >220 mm Hg. Controls were not surfactant depleted and volume-controlled ventilated.	^{99m}Tc-DTPA, MS	HFJV at 2 Hz led to the smallest half-life time, the highest mean airway pressures, and the lowest PaO_2 in comparison to CMV and HFJV at 15 Hz.

For abbreviations see Table 7.

tension of the plasma is present and then a pressure of 25–40 cm H_2O (depending on the radius of the alveoli) has to be generated for each inspiration. This is a well-known symptom in immature newborn babies with respiratory distress syndrome (RDS) and in adults with respiratory failure. In alveoli of different radii, an equal lowering of surface tension would not, however, produce stabilization of the alveolar system. It would, according to the law of Laplace ($P = 2\sigma/r$; P = pressure in the bubble, σ = surface tension, r = radius of the bubble), lead instead to the collapse of the smaller bubble or alveoli and to their emptying into the larger ones. Since alveoli in vivo do not exhibit such behavior one may conclude that the second remarkable quality of the alveolar lining layer is that it can change the surface tension, depending on the size of the alveoli.

Stabilization of Small Airways

As early as 1970, Macklem et al. drew attention to the significance of stabilization of the peripheral airways by surfactant and hinted that its lack might cause airway obstruction or collapse of the small bronchioli with air trapping. Recently, this was shown in an animal model in our laboratory in which the bronchial surfactant was damaged, and it was demonstrated that the pressure needed to open up collapsed bronchioli is approximately 20 cm H_2O. In the same study it was also demonstrated that severe impairment of bronchial surfactant can be successfully treated with exogenous surfactant replacement (Lachmann 1985).

Besides its role in mechanical stabilization, bronchial surfactant also has a transport function for mucus and inhaled particles. This has been proven in vitro in a study showing that particles on a surface film move only in one direction if the surface film is compressed and then dilatated – comparable to the compression and expansion during inspiration and expiration (Lachmann 1985; Rensch and von Seefeld 1984). Furthermore, bronchial surfactant also acts as an antiglue factor, preventing the development of large adhesive forces between mucus and the bronchial wall (Reinfenrath 1983).

Protection Against Lung Edema

Another function of the pulmonary surfactant system is stabilization of the fluid balance in the lung and protection against lung edema (Guyton et al. 1980). In general, alveolar flooding will not occur as long as the suction force in the pulmonary interstitium exceeds the pressure gradient generated by surface tension in the alveolar air-liquid interface. Since the pressure gradient is inversely related to the radius of the alveolar curvature there is, for each combination of interstitial resorptive force and average surface tension, a critical value for surface tension and alveolar radius below which alveolar flooding occurs.

Functional Changes Due to a "Disturbed" Surfactant System

When considering the physiological functions of the alveolo-bronchial surfactant system it can easily be understood that alterations in its functional integrity will lead to (Lachmann 1989):

- Decreased lung distensibility and thus to increased work of breathing and increased oxygen demand by the respiratory muscles
- Atelectasis
- Transudation of plasma into the alveoli with decreased diffusion for oxygen and CO_2
- Enlargement of functional right-to-left shunt due to perfusion of nonventilated alveoli (the von Euler-Liljestrand reflex does not "work" in surfactant deficient alveoli) resulting in hypoxemia and acidosis

Methods for In Vivo Investigation of the Surfactant System

The methods used to investigate the integrity of the pulmonary surfactant system in vivo include: pulmonary compliance measurements, technetium-99m-diethylene triamine pentaacetate (^{99m}Tc-DTPA) clearance and, indirectly, via monitoring of blood gases.

Pulmonary Compliance Measurements

The fact that the surfactant system is responsible for one-half to two-thirds of the total retraction force of the lungs makes lung mechanics studies very important. Moreover, recording of P-V diagrams is the only direct in vivo test for characterization and indication of damage to the surfactant system. To quantify these changes in the P-V diagram, different indices for both the inspiratory loop and expiratory loop were introduced (Clements et al. 1961; Gruenwald 1963; Rüfer 1967). However, there exist a few pathological changes in the lung in which the expiratory loop cannot be used for characterization of the surfactant system, e.g., if there is a combination of a surfactant deficiency with a massive alveolar edema present, part of the edema fluid can block the airways during expiration resulting in air trapping. This can mistakenly be interpreted as a high expiratory stability.

Furthermore, the P-V diagram enables differentiation between surfactant deficiency, pulmonary edema, pneumonia, and/or fibrosis. For example, when it is established that the cause of decreased lung compliance is due to a surfactant deficiency, it is still possible to open up the lungs by administration of a very high inspiratory pressure and keep them stable during expiration by a high PEEP. A similar situation arises in lungs with edema or pneumonia, but, due to the fact that these lungs are filled by plasma or exudate, the total volume which can be forced in at a certain pressure will be less than that of a purely surfactant deficient lung. To differentiate between different types of restrictive lung diseases, e.g., pneumonia and fibrosis, one has additionally to evaluate the blood gases at different intrapulmonary pressures. An increase of PEEP or of mean airway pressure in a pneumonia lung will always be followed by an increase in PaO_2, whereas in a fibrotic stage PaO_2 will decrease or will not change.

^{99m}Tc-DTPA Clearance Measurement

^{99m}Tc-DTPA is a small (molecular weight 492) and water-soluble molecule which, after deposition on the alveolar surface, is transferred into the bloodstream across various biological barriers. These barriers are: the surfactant lining, the alveolar epithelium, the basal lamina layer, and the endothelium. Clearance of ^{99m}Tc-DTPA from the lung measures the overall permeability of these layers. However, it could be demonstrated that the ^{99m}Tc-DTPA clearance rate depends mainly on the functional integrity of the surfactant system. Lungs with a damaged surfactant system are known to have a very high clearance rate (Evander et al. 1987; Wollmer et al. 1989a,b).

When ^{99m}Tc-DTPA is administered via an air jet nebulizer as an aerosol, whose particles favor alveolar deposition, a gamma camera is used to measure the amount of activity in the lungs over a certain period of time. After measurement, clearance curves can be analyzed in freely selected lung regions. This ^{99m}Tc-DTPA clearance technique has proven to be a very sensitive and noninvasive method to study the integrity of the pulmonary surfactant system.

Surfactant System and Arterial Oxygen Tension

Monitoring of PaO_2 is an easy method to obtain indirect parameters from which conclusions can be drawn about the integrity of the surfactant system. If a connection is suspected between hypoxemia and decreased function of the pulmonary surfactant system it can be proved by letting the patient breath 100% oxygen. In healthy lungs, the PaO_2 should increase to at least 500 mmHg. A damaged surfactant system will result in a $PaO_2 < 500$ mmHg due to atelectasis and intrapulmonary shunting. If the application of continuous positive airway pressure (CPAP) or positive end-expiratory pressure (PEEP) results in an improvement of the PaO_2, and this improvement is dependent on the height of the end-expiratory pressure, it means that collapsed terminal airways and/or alveoli due to the damaged surfactant system were reopened. This further means that each tendency of alveolar collapse and atelectasis that can be compensated for by a counter pressure (CPAP, PEEP) indicates surfactant deficiency. In other words, every application of CPAP or PEEP, with the intention of increasing functional residual capacity (FRC), decreasing the intrapulmonary shunt, and improving gas exchange, can only be interpreted as compensating for the increased retraction forces due to a damaged surfactant system. The degree of damage to this system is proportional to the amount of CPAP or PEEP required.

In Vitro Evaluation of Surfactant

For in vitro evaluation, biochemical measurements of lung extracts and/or fluid can be performed. These measurement methods can include using radio-labeled surfactant precursors and measuring the amount and composition of alveolar phospholipids. Surface tension measurements of lung extracts and/or lung lavage fluids can be performed using the Wilhelmy balance developed by Clements (1957) and the pulsating bubble surfactometer (Enhorning 1977). These two methods both have their advantages and disadvantages but are able to give a valid evaluation of the physical properties of the pulmonary surfactant system.

Mechanism of How Artificial Ventilation Affects the Surfactant System

The manner in which the surfactant system is affected by artificial ventilation is not exactly known but one hypothesis is that alveolar surfactant might move along the surface of the acinus towards the airways resulting in a shortage of surface-active material at the alveolar level.

In normal breathing, during end-expiration the surfactant molecules are compressed on the small alveolar area (leading to a low surface tension or a high surface pressure) thus preventing the alveoli from collapse. If the surface of the alveolus is smaller than the surface of the molecules, the molecules are squeezed out of the surface, forced towards the airways, and then lost for the alveoli.

During the following inflation of alveoli, the surface is replenished with surfactant molecules that were in the hypophase. During the next expiration, the same mechanism continues to work and again surfactant molecules are forced into the airways; this is a continuing cycle (Figs. 1 and 2).

The amount of new surfactant that must be secreted is proportional to the loss of surface-active molecules during the breathing cycle. Surfactant molecules secreted on the alveolar lining may be lost into the airways rather rapidly with a large tidal volume and/or high rates, as demonstrated by Faridy (1976a). When secretion and new production by alveolar type II cells keep pace with consumption, no surfactant deficient or depleted situation can occur, as in a normal healthy lung. From the above described mechanism, it becomes clear that the rate of loss of surfactant is greater when the alveoli are highly compressed and then highly inflated, because the smaller the air space the lower the surface tension must be if air space stability is maintained. The consumption

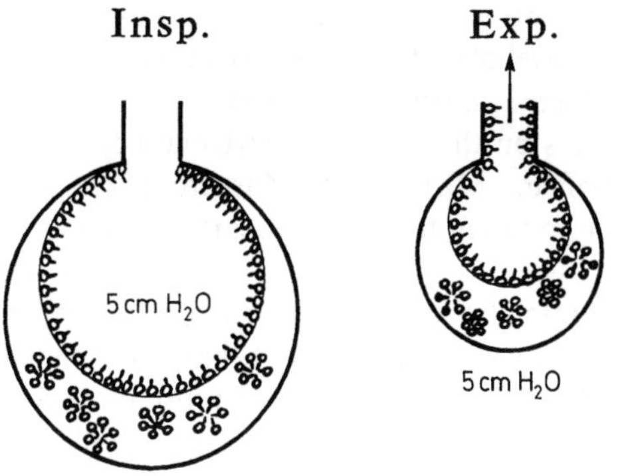

Fig. 1. Balance between synthesis, release, and consumption of surfactant in the healthy lung. The pressure values given represent the intrapulmonary pressure needed to open up this alveolus. At the surface and in the hypophase (micelles), there are sufficient molecules of surfactant. These micelles deliver the surfactant necessary to replace the molecules squeezed out during expiration

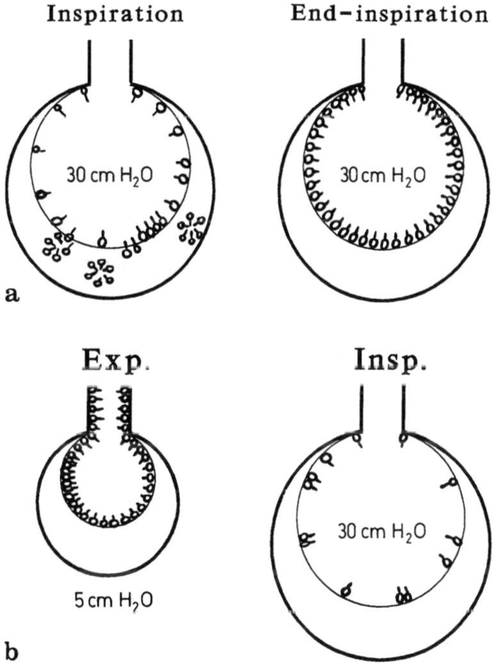

Fig. 2. **A** Imbalance between synthesis, release, and consumption of surfactant due to artifical ventilation. At the beginning of inspiration, there exists an apparent deficiency of surfactant molecules, but there is a respreading of molecules stored in the hypophase to the surfactant layer. At the end of inspiration there is, in principle, enough surfactant on the surface. **B** With the next expiration, surface active molecules are further squeezed out and no surface active molecules are left in the hypophase for respreading, creating the situation where a serious surfactant deficiency follows

becomes greater and the new production and secretion of surfactant must also increase in order to prevent a surfactant deficient state.

This mechanism explains how loss of surfactant by artificial ventilation can be caused by the rhythmic compression (expiration) and decompression (inspiration) of the alveolar lining, especially when the compression is far below the static state of the surfactant layer, which is normally equal to or just above the FRC level. As shown by Wauer and Lachmann (1972), the use of negative end-expiratory pressure (NEEP) or the ventilation of a lung with open thorax exacerbates this process and therefore increases the loss of surface-active molecules (Benzer 1969). PEEP, on the other hand, keeps the end-expiratory volume of the alveoli above the critical level of static state of the surfactant film, thereby preventing further loss of surfactant during expiration.

The effect of large inflations or sighs on the release of surfactant from the type II cells could be due to a "stretch-effect." Massaro and Massaro (1983), used the volume and density of the lamellar bodies in the cells to clearly demonstrate this effect.

The new modes of ventilation, including for instance high frequency ventilation (HFV, HFO) and inversed I/E ratio ventilation (IRV), have one major advantage over the conventional modes of volume controlled ventilation. The P-V swings during the ventilation cycle are much smaller during HFV and IRV. These new modes keep the alveoli inflated (due to an auto-PEEP) at a volume above the static state of the surfactant system thus preventing the nonphysiological consumption rate of surfactant due to artificial ventilation.

Conclusion

Although artificial ventilation remains one of the major breakthroughs in modern health care it is clear that it should be applied cautiously. From the reviewed studies, which all seem to be diffferent in intention and methods used, the same conclusion can be drawn; namely, that when lungs are ventilated with large volume and pressure changes the pulmonary surfactant system is depleted or is in some other ways, damaged. This results in decreased pulmonary compliance which in turn creates the condition in which secondary lung edema can develop. This leads to further damage and inactivation of the alveolar surfactant system. The ventilator mode which is then necessary to ventilate these lungs is potentially more damaging than the ventilator setting that caused it. In a diseased lung these pathophysiological changes are probably more pronounced and severe than in healthy ventilated lungs. The results of these studies provide the rationale for optimal ventilator settings (adequate gas exchange and minimal cardiocirculatory interference), which should produce smaller P-V swings during the ventilatory cycle and keep the lung volume equal or just above the FRC level to prevent a significant depletion of surface-active material. One may also speculate that ventilator induced changes in lung mechanics may be prevented by exogenous surfactant instillation.

Acknowledgement. We thank Dr. C. Vilstrup (Lund University, Sweden) for valuable discussions.

References

Benzer H (1969) Respiratorbeatmung und Oberflächenspannung in der Lunge. In: Frey R, Kern F, Mayrhofer O (eds) Anaesthesiologie und Wiederbelebung, 38. Springer, Berlin Heidelberg New York

Bos JAH, Schairer W, Schaffers JT, Tenbrinck R, Tenhave-Opbroek AAW, Bakker WH, Wollmer P, Lachmann B (1989) Effect of high frequency jet ventilation (HFJV) on the pulmonary clearance of 99mTc-DTPA in respiratory failure in rabbits. Br J Anaesth 63:59S–64S
Clements JA (1957) Surface tension of lung extracts. Proc Soc Exp Biol Med 95:170–172
Clements JA, Hustead RE, Johnson RP, Gribnetz I (1961) Pulmonary surface tension and alveolar stability. J Appl Physiol 16:444–450
Delemos RA, Coalson JJ, Gerstmann DR, Null DM, Akerman NB, Escobedo MB, Robotham JL, Kuehl TJ (1987) Ventilatory management of infant baboons with hyaline membrane disease: the use of high frequency ventilation. Pediatr Res 21:594–602
Enhorning G (1977) Pulsating bubble technique for evaluating pulmonary surfactant. J Appl Physiol 43:198–203
Ennema JJ, Reijngoud DJ, Wildevuur CRH, Egberts J (1984a) Effects of artificial ventilation on surfactant phospholipid metabolism in rabbits. Respir Physiol 58:15–28
Ennema JJ, Reijngoud DJ, Egberts J, Mook PH, Wildevuur CRH (1984b) High-frequency oscillation affects surfactant phospholipid metabolism in rabbits. Respir Physiol 58:29–39
Evander E, Wollmer P, Jonson B, Lachmann B (1987) Pulmonary clearance of inhaled ^{99m}Tc-DTPA: effects of surfactant depletion by lung lavage. J Appl Physiol 62:1611–1614
Evander E, Wollmer P, Jonson B (1990) Pulmonary clearance of ^{99m}Tc-DTPA: effects of ventilatory pattern. Clin Physiol 10:199–209
Faridy EE (1976a) Effect of distension on release of surfactant in excised dogs' lungs. Respir Physiol 27:99–114
Faridy EE (1976b) Effect of ventilation on movement of surfactant in airways. Respir Physiol 27:323–334
Faridy EE, Permutt S, Riley RL (1966) Effect of ventilation on surfactant forces in excised dogs' lungs. J Appl Physiol 21:1453–1462
Forrest JB (1972). The effect of hyperventilation on pulmonary surface activity. Br J Anaesth 44:313–319
Frantz ID III, Stark AR, Davis JM, Davies P, Kitzmiller TJ (1982) High frequency ventilation does not affect pulmonary surfactant, liquid, or morphological features in normal cats. Am Rev Respir Dis 126:909–913
Greenfield LJ, Ebert PA, Benson DW (1964) Effect of positive pressure ventilation on surface tension properties of lung extracts. Anaesthesia 25:312–316
Gruenwald PA (1963) A numerical index of the stability of lung expansion. J Appl Physiol 18:665–667
Guyton AC, Moffatt DS, Adair TA (1980) Role of alveolar surface tension in transepithelial movement of fluid. In: Robertson B, Van Golde LMG, Batenburg JJ (eds) Pulmonary surfactant. Elsevier, Amsterdam, pp 171–185
Hildebran JN, Goerke J, Clements JA (1981) Surfactant release in excised rat lung is stimulated by air inflation. J Appl Physiol (Respir Environ Exercise Physiol) 51:905–910
Lachmann B (1985) Possible function of bronchial surfactant. Eur J Respir Dis 67:49–61
Lachmann B (1989) Surfactant replacement. Appl Cardiopulm Pathophysiol 3:3–11
Lachmann B, Freyse EJ, Grossmann G, Robertson B (1981) Lung-thorax compliance in the artificially ventilated premature rabbit neonate in relation to variations in inspiration:expiration ratio. Pediatr Res 15:833–838
Lachmann B, Jonson B, Lindroth M, Robertson B (1982) Modes of artificial ventilation in severe distress syndrome. Crit Care Med 10:724–732
Macklem PT, Proctor DF, Hogg JC (1970) The stability of peripheral airways. Respir Physiol 8:191–203
Man GCW, Ahmed IH, Logus JW, Man SFP (1987) High-frequency oscillatory ventilation increases canine epithelial permeability. J Appl Physiol 63:1871–1876
Massaro GD, Massaro D (1983) Morphologic evidence that large inflations of the lung stimulate secretion of surfactant. Am Rev Respir Dis 127:235–236
McClenahan JB, Urtnowski A (1967) Effect of ventilation on surfactant and its turnover rate. J Appl Physiol 23:215–220
McCulloch PR, Forkert PG, Froese AB (1988) Lung volume maintenance prevents lung injury during high frequency oscillatory ventilation in surfactant-deficient rabbits. Am Rev Respir Dis 137:1185–1192
Mead J, Collier C (1959) Relation of volume history of lungs to respiratory mechanics in anesthetized dogs. J Appl Physiol 14:669–678

Nilsson R, Grossmann G, Robertson B (1978) Lung surfactant and the pathogenesis of neonatal bronchiolar lesions induced by artificial ventilation. Pediatr Res 12:249–255

Obara H, Maekawa N, Hamatani S, Iwai S (1987) Effect of combined high-frequency oscillatory ventilation on rabbit alveolar type II cells. Crit care Med 15:692–695

Oyarzùn MJ, Clements JA (1977) Ventilatory and cholinergic control of pulmonary surfactant in the rabbit. J Appl Physiol (Respir Environ Exercise Physiol) 43:39–45

Oyarzun MJ, Clements JA, Baritussio A (1980) Ventilation enhances pulmonary alveolar clearance of radioactive dipalmitoyl phosphatidylcholine in liposomes. Am Rev Respir Dis 121:709–721

Price HL, Connor EH, Dripps RD (1954) Some respiratory and circulatory effects of mechanical respirators. J Appl Physiol 6:517

Reinfenrath R (1983) Surfactant action in bronchial mucus. In: Cosmi EV, Scarpelli EM (eds) Pulmonary surfactant system. Elsevier, Amsterdam, pp 339–347

Rensch H, von Seefeld H (1984) Surfactant–mucus interaction. In: Robertson B, van Golde LMG, Batenburg JJ (eds) Pulmonary surfactant. Elsevier, Amsterdam, pp 203–214

Rüfer R (1967) Der Einflu047 oberflächenaktiver Substanzen auf Entfaltung und Retraktion isolierter lungen. Pflugers Arch Gesmate Physiol 298:170–184

Solimano A, Bryan C, Jobe A, Ikegami M, Jacobs H (1985) Effects of high-frequency and conventional ventilation on the premature lamb lung. J Appl Physiol 59:1571–1577

Thet LA, Alvarez H (1982) Effect of hyperventilation and starvation on rat lung mechanics and surfactant. Am Rev Respir Dis 126:286–290

Thet LA, Clerch L, Massaro GD, Massaro D (1979) Changes in sedimentation of surfactant in ventilated excised rat lungs. J Clin Invest 64:600–608

Wauer R, Lachmann B (1972) Die Ventilette, ein Notfallbeatmungsgerät für Neugeborene und Säuglinge - ein Erprobungsbericht. padiatr Grenzgeb 11:411–422

Webb H, Tierney DF (1974) Experimental pulmonary edema due to intermittent positive pressure ventilation with high inflation pressures. Protection by positive end-expiratory pressure. Am Rev Respir Dis 110:556–565

Wollmer P, Evander E, Jonson B (1989a) Assessment of surfactant function by measurement of the pulmonary clearance of inhaled ^{99m}Tc-DTPA. In: Lachmann B (ed) Surfactant replacement therapy in neonatal and adult respiratory distress syndrome. Springer, Berlin Heidelberg New York; pp 66–76

Wollmer P, Evander E, Jonson B, Lachmann B (1989b) Pulmonary clearance of inhaled ^{99m}Tc-DTPA and surfactant function: In: Ekelund L, Jonson B, Malm L (eds) Surfactant and the respiratory tract. Elsevier, Amsterdam, pp 97–102

Wyszogrodski I, Kyei-Aboagye K, Taeusch HW Jr, Avery ME (1975) Surfactant inactivation by hyperventilation: conservation by end-expiratory pressure. J Appl Physiol 38:461–466

Part 7: The Respiratory Pump

Assessment of Dyspnea and Respiratory Muscle Function

C.-P. Criée, G. Laier-Groeneveld and U. Hüttemann

Dyspnea (breathlessness or shortness of breath) is a sensation that almost everyone has experienced and so intuitively understands. With respect to pathological dyspnea, several questions need to be answered: Is the pathological dyspnea of patients with respiratory disease the same as that experienced by those with cardiac disease? Are these sensations similar to dyspnea induced by increased ventilation or flow-resistive loading in normal subjects? Although there is disagreement about whether there is only one or different kinds of dyspnea [7], no difference in the dyspnea of normals and patients has been found [16]. It is now generally accepted that dyspnea means a sensation of labored or difficult breathing [1, 5, 7, 16]. This is almost identical to the definition given by J.C. Meakins in 1934, in a clinical lecture: "Dyspnoea is the consciousness of the necessity for increased respiratory effort" [27]. An increased respiratory effort indubitably involves the respiratory muscles, especially the inspiratory muscles, which contract stronger during increasing effort. A hypothesis to explain the mechanism of dyspnea by inspiratory muscle function is that of "length-tension inappropriateness" put forward initially by Campbell and Howell in 1963 [6]. They postulated that dyspnea arises in situations in which the ventilation achieved is inappropriately small in relation to the pressure developed by the inspiratory muscles.

To assess the clinical relevance of this hypothesis, we studied 55 patients with different degrees of ventilatory impairment during quiet breathing. Inspiratory pressure was measured noninvasively using the airway occlusion method. If inspiratory airflow is prevented by occluding the airways with a valve in front of the mouthpiece, the lung volume does not increase and the inspiration is quasistatic. The negative pressure on the lung surface generated by contraction of the inspiratory muscles is transmitted all the way up to the mouth without being influenced by flow resistance or compliance of the respiratory system. Here, it can readily be measured at the mouthpiece and is termed mouth occlusion pressure. Since mouth pressure waves are distorted by responses to occlusion with a latency of 150 ms during normal breathing, Whitelaw et al. [35] recommended measuring mouth pressure 100 ms after the onset of inspiration, the $P_{0.1}$. To measure the $P_{0.1}$, a magnetic valve in front of the mouthpiece is occluded immediately with the onset of inspiration and reopens automatically after 120 ms. While the valve is occluded, inspiratory flow is zero and mouth pressure becomes more negative (Fig. 1). Although subatmospheric, $P_{0.1}$ is usually expressed with a positive sign. Using a mechanical switch, occlusion of the valve is induced at irregular intervals, between three and six times per

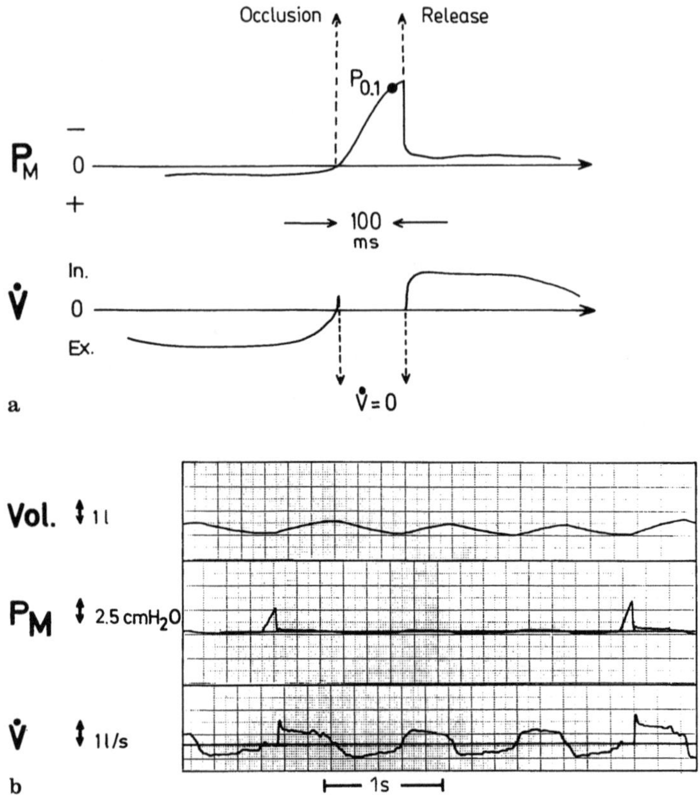

Fig. 1. A Respiratory flow ($\dot{V}$), mouth pressure (*PM*), and tidal volume (Vol.) during an occlusion of 110 ms duration. The flow during occlusion is zero and suddenly increases following release of the magnetic valve. *Closed circle*, pressure 100 ms after the onset of inspiration ($P_{0.1}$). **B** Original registration showing that occlusion does not disturb the normal breathing pattern. (From [8]).

minute, in order to avoid cortical responses and disturbance of the normal breathing pattern. Studies in anesthetized humans and animals and in trained conscious volunteers have shown that the $P_{0.1}$ is proportional to the pressure at any fixed time later in inspiration. This is the justification for accepting $P_{0.1}$ as being representative of the inspiratory pressure development throughout the entire breath [28].

Since $P_{0.1}$ reflects inspiratory pressure development and both mean inspiratory flow, V_T/T_I (V_T, tidal volume; T_I, duration of inspiration), and minute ventilation, V_E, reflect the resulting ventilation, $P_{0.1}/V_E$ and $P_{0.1}/V_T/T_I$ are adequate indices to assess the "length-tension inappropriateness." Compared to normal subjects, patients exhibiting dyspnea during walking (grades 3 and 4 of the MRC scale of breathlessness) showed, on average, a three fold increase in both indices; they were increased more than five fold in patients dyspneic at rest [11]. Since the determination of $P_{0.1}$ does not require cooperation and does not disturb the patient's comfort, we were able to study 20 patients during weaning from mechanical ventilation [11]. Ten patients, who tolerated spontaneous breathing for less than 15 min due to intolerable orthopnea (Fig. 2), showed, on the average, a significant increase in both indices compared to ten patients who tolerated spontaneous breathing for an unlimited period of time and could be extubated successfully (Fig. 2). Compared to normal subjects, the "length-tension inappropriateness" of inspiratory muscles was increased more than ten-fold in patients exhibiting intolerable dyspnea (Fig. 2). During spontaneous breathing the tube-mediated resistance to airflow is an additional burden for a patient's respiratory muscles. We showed that extubation from endotracheal tubes ranging in size from 7 mm to 7.5 mm was followed by a 47% decrease in $P_{0.1}$ which resulted in a decrease of $P_{0.1}/V_E$ and $P_{0.1}/V_T/T_I$ by more than 50% on average (Fig. 3) [10]. Therefore, to prevent inspiratory muscle fatigue and dyspnea, the period of spontaneous breathing preceding extubation should be as short as possible.

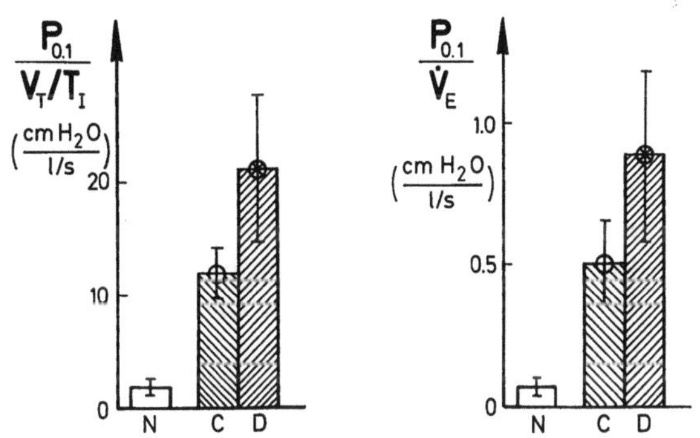

Fig. 2. $P_{0.1}$ in relation to mean inspiratory flow ($P_{0.1}/V_T/T_I$) and minute ventilation ($P_{0.1}/V_E$) during quiet breathing in intubated patients who tolerated spontaneous breathing for less than 15 min due to intolerable orthopnea (*D*) and intubated patients who tolerated spontaneous breathing for an unlimited period of time and who could be extubated successfully(*C*); *N*, mean values ± 1 SD in normal subjects. (From [11])

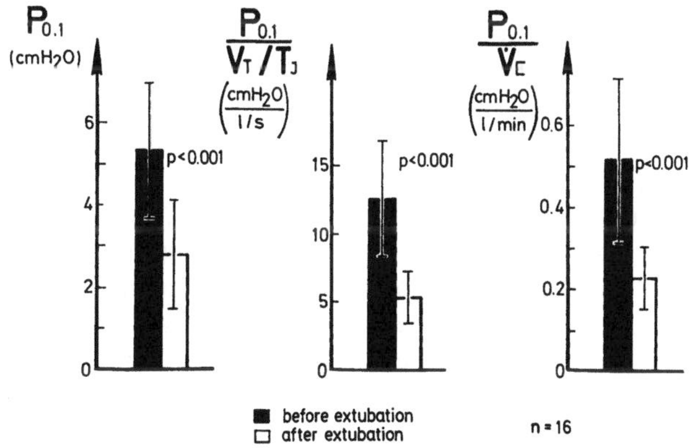

Fig. 3. Mean values ± 1 SD of $P_{0.1}$, $P_{0.1}/V_T/T_I$, and $P_{0.1}/V_E$ in 16 patients before (*closed columns*) and after (*open columns*) extubation

So far our clinically oriented studies support the hypothesis of Campbell and Howell. In more experimentally oriented studies, psychophysical techniques were used. Psychophysics is the quantitative study of the relationship between sensory stimuli and the evoked sensory response. These techniques have been reviewed recently by Killian [20, 21]. Using the technique of load detection Killian et al. [22] demonstrated that the perceived magnitude of added loads is not a function of the load itself, but is directly related to the inspiratory pressure and its duration, following a power law as in other sensory modes. A more popular technique uses scales in order to quantify the intensity of dyspnea. The revised Borg scale ranges from 0 to 10 and has simple verbal expressions tagged to numbers such as "very, very slight" up to "maximal." These descriptions are such that a doubling of the numerical rating corresponds to a twofold increase in sensation intensity. Using the Borg scale, the intensity of dyspnea in normal subjects during exercise and flow-resistive loading was closely related to the $P_{0.1}$ [1], the pleural pressure and its duration, inspiratory flow, and breathing frequency [15]. Thus, these studies reveal the close relationship between the sensation of dyspnea and the force developed by the inspiratory muscles, measured as inspiratory pressure.

Inspiratory force normally reflects respiratory effort, but effort increases disproportionately to force when a muscle is weakened. Since dyspnea occurs in patients with muscle weakness, in spite of normal inspiratory pressures the sense of respiratory effort is more likely to promote the sensation of dyspnea than the sense of force [16]. This is supported by studies in normal subjects during flow-resistive loading. For a given pressure, dyspnea was less for a subject with strong respiratory muscles than for another with weaker muscles. The interindividual variability was less when the intensity of dyspnea was correlated to pressure, expressed as a fraction of maximal inspiratory pressure (reflecting effort) rather than to pressure expressed in absolute values (reflecting force) [19]. Corresponding to these results Bradley et al. [3] showed a very close correlation between the sensation of inspiratory effort rated on the Borg scale and esophageal pressure swings expressed as a percentage of maximal inspiratory pressure in normal subjects during flow-resistive loading.

O'Conell and Campbell [29] were the first to show that dyspneic patients with chronic obstructive lung disease (COLD) generated higher pressures, expressed as percent of maximum, than the patients who were not dyspneic; however, the presence or absence of dyspnea correlated poorly with either the maximal pressure or the dynamic pressure swings alone. Based on these results, we decided to correlate $P_{0.1}$ to its maximum. The method of assessing maximal inspiratory muscle force by measuring mouth pressure, during maximal inspiratory efforts from residual volume against an occluded valve is very old and was first described in 1730 [31]. The maximal pressure achieved during complete inspiration is termed maximal static inspiratory pressure (PI_{max}); normal values have been reported by several authors [8]. The maximal pressure achieved 100 ms after the onset of a maximal inspiratory effort is the $P_{0.1max}$. Since $P_{0.1}$ reflects actual inspiratory pressure generation and $P_{0.1max}$ is representative of maximal inspiratory pressure generation, the $P_{0.1}/P_{0.1max}$ is an adequate index for assessing the relative force of the inspiratory muscles and hence respiratory effort. We first tested seven normal subjects with different alinear tubes inserted between the mouthpiece and pneumotachograph. During the last minute, prior to stopping flow-resistive loading, subjects generated a mean $P_{0.1}$ of 67% ± 18% of $P_{0.1max}$, the lowest pressure being 41% of $P_{0.1max}$. Tests were never discontinued before 15 min when $P_{0.1}$ was less than 35% of $P_{0.1max}$. Almost identical results were found during flow-resistive loading and additional exercise [8]. All subjects complained of dyspnea as the only reason for stopping the test.

In 55 patients with COLD we found a linear correlation between $P_{0.1}$ and the resistance to airflow during quiet breathing. $P_{0.1max}$ (and PI_{max}) was inversely correlated to residual volume [8]. This means that actual pressure development is increased in order to overcome the increased airflow resistance and that maximal pressures are reduced due to hyperinflation of the lungs [8]. The 30 COLD patients were studied during 5 min of exercise; 15 patients discontinued exercise between the first and fifth minute because of dyspnea, while the other 15 patients completed the 5 min. In all patients discontinuing exercise, $P_{0.1}$ exceeded 36% of $P_{0.1max}$; the average increase was 45% ± 9%. In contrast, patients with no exercise limitation had, on average, a $P_{0.1}$ of only 23% ± 7% of the $P_{0.1max}$ (Fig. 4) [8].

Similar results were found in 25 patients with interstitial lung disease. Actual inspiratory pressure development ($P_{0.1}$) was increased in order to overcome the elastic resistance to inflation of the lungs and maximal inspiratory pressures were reduced most likely due to impaired force-pressure translation [8]. In all the patients who stopped exercise prematurely, the mean $P_{0.1}$ during the last minute exceeded 40% of $P_{0.1max}$. In contrast, patients who completed exercise showed a significantly lower increase in $P_{0.1}/P_{0.1max}$ in the last minute (on average 23% ± 7%) [8].

We concluded that, in patients with different lung diseases and in normal subjects during flow-resistive loading, the increased demand on inspiratory muscles, resulting in a mean $P_{0.1}$ exceeding 36% of $P_{0.1max}$, leads to dyspnea and exercise limitation.

The $P_{0.1}/P_{0.1max}$ in 25 patients with COLD during tidal breathing is shown in Fig. 5 [9]. Five patients were treated in our intensive care unit for orthopnea and ventilatory failure (mean ± SD PCO_2: 70 ± 7 mmHg); they were not intubated. Five patients were studied during recovery from acute respiratory failure (mean ± SD PCO_2: 51 ± 5 mmHg). Fifteen outpatients were in stable condition without ventilatory failure. While normal subjects generated only 1%–2% of $P_{0.1max}$ during quiet breathing, acutely ill patients developed, on average, 22% of $P_{0.1max}$ 22 times per minute in order to achieve a minute ventilation of 8.7 l/min only. When they increased their ventilation to 11 l/min they were most dyspneic and generated 34% of their maximal pressure during each breath, which is close to the limit leading to inspiratory muscle fatigue. We noticed that patients with orthopnea showed the least efficient relationship

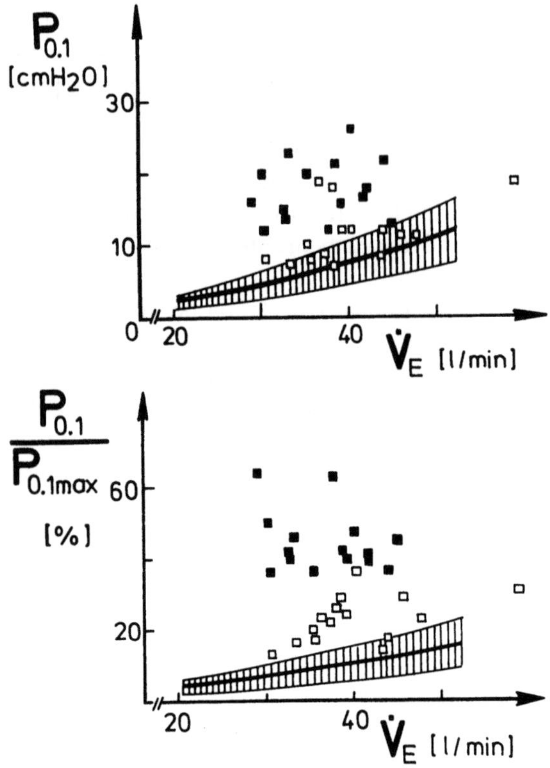

Fig. 4. $P_{0.1}$ and $P_{0.1}$ as a percentage of its maximum ($P_{0.1}/P_{0.1max}$) in relation to minute ventilation (V_E) during exercise in patients with COLD. *Closed squares*, mean values during the last minute of exercise in patients who discontinued exercise because of dyspnea; *open squares*, mean values in patients who completed exercise; *hatched area*, mean values ± 1 SD in normal volunteers. (From [8])

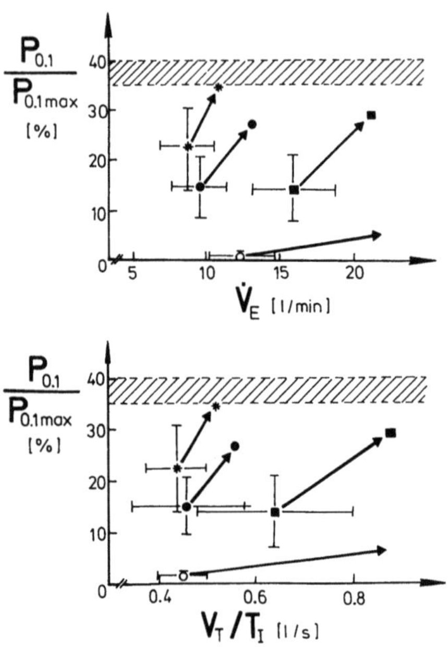

Fig. 5. Correlation of $P_{0.1}$ as percentage of its maximum and V_E and V_T/T_I (see Fig. 2 legend) at rest and during voluntary hyperventilation. *, 5 patients treated in our ICU for orthopnea and ventilatory failure; they were not intubated. ●, 5 patients studied during recovery from acute respiratory failure: ■, 15 outpatients who were in stable condition without ventilatory failure; ○, normal subjects. *Arrows*, increase in $P_{0.1}/P_{0.1max}$, V_E and V_T/T_I during voluntary hyperventilation; *hatched areas*, pressures which presumably would lead to inspiratory muscle fatigue. (From [9])

between inspiratory muscle demand, which reflects respiratory effort, and resulting ventilation. Furthermore, we concluded that in patients with COLD and in acute respiratory failure ventilation is limited by the increased inspiratory pressures that are capable of being generated indefinitely by the inspiratory muscles [9].

Our clinical studies demonstrate that intolerable dyspnea arises when $P_{0.1}$ exceeds about 35% of $P_{0.1max}$, which is near the limit expected before the onset of muscle fatigue. However, as recently reviewed by Fitting [16], based on experimental studies there is disagreement whether dyspnea is increased by inspiratory muscle fatigue at all. Although dyspnea is very closely linked to inspiratory muscle function, it depends, like other subjective sensations, on previous experience, individual personality, and psychological factors [1]. Keeping this in mind, it is not surprising that Leblanc et al. [25], in an excellent study with normal subjects and patients suffering from lung disease, obesity, muscular weakness, and cardiac disease, could explain only 69% of the variance in dyspnea by a multiple linear regression equation that included almost all variables of inspiratory muscle function.

The close relationship to muscle function implies that dyspnea should decrease by lowering inspiratory pressure generation or by increasing muscle strength. Reducing the demand on inspiratory muscles may be relatively simple when the cause of the increased demand is treatable, as in asthma; it is very difficult in chronic lung disease, neuromuscular disorders, and scoliosis.

Several attempts have been made to increase muscle strength. There is little doubt that aminophylline enhances skeletal muscle contractility. However, two recent studies by Brophy et al. [4] support our view [12] that these effects, at therapeutic concentrations, are too small to be statistically and clinically significant. The effect of training the inspiratory muscles has recently been reviewed by Worth [36]. Training can improve muscle strength and endurance and may reduce the "fear of dyspnea." Nonetheless, we should be aware of the fact that exercising a damaged or regenerating muscle may produce further irreversible damage. Before inspiratory muscle training can be recommended on a general basis additional studies are needed [36].

In 1977 Rochester et al. [33] reported a most interesting study. When patients with chronic ventilatory failure used a tank respirator their diaphragmatic activity fell to about 10% of the level measured during spontaneous breathing. Coincident with the loss of diaphragmatic activity, the patients obtained relief of dyspnea. Cropp et al. [14] studied five patients with COLD during 4–8 h of daily mechanical ventilation for 3 consecutive days. Patients experienced improvement in their sensation of dyspnea both during assisted ventilation and for several hours subsequent to its discontinuation. Thus, the effect on dyspnea is still present for some time following cessation of mechanical ventilation. This, however, has been known for as many as 10–30 years [17, 32, 34]. An improvement in the degree of dyspnea and exercise performance and of arterial blood gases during spontaneous breathing are well-known effects of mechanical ventilation used daily for a minimum of several hours (intermittent ventilation). Providing rest for overloaded inspiratory muscles, which allows recovery from fatigue and hence increases muscle contractility, is the putative effect of intermittent ventilation. This is supported by studies demonstrating an increase in (PI_{max}) [2, 13, 18, 23, 26] and maximum voluntary ventilation (MVV) [13, 23, 26] by this method. We studied the effects of noninvasive intermittent ventilation (NIV) via a nasal mask. Since 1985, as an alternative to tracheostomy and negative pressure ventilation used in the studies mentioned above, a nasal mask, first described in Lyon by Rideau [30], has been employed at the Croix Rousse Hospital. The mask is made of a silicone paste and is individually molded for each patient. About 100 patients have been treated so far with NIV by Robert et al. [32]. Thanks to the Lyon group we learned how to apply this method and have now developed a simple technique allowing production of individual masks using modern dentistry techniques and materials which ensure almost perfect stability and fit (Fig. 6) [24]. Our patients use NIV at home for about 8 per 24 h during the night. A simple volume cycled ventilator is adjusted to maintain normal oxygen pressure and mild hypocapnia [24]. We have analyzed the results from 22 patients with chronic ventilatory failure and chronic muscular weakness. There were 13 patients who suffered from restrictive ventilatory impairement due to neuromuscular disease, scoliosis, and sequelae of tuberculosis; 9 patients suffered from COLD. Corresponding to the studies mentioned above, arterial blood gases improved during spontaneous breathing within 6 weeks (Table 1). Almost all patients obtained relief from dyspnea (Table 2). In this context the most interesting finding was the significant increase in PI_{max} (Table 1) and in $P_{0.1max}$, both reflecting the increased strength of the inspiratory muscles. Since $P_{0.1}$ remained constant, we concluded that, in spite of unaltered demand on inspiratory muscles, respiratory effort was reduced due to increased muscle strength, which again supports the close relationship to the sense of dyspnea.

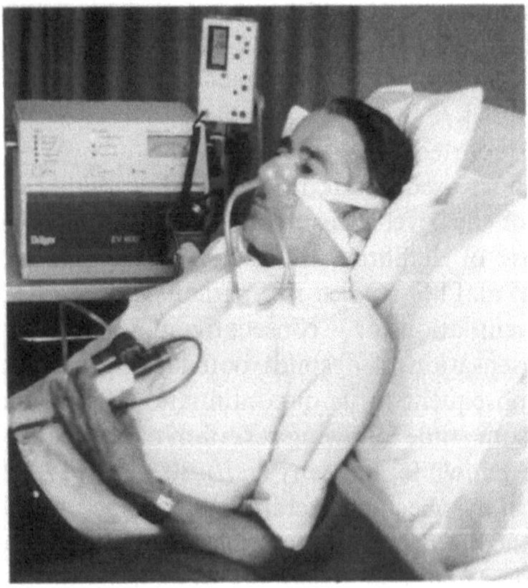

Fig. 6. A patient suffering from COLD using an individually molded mask during noninvasive intermittent ventilation (NIV)

Table 1. Noninvasive intermittent ventilation

	n	Age (years)	PCO_2 (torr)	PO_2 (torr)	VC (l)	PI_{max} (cm H_2O)
	13		56 ± 11	53 ± 10	0.87 ± 0.32	44 ± 20
Restrictive		50 ± 13	***	***	**	**
	13		45 ± 4	71 ± 7	1.01 ± 0.3	57 ± 22
	Σ = 22					
	9		52 ± 7	56 ± 6	1.8 ± 0.57	45 ± 12
COLD		57 ± 6	*	**	n.s.	**
	9		46 ± 6	65 ± 7	2.06 ± 0.45	61 ± 13

$*p < 0.05$; $**p < 0.02$; $***p < 0.0001$
Mean values ± 1 SD for arterial oxygen pressure (PO_2) and arterial carbon dioxide pressure (PCO_2) during spontaneous breathing, and for vital capacity (VC) and maximal static inspiratory pressure (PI_{max}) in 22 patients prior to treatment and during noninvasive intermittent ventilation.

Table 2. Dyspnoea-limited exercise

Exercise Change

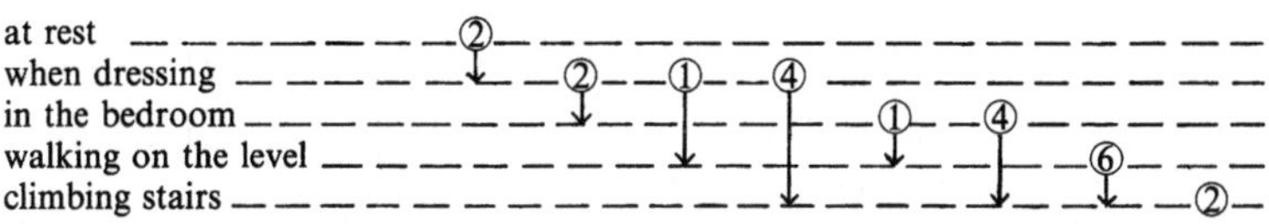

Changes in dyspnea-limited exercise during noninvasive intermittent ventilation. Circles include the number of patients and indicate the dyspnoea level before and arrows indicate the dyspnea level during therapy

Acknowledgement. We are most grateful to Mrs. I. Schaffrinski and to Miss S. Taschemski for careful preparation and translation of the manuscript.

References

1. Altose MD (1985) Assessment and management of breathlessness. Chest 88 [Suppl]:77S–83S
2. Ambrosino N, Zocchi L, Rampulla C, Buonocore M, Fracchia C, Colombini V, Brega S (1988) Intermittent negative ventilation in patients with severe chronic obstructive pulmonary disease. Eur Respir J 1 [Suppl]:65S
3. Bradley TD, Chartraud DA, Fitting JW, Killian KJ, Grassino A (1986) The relation of inspiratory effort sensation to fatiguing patterns of the diagphragm. Am Rev Respir Dis 134:1119–1124
4. Brophy CJ, Moxham J, Green M (1988) The effect of aminophylline on respiratory muscle contractility. In: Criée C-P, Hüttemann U (eds) The respiratory pump. Prax Klin Pneumol 42 [Suppl 2]:839–841
5. Burki NK (1987) Dyspnea. Lung 165:269–277
6. Campbell EJM, Howell JBL (1963) The sensation of breathlessness. Br Med Bull 19:36–40
7. Cockcroft A, Adams L (1986) Measurement and mechanism of breathlessness. Bull Eur Physiopathol Respir 22:85–92
8. Criée C-P (1988) Analysis of inspiratory mouth pressures. In:Criée C-P, Hüttemann U (eds) The respiratory pump. Prax Klin Pneumol 42 [Suppl 2]:820–826

9. Criée C-P, Neuhaus KL, Wilhelms E, Kreuzer H (1982) Mouth occlusion pressure in patients with chronic obstructive lung disease in stable state and in acute respiratory failure. Bull Eur Physiopathol Respir 18 [Suppl 4]:155–164
10. Criée C-P, Neuhaus KL, Wilhelms E, Homann K, Kreuzer H (1982) The effects of intubation on pulmonary mechanics. Bull Eur Physiopathol Respir 18 [Suppl 4]:213–219
11. Criée C-P, Neuhaus KL, Wilhelms E, Homann K, Kreuzer H (1984) Die effektive inspiratorische Impedanz–ein einfacher Index zur Abschätzung der mechanischen Eigenschaften des respiratorischen Systems. Atemw Lungenkrkh 10:260–265
12. Criée C-P, Wilhelms E, Neuhaus KL (1987) Atemmuskulatur II: Diagnostik der Ermüdung–Pharmakotherapie–Training. Atemew Lungenkrkh 4:121–127
13. Cropp A, Dimarko AF (1987) Effects of intermittent negative pressure ventilation on respiratory muscle function in patients with severe chronic obstructive pulmonary disease. Am Rev Respir Dis 135:1056–1061
14. Cropp AJ, Dimarco AF, Altose MD (1984) Effects of intermittent assisted ventilation in patients with severe COPD. Am Rev Respir Dis 129 [Suppl]:A34
15. El-Manshawi A, Killian KJ, Summers E, Jones NL (1986) Breathlessness during exercise with and without resistive loading. J Appl Physiol 61:896–905
16. Fitting J-W (1988) Dyspnoea and respiratory muscle function. In:Criée C-P, Hüttemann U (eds) The respiratory pump. Prax Klin Pneumol 42 [Suppl 2]:836–838
17. Garay SM, Turino GM, Goldring RM (1981) Sustained reversal of chronic hypercapnia in patients with alveolar hypoventilation syndromes. Am J Med 70:269–274
18. Gutiérrez M, Beroiza T, Contreras G, Diaz O, Cruz E, Moreno R, Lisboa C (1988) Weekly cuirass ventilation improves blood gases and inspiratory muscle strength in patients with chronic air-flow limitation and hypercarbia. Am Rev Respir Dis 138:617–623
19. Jones GL, Killian KJ, Summers E, Jones NL (1985) Inspiratory muscle forces and endurance in maximum resistive loading. J Appl Physiol 58:1608–1615
20. Killian KJ (1985) The objective measurement of breathlessness. Chest 88 [Suppl]:84S–89S
21. Killian KJ (1988) Assessment of dyspnoea. Eur Respir J 1:195–197
22. Killian KJ, Bucens DD, Campbell EJM (1982) Effect of breathing patterns on the perceived magnitude of added loads to breathing. J Appl Physiol 52:578–584
23. Kinnear W, Hockley S, Harvey F, Shneerson F (1988) The effects of one year of nocturnal cuirass-assisted ventilation in chest wall disease. Eur Respir J 1:204–208
24. Laier-Groeneveld G, Hüttemann U, Criée C-P (1989) Die intermittierende nichtinvasive Selbstbeatmung–Beatmung auf der Normalstation als effektive Therapie der ventilatorischen Insuffizienz. Intensivmedizin 26:392–397
25. Leblanc P, Bowie DM, Summers E, Jones NL, Killian KJ (1986) Breathlessness and exercise in patients with cardiorespiratory disease. Am Rev Respir Dis 133:21–25
26. Marino W, Braun NMT (1982) Reversal of the clinical sequelae of respiratory muscle fatigue by intermittent mechanical ventilation. Am Rev Respir Dis 125 [Suppl]:85
27. Meakins JC (1934) Dyspnea. JAMA 103:1442–1445
28. Milic-Emili J, Grassino AE, Whitelaw WA (1981) Measurement and testing of respiratory drive. In:Hornbein TF (ed) Lung biology in health and disease, vol 17:regulation of breathing, part II. Dekker, New York, pp 689–704
29. O'Connell JM, Campbell AH (1976) Respiratory mechanics in airways obstruction associated with inspiratory dyspnoea. Thorax 31:669–677
30. Rideau Y (1986) Management of wheelchair muscular dystrophy patient:prevention of death (abstract). 4th international congress on neuromuscular diseases, Los Angeles, 1986
31. Ringqvist T (1966) The ventilatory capacity in healthy subjects. Scand J Clin Lab Invest 18 [suppl 88]:1–179
32. Robert D, Laier-Groeneveld G, Leger P (1988) Mechanical assistance. Prax Klin Pneumol 42:846–849
33. Rochester DF, Braun NMT, Laine S (1977) Diaphragmatic energy expenditure in chronic respiratory failure. Am J Med 63:223–232
34. Sawicka EH, Loh L, Branthwaite MA (1988) Domiciliary ventilatory support:an analysis of outcome. Thorax 43:31–35
35. Whitelaw WA, Derenne J-P, Milic-Emili J (1975) Occlusion pressure as a measure of respiratory center output in conscious man. Respir Physiol 23:181–199
36. Worth H (1988) Training of the inspiratory muscles. Prax Klin Pneumol 42 [Suppl 2]:842–845

Muscle Fatigue in Acute Respiratory Failure

G.W. Sybrecht

In 1757 Albrecht von Haller, master physiologist of his time, published his famous work "De partibus corporis humani sensilibus et irritabilibus", in which the foundation of our understanding of muscle contractility was laid down. Since then enormous contributions have been made to our understanding of the physiology of respiration, which during von Haller's days was very limited. The astonishing fact, however, is that even today, with the accumulated knowledge of research into the control and function of gas exchange, relatively little is known about how the respiratory muscles work and especially how their action is controlled and integrated when they are loaded with a fatiguing burden. Although there has been great progress since 1951, when Fenn and Rahn stated that they could only find 200 references on the function of the respiratory muscles, and especially since 1977, when diaphragmatic fatigue in humans was first documented [1], there is still a lack of understanding in the function of the vital respiratory pump. This article deals with some aspects of respiratory muscle function that are pertinent to the practice of today's medicine.

In order to understand respiratory muscle function it is necessary to visualize two pumps in action: (1) the respiratory muscles, which maintain convective gas transport to the gas exchanging pulmonary regions and (2) the heart, which pumps blood through the vascular system. Both pumps are finely controlled in order to maintain homeostasis. The regulation of ventilation ensures that a narrow range of blood gas values, independent of work, metabolic changes, and varying inspiratory oxygen pressures, are maintained to preserve the ionic charges of key proteins which preserve the homeostasis of the "milieu interne."

Under normal conditions the respiratory muscles have no problems overcoming elastic, resistive, and inertia forces to produce an adequate alveolar ventilation, which delivers fresh gas from the atmosphere to the gas exchanging areas of the lung. Work is mainly performed both by the inspiratory muscles and those that ensure patency of the extra- and intrathoracic airways even during expiration, which at rest is passive. As pointed out above, until very recently it seemed highly unlikely, in view of the huge capacity of ventilation, that overloaded respiratory muscles might develop fatigue, rendering them unable to cope with the ventilatory demand of the body. If this should happen, the ratio of ventilatory demand to ventilatory capacity must be markedly increased. With this concept in mind it is plausible that respiratory muscle failure or fatigue occurs during very high ventilatory demands, e.g., strenuous exercise or in the presence of mechanical disadvantages of the respiratory muscles, e.g., increased impedance of the respiratory system or increased lung volumes. The two latter conditions do coincide in chronic airway obstruction. There are, however, other clinical settings with increased loads, e.g., restrictive ventilatory deficits from a variety of causes, such as pneumonia, interstitial lung diseases, pulmonary edema, adult respiratory distress syndrome, or obstructive ventilatory disturbances, such as breathing through a tracheal tube when intubated or acute bronchospasm.

The ventilatory capacity, on the other hand, may be markedly decreased by the functional status of the working respiratory muscles, e.g., secondary due to impaired perfusion, as in shock, or inadequate oxygenation due to decreased saturation of the arterial blood, or secondary to hypophosphatemia resulting in an impaired energy supply. Also postoperatively especially after abdominal surgery, the involvement of the respiratory muscles may result in compromised function. It is evident that the concurrence of a number of these disturbances predisposes to respiratory pump failure with the consequence of acute respiratory acidosis. The predisposing factors can be summarized as those interfering with energy supply (cardiac output, O_2 saturation, electrolyte imbalance: Na^+, K^+, PO_4^{2-}, HCO_3^-), work of breathing (absolute lung volume, respiratory impedance, minute ventilation), and functional status of the inspiratory muscles themselves.

In order to quantify the relation between the actual tidal respiratory muscle pressure and the generating capacity the Rohrer-Campbell analysis can be used [2]. Figure 1 illustrates how absolute lung volume, the statics of the respiratory system, and pleural pressure, as generated by the respiratory muscles, are interrelated. Under physiologic conditions the lowest (subatmospheric) pleural pressures against a closed airway using maximum inspiratory efforts are depicted by the curve P_{plmin}. $P_{\text{st(w)}}$ represents the curve which is obtained during relaxation of respiratory muscles and reflects the recoil of the chest wall, whereas the $P_{\text{st(l)}}$ curve identifies the elasticity of the lung during quasi-static inflation. The difference between $P_{\text{st(w)}}$ and the dynamic inspiratory pleural pressure

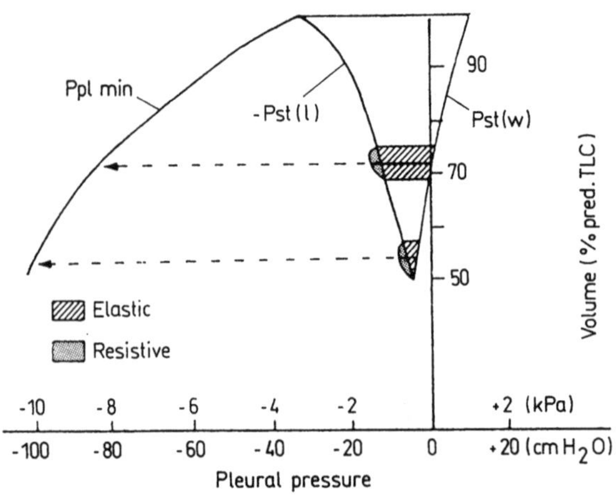

Fig. 1

(horizontal difference) indicates the actual tidal requirement, whereas the distance between $P_{st(w)}$ and P_{plmin} (horizontal sum of continuous and dashed line) identifies the pressure generating capacity. Note that only a fraction of this capacity is necessary to overcome resistive and elastic forces. The hatched area depicts the work of breathing. In comparison the same analysis for a patient with a marked increase in lung volume (emphysema) and one with severe loss of pressure generating capacity (muscle weakness) is presented in Figs. 2 and 3. Note the increase in TLC in the patient with emphysema and the fact that end-tidal volume occurs at a positive $P_{st(w)}$, indicating increased inspiratory muscle action. Although the absolute pressures generated at the increased lung volume are less than in normals, the ratio of pressure actually demanded to the

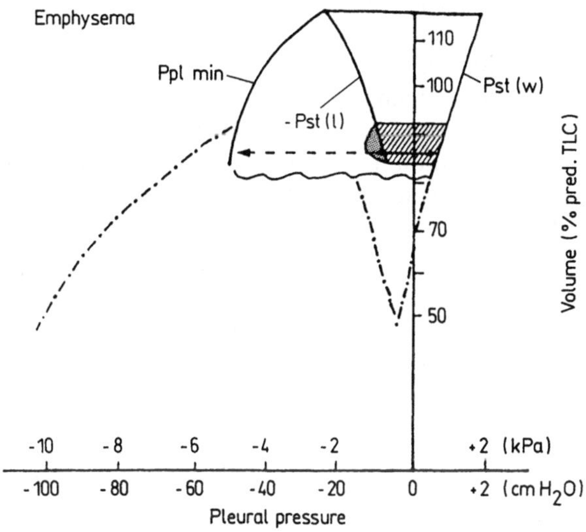

Fig. 2

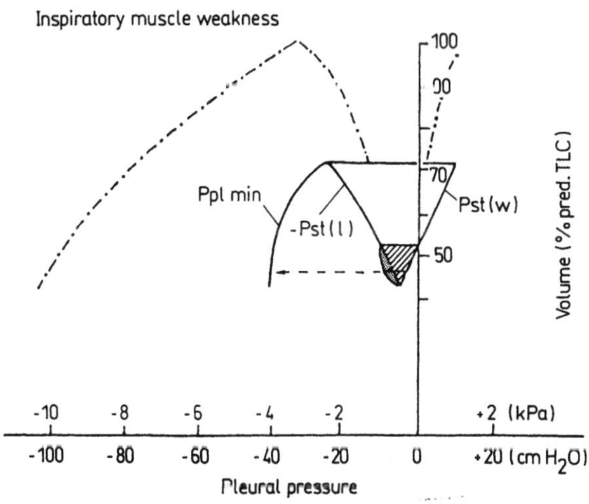

Fig. 3

potential capacity is increased, indicating a loss of reserve that could normally be recruited for exercise-induced or otherwise increased CO_2 production.

In patients with muscular weakness the pressure demand vs capacity ratio is changed due to the loss of capacity with enhanced fatigue as a consequence. It should be mentioned that there are some changes in the mechanical properties of the respiratory system of these patients; they develop both stiffer lungs due to low lung volume breathing and less compliant chest walls [4]. The presence of deficits like these, described in chronic airway obstruction and in respiratory muscle weakness, predisposes to increased arterial partial pressure for CO_2 and, with impaired pulmonary gas exchange present to, hypoxemia. The latter contributes potentially to decrease the pressure generating capacity further.

The above reasoning, using the Rohrer-Campell analysis, does not explain or take into account the timing of respiration under these conditions. It is almost always characterized by tachypnea. Bellemare and Grassino [5] developed the notion that, if the tension-time index is greater than 0.15 fatigue, of the inspiratory muscles will occur with impending acute respiratory failure. This analysis shows that very short duty cycles (T_I/T_{TOT}) are possible when high tidal transdiaphragmatic pressures, in relation to maximum transdiaphragmatic pressures, are to be generated. Resistive loading or deteriorating airway function in obstructive pulmonary disease may result in tension-time products, i.e., tension-time indices that are higher, indicating a fatiguing load.

Recently it has been proposed that a distinction should be made between manifest respiratory muscle fatigue and a state characterized by tachypnea to be called incipient fatigue [6]. The issue, however, is unresolved and for clinical purposes incipient fatigue with tachypnea as a key sign may occur before overt fatigue is present. It has been shown that in response to acute flow-resistive loads endogenous opioids are released in order to prevent the manifestation of respiratory muscle fatigue [7]. For the practicing physician it seems therefore prudent not to antagonize these opioids by administering naloxone. In the presence of clinical signs of respiratory muscle fatigue – these signs are well established and summarized in a paper by Cohen et al. [8] – all therapeutic measures taken should aim for the prevention of overt fatigue with resulting respiratory acidosis. In order to prevent this life-threatening situation the events and underlying mechanisms leading to this threat need to be diagnosed. This means that all aspects mentioned that will predispose a patient to respiratory pump failure need to be studied both clinically at the bedside and by using specific tests. Although a number of such diagnostic tests have been advocated, it should be stressed that the status and capacity of the respiratory muscles can be reliably defined using physical examination and simple bedside tests like mouth occlusion pressure and the spirogram [9]. The same applies for the weaning of patients who have been ventilated for acute respiratory pump failure.

Once the diagnosis of respiratory muscle fatigue, incipient or overt, with impending or manifest respiratory failure has been established, how can this condition be treated or reversed? A rational approach needs to take into account the underlying pathology. The first therapeutic goal, however, is to maintain or reestablish tissue oxygenation. This can be achieved by producing an arterial oxygen saturation of > 90%, i.e., a PaO_2 > 8.0 kPa, a hemoglobin concentration of > 10 g/dl, and an adequate cardiac output. Secondly, any acidemia needs to be abolished, i.e., the pH should be greater than 7.34 but not greater than 7.40. It is important to realize that the absolute value of the CO_2 tension is secondary to the pH value, and there should not be an attempt to normalize this PCO_2 value using a setting of mechanical ventilation that is potentially dangerous, i.e., which results in barotrauma of the lung.

Mechanical ventilation, on the other hand, is needed to reach the aforementioned goals. By using mechanical ventilation the work of breathing for the respiratory muscles can be minimized therefore allowing recovery of these muscles during rest. The appropriate technique for applying mechanical ventilation has been described for various clinical settings. An important precaution, however, noted by Ward et al., is the use of airway pressure-time curves in order to assess the extra efforts needed by patients when the ventilator setting, especially inspiratory flow rate, is inadequate [10].

Various pharmacologic compounds have been advocated in this situation, especially theophylline, which has been called the digitalis of the diaphragm. This drug can be used to improve inspiratory muscle contractility, but the use of this drug with its narrow therapeutic range and pure hepatic elimination is not easy and monitoring is mandatory. Catecholamines, especially dopamine, have also been documented to improve transdiaphragmatic pressure development. This drug's influence on cardiac output and the distribution of blood flow needs to be considered [11].

Applying these aforementioned principles allows the intensive care unit team to further treat the underlying disease that has led to respiratory muscle fatigue, thereby restoring the patients ability to be weaned off the ventilator once his status has improved. Complications of these clinical conditions are not rare and, depending on the nature of the first insult, multiorgan failure may be the unfortunate end result. This needs to be avoided. It should be stressed that respiratory muscle failure due to a variety of clinical conditions, if not recognized and managed competently, is the first step in a sequence of events that lead to a catastrophic clinical situation. It seems therefore prudent to look for early signs of respiratory muscle dysfunction and for the conditions that predispose a patient to this very dangerous clinical condition.

References

1. Roussos CS, Macklem PT (1977) Diaphragmatic fatigue in man. J Appl Physiol 43 (2): 189–197
2. Campbell EJM (1958) The respiratory muscles and the mechanics of breathing. Lloyd-Luke, London
3. Gribbin HR, Gardiner IT, Heinz GJ, Gibson GJ, Pride NB (1983) Role of impaired inspiratory muscle function in limiting the ventilatory to carbon dioxide in chronic airflow obstruction. Clin Sci 64:487–495

4. Pride NB (1984) Interactions between chest wall, respiratory muscles and lung function in disease. Bull Eur Physiopathol Respir 20:423–428
5. Bellemare F, Grassino A (1982) Effect of pressure and timing of contraction on human diaphragm fatigue. J Appl Physiol (Respir Environ Exercise Physiol) 53:1190–1195
6. Rochester DF (1988) Does respiratory muscle rest relieve fatigue or incipient fatigue. Am Rev Respir Dis 138:516–517
7. Scardella AT, Parisi RA, Phair DK, Santiago TV, Edelman NH (1986) The role of endogenous opioids in the ventilatory response to acute flow-resistive loads. Am Rev Respir Dis 133:26–31
8. Cohen C, Zagelbaum G, Gross D, Roussos C, Macklem PT (1982) Clinical manifestations of inspiratory muscle fatigue. Am J Med 73:308–316
9. Minde FW, Sybrecht GW (1986) Spontanatmungsfähigkeit bei Beatmung: Beurteilung mittels Spirogramm und Mundokklusionsdruck. Atemw Lungenkrkh 12 (6):275–280
10. Ward ME et al. (1988) Optimizing of respiratory muscle relaxation during mechanical ventilation. Anesthesiology 69:29
11. Aubier M, Murciano D, Menu Y, Boczkowski, Mal H, Pariente R (1989) Dopamine effects on diaphragmatic strength during acute respiratory failure in chronic obstructive pulmonary disease. Ann Intern Med 110:17–23

Coordination of Respiratory Muscles

S.H. Loring

Coordination of respiratory muscles is an important feature of normal breathing, and it may be critical for survival in subjects with disease of the lungs or chest wall. For simplicity, we sometimes think of inspiratory and expiratory muscles as single units, and we speak of inspiratory drive and expiratory drive as if they were single variables that could be characterized by a single number. Recent work on respiratory muscles has provided us with a different picture of a complex respiratory pump with fine neural control. Here, we will consider those features of the chest wall that make respiratory muscle coordination essential, and we will also consider some of the ways respiratory muscles are coordinated.

One feature of the respiratory pump that makes coordination essential is its structural complexity. All the muscles of the trunk act on structures that surround the lungs. Only some of those muscles are important for respiration. Moreover, all of the so-called muscles of respiration have important nonrespiratory functions. This multiplicity of function has importance for the muscles' respiratory action. For example, many trunk muscles are primarily postural, and only secondarily respiratory. By this I mean that they may be very effective at their postural tasks and relatively ineffective at ventilating the lungs. Such is the case for the intercostal muscles. These muscles clearly have an important postural function; the internal intercostals of one side and external intercostals of the other are activated together to rotate the trunk. Their respiratory action is much less obvious, and De Troyer and colleagues suggested that, in dogs, the intercostal muscles "might be more involved in postural movements than in respiration" (De Troyer et al. 1985b; Decramer et al. 1986). Even the diaphragm has important nonrespiratory functions, such as its expulsive function in vomiting, defecation and parturition, and its postural function in stabilizing the trunk during lifting and other tasks. Clearly, the respiratory controller has to "make do" with many postural trunk muscles that are less than optimally suited to their respiratory task.

The respiratory action of a given muscle may be limited not only by its strength and mechanical advantage but also by its degree of activation in respiratory tasks. An example of limited activation is that of the parasternal intercostal muscles. McKenzie and Gandevia found that these inspiratory muscles cannot be fully activated in a voluntary inspiratory effort. By contrast, they can be fully activated in postural efforts involving trunk flexion (McKenzie et al. 1988). Thus, the contribution of the parasternal intercostals is limited not by the muscle's strength but by the degree to which they can be activated in inspiratory efforts. The same is true for the diaphragm in maximal inspiratory efforts at low lung volumes (Hershenson et al. 1988).

The word "coordination" encompasses many ideas, and we will consider two ideas in particular. The first idea is that of the distribution of muscular activation: Which muscles are active at any instant and to what degree? This distributive function of the respiratory controller balances the activity of the various respiratory muscles to make the respiratory pump function as a unified structure without undue distortion. The second idea included in coordination is that of timing: the modulation of neural drive to various muscles to produce smoothly varying airflow. We will deal with the timing aspects of respiratory muscle coordination below.

Coordination of respiratory muscles is essential because of the ease with which the chest wall can be distorted by an imbalance of muscular forces. Certainly, the diaphragm causes distortion. Danon and colleagues studied breathing in high cervical tetraplegic subjects and showed that the diaphragm acting alone produced profound distortion of the chest wall (Danon et al. 1979). This distortion, belly out and rib cage in, could not be abolished by abdominal binders that simulated the normal abdominal muscle tone (Strohl et al. 1984). Inspiratory muscles of the rib cage, when active alone, produce an opposite distortion accompanied by inspiration (De Troyer et al. 1985a). Intercostal and other respiratory muscles also cause distortion of the thorax when their activity is not balanced by that of other muscles (Danon et al. 1979; Sampson and De Troyer 1982; Mier et al. 1985; De Troyer et al. 1985a; Ringel et al. 1985; Mortola and Sant'Ambrogio 1978). Thus, the inspiratory and expiratory neural outflow must be distributed rather precisely to achieve undistorted motion of the chest wall (De Troyer and Estenne 1984).

What is the mechanical basis for the easy distortability of the chest wall? Part of this basis is the serial arrangement of many of the muscles of respiration. Consider the diaphragm and the inspiratory intercostal muscles of the rib cage. These muscles are so arranged that they both shorten during inhalation, but if during an inspiratory effort one muscle pulls too hard, it will shorten and the other muscle lengthen. This is like two muscles, hooked end-to-end, acting in series on a load.

We studied the repiratory muscles of normal subjects and found that the rib cage muscles, the diaphragm, and the muscles of the abdominal wall could be thought of as acting in series during various static respiratory efforts (Hershenson et al. 1988). Not surprisingly, the muscles acting in series were not always of equal strength. In particular, the diaphragm was potentially able to overwhelm the inspiratory muscles of the rib cage during inspiratory efforts. The diaphragm did not overwhelm the rib cage muscles, however, and even in maximal inspiratory efforts, the diaphragm did not shorten excessively, causing collapse of the rib cage and lengthening the rib cage muscles. Instead the subjects naturally made their maximal inspiratory efforts with a less than maximal activation of the diaphragm. It is as if their respiratory controller would not allow one muscle or muscle group to overwhelm other muscles in the series.

There are other examples of muscles in series. For example, some evidence suggests that the parasternal intercostal muscles and the external intercostal muscles, both of which expand the rib cage, may be arranged in a similar way (De Troyer and Farkas 1989a). We speculate that lack of distortion of the chest wall is paramount for the respiratory controller in determining the distribution of activation among the various respiratory muscles.

The distribution of activation is critical not only among, but also within the various respiratory muscles. The intercostal muscles must be smoothly activated over many interspaces, or else the ribs of one interspace move together, the interspace narrows, and the adjacent interspaces widen (De Troyer et al. 1983). De Troyer has shown that the intercostal muscles of dogs, when active in one to three interspaces, have very slight and often unexpected respiratory effects (De Troyer et al. 1983). However, the normal activation of the intercostal muscles is over many interspaces, and the activation tends to be strongest in those areas where we might expect the intercostals to have the greatest mechanical advantage, in the upper interspaces for the inspiratory intercostal muscles and over the lowest interspaces for the expiratory intercostal muscles (Taylor 1960; De Troyer and Ninane 1986). Our own studies suggest that when active in many interspaces simultaneously, the intercostal muscles have a significant respiratory action, and this action is qualitatively different from what one would predict from observing intercostal muscle action in a single interspace or a few interspaces. For this muscle, coordinated action is essential for normal function.

Other respiratory muscles, too, comprise several parts in series, each of which must be activated to produce a concerted action. The costal and crural portions of the diaphragm must be coactivated for normal diaphragmatic function (De Troyer et al. 1983), as must the various portions of the parasternal muscles (De Troyer and Farkas 1989b).

The other major feature of coordinated breathing is timing. In addition to respiratory frequency and the divisions of the breath period, T_I and T_E, which we will not consider here, timing also includes the small differences in onset and termination of inspiratory or expiratory activity. A clear example of such coordinated timing is seen in upper airway musculature. Strohl and colleagues have shown that the alae nasi are activated slightly before the diaphragm and before the onset of inspiratory flow (Strohl et al. 1980). The pattern of activity of airway muscles is different from that of the diaphragm and other inspiratory muscles. Whereas the diaphragm electromyograph (EMG) builds throughout inspiration, the upper airway dilator muscles become highly activated early in inspiration and this activity persists (Oliven et et al. 1989). Presumably, this pattern of activation opens and rigidifies the airway before the onset of inspiratory airflow can cause narrowing or collapse (Remmers et al. 1978).

Another aspect of timing is the gradual reduction of inspiratory muscle activity during the early part of expiration (De Troyer and Estenne 1984). This early expiratory decrescendo of inspiratory activity acts to smooth the transition of airflow and to reduce the sudden accelerations and shape changes that would occur as a result of sudden changes in muscular activation. There is a similar decrescendo of expiratory activity during inspiration in dogs (De Troyer et al. 1989). The time and distribution of respiratory muscle activity in dogs depends not only on body position (Farkas et al. 1988) and mechanical factors but also on the nature of the chemical stimulus (Smith et al. 1989a, b; Fregosi and Bartlett 1989). This influence of chemical stimuli on respiratory muscle coordination may be by way of mechanoreceptors, although the mechanisms are still obscure (Smith et al. 1989b).

One of the most important features of respiratory muscle coordination is the adjustment of muscle activity with changes in posture. We know more about the effects of postural changes on breathing in dogs than in humans, but the patterns seem similar. In the supine position, in which the abdominal wall is unstressed, the abdominal viscera push the diaphragm gently into the thorax. In this position, humans breathe with minimal or no activity of the abdominal muscles (Strohl et al. 1981; Loring and Mead 1982). Perhaps it was because most early observations were made in supine animals and people that it became dogma that inspiration was active and expiration was passive. This is not so in the upright posture, where subjects normally use the abdominal muscles to maintain belly wall shape and lung volume (Loring and Mead 1982; Strohl et al. 1981). Without abdominal muscle tone, the abdomen of the upright person protrudes and the diaphragm shortens excessively, putting the inspiratory muscles on an unfavourable portion of their length-tension characteristic.

Abdominal muscles are not recruited uniformly, but are more active in the dependent regions where the transabdominal pressure difference is greatest (Strohl et al. 1981). In the upright position, expiratory abdominal muscles are also important for speech, providing the elevated intrathoracic pressures necessary for vocalization at low lung volumes (Hoit et al. 1988). There is some evidence that muscles of the rib cage also are more active in the upright postures than supine (Druz and Sharp 1981; De Troyer and Estenne 1984).

Phasic activity of abdominal muscles during expiration has important ventilatory effects, providing a substantial part of the tidal volume by driving the respiratory system below its relaxation volume. In this way, expiratory muscles spare the inspiratory muscles not only by assuring that the latter are operating at a favorable muscle length (Banzett and Mead 1985; Fitting et al. 1989) but also by actually sharing in the work of ventilation (Banzett and Mead 1985). Thus, expiratory muscle recruitment is seen as an important strategy during inspiratory resistive loading (Martin and De Troyer 1982) and in disease.

In disease respiratory muscle coordination becomes critical, and failure of this coordination can result in respiratory failure. Sleep apnea syndrome with airway obstruction is an example of a failure of respiratory muscle coordination and timing leading to morbidity (Remmers et al. 1978). With respiratory muscle fatigue, coordination may become deranged, with rib cage muscles and the diaphragm taking turns in displacing successive tidal volumes (Roussos et al. 1979). This "respiratory alternans" has been used as an indication of impending respiratory failure (Cohen et al. 1982). Diseases such as parkinsonism, that affect skeletal muscle coordination, can have profound effects on ventilatory performance (Tzelepis et al. 1988).

In summary, the respiratory pump is a mechanically complex assemblage of structures and muscles that are called upon to perform many diverse functions. Coordinating the muscles of respiration is a complex task that depends on mechanical and chemical inputs. The activation of the muscles must provide for balance between different muscles and parts of muscles to keep shape distortion to a minimum. Coordination also provides for modulation of muscle activities to optimize the mechanical efficiency or effectiveness of respiratory muscles.

Many questions remain: What are the receptors that are important for coordination? What are the principles that govern the nature of coordination? Where in the central nervous system does coordination occur, and how much of respiratory muscle coordination is learned? Is it possible that the respiratory adjustments to many common perturbations, like postural change and exercise, are *learned* as much as walking is learned? The answers should be very interesting.

References

Banzett RB, Mead J (1985) Reflex compensation for changes in operational length of inspiratory muscles. In: Roussos C, Macklem PT (eds) The thorax, part A. Dekker, New York, p 595

Cohen CA, Zagelbaum G, Gross D, Roussos CH, Macklem PT (1982) Clinical manifestations of inspiratory muscle fatigue. Am J Med 73:308–316

Danon J, Druz WA, Goldberg NB, Sharp JT (1979) Function of the isolated paced diaphragm and the cervical accessory muscles in C1 quadriplegics. Am Rev Respir Dis 119:909–919

De Troyer A, Estenne M (1984) Coordination between rib cage muscles and diaphragm during quiet breathing in humans. J Appl Physiol 57:899–906

De Troyer A, Estenne M (1985) Rib cage mechanisms in simulated diaphragmatic paralysis. Am Rev Respir Dis 132:793–799

De Troyer A, Farkas GA (1989a) Passive shortening of canine parasternal intercostals during breathing. J Appl Physiol 66:1414–1420

De Troyer A, Farkas GA (1989b) Mechanical arrangement of the parasternal intercostals in the different interspaces. J Appl Physiol 66:1421–1429

De Troyer A, Ninane V (1986) Repiratory function of intercostal muscles in supine dog: an electromyographic study. J Appl Physiol 60:1692–1699

De Troyer A, Sampson M, Sigrist S, Macklem PT (1983) Action of costal and crural parts of the diaphragm on the rib cage in dog. J Appl Physiol 53:30–39

De Troyer A, Kelly S, Zin WA (1983) Mechanical action of the intercostal muscles on the ribs. Science 220:87–88

De Troyer A, Estenne M, Ninane V (1985a) Rib cage mechanics in simulated diaphragmatic paralysis. Am Rev Respir Dis 132:793–799

De Troyer A, Kelly S, Macklem PT, Zin WA (1985b) Mechanics of intercostal space and actions of external and internal intercostal muscles. J Clin Invest 75:850–857

De Troyer A, Gilmartin JJ, Ninane V (1989) Abdominal muscle use during breathing in unanesthetized dogs. J Appl Physiol 66:20–27

Decramer M, Kelly S, De Troyer A (1986) Repiratory and postural changes in intercostal muscle length in supine dogs. J Appl Physiol 60:1686–1691

Druz WS, Sharp JT (1981) Activity of respiratory muscles in upright and recumbent humans. J Appl Physiol 51:1552–1561

Farkas GA, Baer RE, Estenne M, De Troyer A (1988) Mechanical role of expiratory muscles during breathing in upright dogs. J Appl Physiol 3:1060–1067

Fitting JW, Easton PA, Arnoux R, Guerraty A, Grassino A (1989) Diaphragm length adjustments with body position changes in the awake dog. J Appl Physiol 66:870–875

Fregosi RF, Bartlett D Jr (1989) Internal intercostal nerve discharges in the cat: influence of chemical stimuli. J Appl Physiol 66:687–694

Hershenson MB, Kikuchi Y, Loring SH (1988) Relative strengths of the chest wall muscles. J Appl Physiol 65:852–862

Hoit JD, Plassman BL, Lansing RW, Hixon TJ (1988) Abdominal muscle activity during speech production. J Appl Physiol 65:2656–2664

Loring SH, Mead J (1982) Abdominal muscle use during quiet breathing and hyperpnea in uninformed subjects. J Appl Physiol (Respir Environ Exercise Physiol) 52:700–704

Martin JG, De Troyer A (1982) The behaviour of the abdominal muscles during inspiratory mechanical loading. Respir Physiol 50:63–73

McKenzie DK, Plassman BL, Gandevia SC (1988) Maximal activation of the human diaphragm but not inspiratory intercostal muscle during static inspiratory efforts. Neurosci Lett 89:63–68

Mier A, Brophy C, Estenne M, Moxham J, Green M, De Troyer A (1985) Action of abdominal muscles on rib cage in humans. J Appl Physiol 58:1438–1443

Mortola JP, Sant'Ambrogio G (1978) Motion of the rib cage and the abdomen in tetraplegic patients. Clin Sci Mol Med 54:25–32

Oliven A, Odeh M, Gavriely N (1989) Effect of salicylate on upper airway dilating muscles in anesthetized dogs. Am Rev Respir Dis 139:170–175

Remmers JE, DeGroot WJ, Sauerland EK, Anch AM (1978) Pathogenesis of upper airway occlusion during sleep. J Appl Physiol (Respirat Environ Exercise Physiol) 44:931–938

Ringel ER, Loring SH, Mead J, Ingram RH Jr (1985) Chest wall distortion during resistive inspiratory loading. J Appl Physiol 58:1646–1653

Roussos CH, Fixley M, Gross D, Macklem PT (1979) Fatigue of inspiratory muscles and their synergic behavior. J Appl Physiol 46:897–904

Sampson MG, De Troyer A (1982) Role of intercostal muscles in the rib cage distortions produced by inspiratory loads. J Appl Physiol (Respir Environ Exercise Physiol) 52:517–523

Smith CA, Ainsworth DM, Henderson KS, Dempsey JA (1989a) Differential responses of expiratory muscles to chemical stimuli in awake dogs. J Appl Physiol 66:384–391

Smith CA, Ainsworth DM, Henderson KS, Dempsey JA (1989b) Differential timing of respiratory muscles in response to chemical stimuli in awake dogs. J Appl Physiol 66:392–399

Strohl KP, Hensley MJ, Hallett M, Saunders NA, Ingram RH Jr. (1980) Activation of upper airway muscles before onset of inspiration in normal humans. J Appl Physiol (Respir Environ Exercise Physiol) 49:638–642

Strohl KP, Mead J, Banzett RB, Loring SH, Kosch PC (1981) Regional differences in abdominal muscle activity during various maneuvers in humans. J Appl Physiol (Respir Environ Exercise Physiol) 51:1471–1476

Strohl KP, Mead J, Banzett RB, Lehr J, Loring SH, O'Cain CF (1984) Effect of posture on upper and lower rib cage motion and tidal volume during diaphragm pacing. Am Rev Respir Dis 130:320–321

Taylor A (1960) The contribution of the intercostal muscles to the effort of respiration in man. J Physiol 151:390–402

Tzelepis GE, McCool FD, Friedman JH, Hoppin FG Jr (1988) Respiratory muscle dysfunction in Parkinson's disease. Am Rev Respir Dis 138:266–271

Part 8:
Artificial Ventilation

Polymorphous Ventilation: A New Ventilation Concept for Distributed Time Constants*

G. Wolff[1], L. Eberhard[1], J. Guttmann[1], W. Bertschmann[1], J. Zeravik[2], and M. Adolph[2]

Background

After a laparotomy the arterial PO_2 is reduced and only comes back to preoperative values after about 5 days. This was already interpreted in the 1930s as being connected with another postoperative finding, the reduction in pulmonary gas volume (Beecher 1933 a, b; Beecher et al. 1933; Bendixen 1964; Bendixen and Laver 1965; Berggren 1942). In the following years many aspects of the anesthesia, surgical procedure, and mechanical ventilation were discussed as possible causes of this hypoxemia, including among others the altered pattern of diaphragmatic movements (Westbrook et al. 1973; Froese and Bryan 1974; Rehder et al. 1975), a change in the surfactant factor (Clemens et al. 1961), and the shift of blood volume. It is now generally accepted that the above mentioned reduction in pulmonary gas volume has something to do with the cause of hypoxemia. This connection is the rational basis of volume controlled ventilation with PEEP, which in the last two decades has been successfully employed with respect to oxygenation. However, it is only in recent years that an understanding of the chain of events has been conclusively elaborated and the speed at which these events develop worked out (Hedenstierna et al. 1985a, b, 1989; Rehder et al. 1985; Tokics et al. 1987): After intubation and mechanical ventilation a sizable volume of dependent lung regions collapses within 3 min. This occurs even in patients who originally had normal lungs. The regional collapse disappears after PEEP is applied and reappears when PEEP is withdrawn, both again in a few minutes. Today, there is no question that mechanical ventilation with PEEP is a powerful therapeutic method. However, it is also accepted that mechanical ventilation has undesirable and dangerous side effects and that – up to now – even the most sophisticated modes of ventilation cannot avoid these adverse effects. It is therefore still worthwhile to look for new and better modes of ventilation.

If the ventilatory pattern is changed from pattern A to pattern B, beneficial and adverse effects are observed. In order to find out which pattern is preferable for the patient, the usual study design suggests that both patterns be investigated

---

* Supported by the Swiss National Science Foundation Nr. 3.956–0.85
[1] Division for Clinical Physiology, Clinic for Cardiac and Thoracic Surgery, Department of Surgery, University of Basel, Kantonsspital, CH-4031 Basel, Switzerland
[2] Division for Anesthesiology and Operative Intensive Care Medicine, Central Clinics, Augsburg, FRG

under steady state conditions, one after the other, and the two sets of results compared. The final decision depends on the balance between the beneficial and the adverse effects of pattern A compared to pattern B.

In the present paper, however, we describe another approach, focusing not on steady states but on changes, i.e., on transient states. The first investigation consists of the endless repetition of three steps starting from reference pattern A. In step 1 pattern B is introduced gradually (as a ramp) and only for 2 min. In step 2 pattern B is gradually withdrawn again in 2 min and there is a return to the reference pattern. Step 3 is a pause of 2 min with the reference pattern. The total sequence of 6 min is repeated again and again. Let us assume that beneficial as well as adverse effects are observed; however, the beneficial effects are longer than the adverse effects; under such conditions the periodic repetition of a change of pattern may be preferable to the continuous application of the changed pattern, because of the favorable kinetic effects as a consequence of different time constants. Observations made during such transient states are described in the following section. In addition some transient states in intermittent mandatory ventilation (IMV) are reported.

PEEP is the best known mechanical measure to increase lung volume. By elevating the external expiratory airway pressure, exhalation is prematurely interrupted, i.e., the following inspiration starts at a higher level of pulmonary gas volume. If the elevated PEEP is continuously applied (PEEP step), the pulmonary gas volume eventually stabilizes at a higher level and the distribution of $\dot{V}_A/\dot{Q}$ is shifted towards higher values (Dantzker et al. 1979; Ralph et al. 1985). Some data on the time course when PEEP increments are applied for 1 h are presented in the section "stepwise changes in PEEP".

During passive expiration flow starts with an early peak before it gradually falls to zero, forming an exponential curve. If expiratory flow is diminished, the preset time period for expiration can become too short, so that the onset of the following inspiration interrupts expiratory gas flow before zero flow is reached. Exhalation, therefore, is prematurely interrupted, i.e, the expiratory tidal volume is smaller than the inspiratory tidal volume. If ventilation with such a pattern is continued, pulmonary gas volume gets larger from breath to breath and airway pressure is gradually increased, until – in a new steady state – the inspiratory and expiratory tidal volumes are again equal and pulmonary gas volume stabilizes. This can occur for a normal expiratory time (TE) if the expiratory flow resistance is increased, as for example in obstructive lung disease. It can also hold true for normal flow resistance if TE is altered to an especially short time, as for example with inverted ratio ventilation. If the increased expiratory flow resistance is inhomogeneously distributed, a given TE allows some fast compartments to empty completely while some slow compartments at the end of expiration still retain gas; the enlargement of pulmonary gas volume is then unequally distributed. Use of the flow pattern as another measure to interfere with expiration is described in the section "The Time Course of Passive Expiration."

In order to clarify these questions we designed a noninvasive measuring system. Its temporal resolution is high enough to allow the results to be assessed breathwise (Brunner and Wolff 1988). During the measurements the short connection tube (connecting the endotracheal tube with the Y-piece) is exchanged with the "measuring head"; the measuring head and the connection tube have the same length and identical volumes. Six of the seven measured analogue signals are picked up in the measuring head (Fig. 1): gas flow (Fleisch pneumotachograph), airway pressure (pressure transducer), and dry fractions of oxygen, carbon dioxide, nitrogen, and argon (mass spectrometer, Centronic MGA 200). The seventh signal is the pressure in the esophageal balloon. The measuring signals are digitalized and reproduced with computer assistance; the results are depicted on the screen breath-by-breath at the bedside; the measuring system and computer remain in the background. Thus, the circle (investigator to ventilator to patient to measuring head to transducers to computer to results on the screen to investigator) is closed. Carbon dioxide delivery and oxygen uptake are analyzed breath-by-breath and averaged per minute; compliance of the total respiratory system and of the lung are analyzed and the accessible pulmonary volume or pulmonary gas volume is estimated by means of the nitrogen washout maneuver. Our measuring system allows us to analyze all data breath-by-breath. Therefore, in IMV it is possible to analyze the mandatory breath (MB) separately from the spontaneous breaths (SBs) and to compute the mean of the MBs and the mean of the SBs separately. Such a study on the transient states within the IMV cycle is reported in the following section.

When we started this study, we realized that the number of patients in Basel with severe acute respiratory insufficiency (ARI, definition of Ralph et al. 1985) had become so small that it was no longer possible to complete such a study in a reasonable time. Therefore, having learned that numerous patients with ARI were being transferred by helicopter to Augsburg and that our colleagues there were interested in investigating ARI patients in detail, we set up a second measuring system in Augsburg and investigated these patients according to a common protocol. Moreover, we needed a respirator with a bidirectional computer interface and a manufacturer interested in modifying the machine for the N_2 washout maneuver; the electronic ventilator (EV-A, Draeger Werk AG,

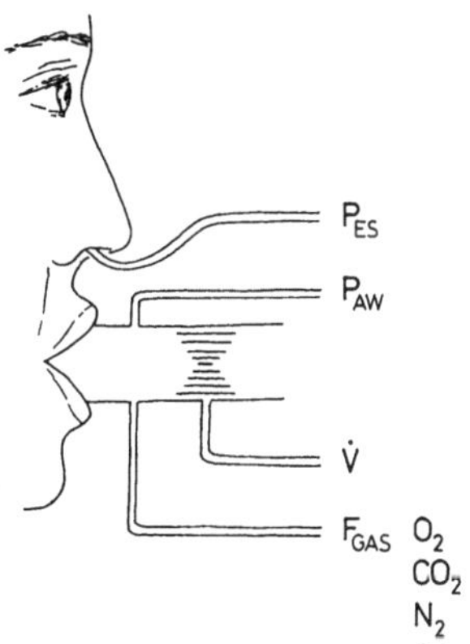

Fig. 1. The measuring head where six signals are taken: airway pressure (P_{AW}), gas flow ($\dot{V}$), and gas composition (fraction of O_2, CO_2, N_2, and argon); P_{ES}, pressure in the esophageal balloon. Patientwards the measuring head is connected with the endotracheal tube (or with the mouthpiece) and machinewards with the Y-piece (or with the atmosphere). The dimensions of the measuring head (volume and length) are the same as those of an otherwise normal connecting tube. The airway resistance of the measuring head is identical to the airway resistance of the Fleisch pneumotachograph no. 2, i.e., the resistance is negligible

Lübeck) came very close to our requirements and we were therefore eager to have the engineers of Draeger Werk AG in our group as well. Participating investigators are listed in the acknowledgements.

Transient Changes in Airway Pressure

PEEP Wave

In 1979 we investigated the exact temporal correlation between a PEEP change in wave form and the consecutive alteration of the arterial O_2 partial pressure (PaO_2) measured with an intra-arterial oxygen probe (Wolff et al. 1979) (Fig. 2). Under volume controlled respiration, PEEP was slowly and steadily raised (by 10 mbar in 2 min), then equally slowly and steadily lowered again to the original level. It was then left unaltered for 2 min. This 6 min sequence, which we called "PEEP wave", was repeated for some hours. Airway pressure and PaO_2 were registered; 90 s after the beginning of the PEEP wave the PaO_2 signal began to rise and 2 min later to fall again. The delay time of the instruments came to about 90 s and therefore the PaO_2 itself appeared to rise and fall with the PEEP without substantial delay. The increase in PaO_2 during the rise of PEEP within the first wave can reach 100 mm Hg. However, during the drop in PEEP the PaO_2 does not return to its initial value but comes to rest about 10 mm Hg higher. Thus, when the PEEP wave was repeated, each new rise of the PaO_2 began at a higher initial value, and the initial values themselves formed a climbing curve towards a new PaO_2 level, which in this case would lie perhaps 80 mm Hg higher than in the beginning. Figure 3 shows PaO_2 and the simultaneously specified cardiac output. The cardiac output fell with every PEEP wave but climbed afterwards to the starting point again. Obviously, the gradual rise of PaO_2 was not conditioned through a corresponding gradual reduction of the cardiac output. We may conclude: (a) that the intrapulmonary function change resulting from the PEEP wave can itself outlast that wave and (b) that the advantages of the PEEP wave can last longer than its disadvantages – whatever mechanisms are involved. Moreover, the shift of low $\dot{V}_A/\dot{Q}$ ratios towards higher ones by a PEEP wave has a larger time constant than the PEEP wave, which is its cause.

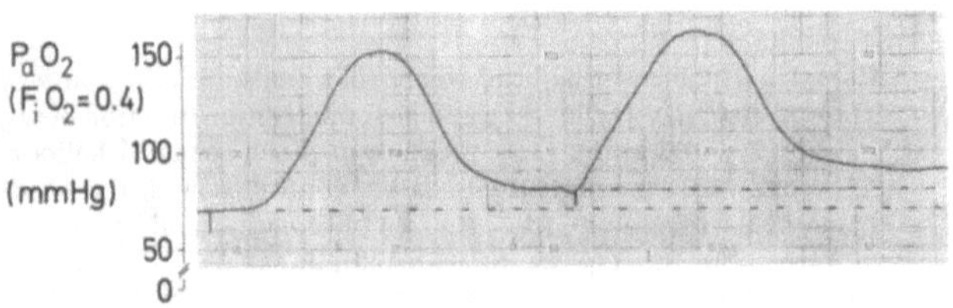

Fig. 2. Continuously measured PaO_2 (intra-arterial electrode in the femoral artery) in a patient with acute respiratory insufficiency. First and second PEEP wave. Rise of PEEP 2 min, decrease of PEEP 2 min, pause 2 min. See text

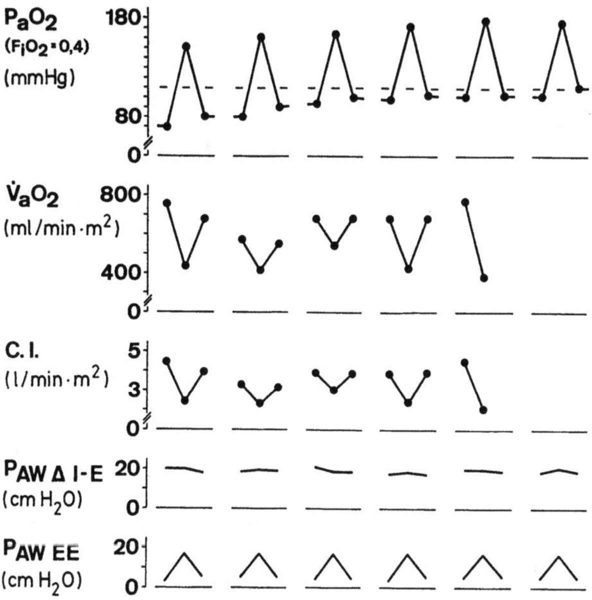

Fig. 3. PaO_2, arterial oxygen transport ($\dot{V}aO_2$), cardiac index (C.I.; thermo dilution technique), inspiratory/expiratory difference in airway pressure ($P_{AW}\Delta I - E$) and PEEP (P_{AWEE}) in the first six PEEP waves. Same run of PEEP waves as in Fig. 2. Basic PaO_2 rises from one PEEP wave to the other, but basic C.I. stays constant. See text

Intermittent Mandatory Ventilation

We followed patients after heart surgery and studied the changeover from controlled ventilation (CPPV) to IMV and from IMV to continuous positive pressure breathing (CPPB) or continuous positive airway pressure (CPAP). We found that during the changeover from CPPV to IMV the pulmonary gas volume (APV) accessible by N_2 washout remains constant (Wolff et al. 1986). During the changeover from IMV to CPAP the APV falls a small but statistically significant amount. The cardiac output rises during the changeover from CPPV to IMV a small but significant amount and remains constant during the changeover from IMV to CPAP. Additionally, we zoomed in on the IMV cycle and analyzed separately MBs and SBs. The end-tidal fraction of CO_2 (FCO_2-et) and the alveolar efficiency of CO_2 elimination (alv. eff CO_2) are larger in SB than in MB (Fig. 4). This shows that under IMV two important goals are reached in the lung, if not simultaneously at least in satisfactory succession. In a sequence of breaths, these are: (1) pulmonary gas volume and oxygenation are maintained with the large MBs applied every 15 s and with PEEP; (2) the match of perfusion and ventilation is more favorable during the SBs taken by the patient every 3 s so that CO_2 elimination in the SBs is increased. Thus, under IMV the oxygenation and the elimination of CO_2 are optimized not in the same but in consecutive breaths, in the SBs and in the MBs. We conclude that it is not

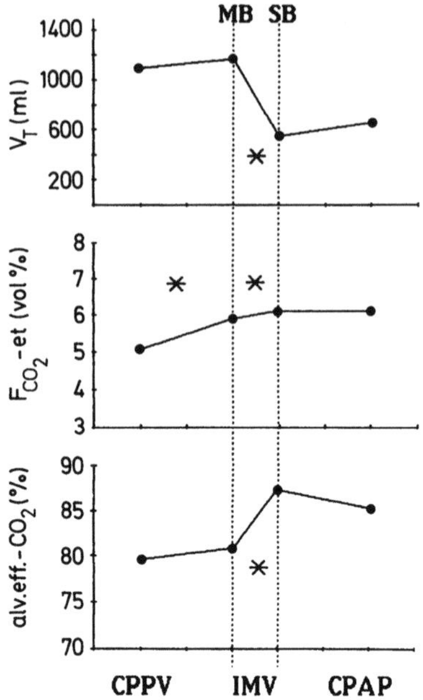

Fig. 4. Tidal volume (V_T), end-expiratory CO_2 fraction (F_{CO_2}*-et*) and alveolar efficiency for CO_2 elimination (*alv. eff. -CO*$_2$). Mean values of ten patients during weaning from a ventilator after open heart surgery. *CPPV*, continuous positive pressure ventilation; *IMV*, intermittent mandatory ventilation; *CPAP*, spontaneous breathing with continuous positive airway pressure. In the spontaneous breath (*SB*) alv. eff. CO_2 is increased by 8% over the mandatory breath (*MB*). See text

necessary that all exercises are completed simultaneously to achieve good breathing form.

Stepwise Changes in PEEP

A Single PEEP Step

Another investigation concentrated on the time course of distensibility (of the total respiratory system) after an increment in PEEP was set. In ARI patients PEEP was at first at an average of 11 mbar and was then increased with an increment of 7 mbar. $\dot{Q}_S/\dot{Q}_T$ was 22% initially and 10% lower (average of paired differences) after 1 h with the higher PEEP. In the same period cardiac output (CO) decreased by 1 l/min starting from 5.8 l/min.

The measured pulmonary gas volume (APV assessed with the N_2 wash out maneuver or $APV_{(n)\ measured}$) and the compliance of the total respiratory system (C) were determined in each investigation so that the two point equation for static distensibility could be used:

$$\Delta P = \Delta V \times 1/C \tag{1}$$

Transformation of Eq. 1 into Eq. 2 yields:

$$\Delta V = \Delta P \times C \tag{2}$$

The APV which should be expected after the change of PEEP ($APV_{(2)\,\mathrm{predicted}}$) can thus be estimated by Eq. 3:

$$APV_{(2)\,\mathrm{predicted}} = APV_{(1)\,\mathrm{measured}} + [C \times (\mathrm{PEEP}_{(2)} - \mathrm{PEEP}_{(1)})] \quad (3)$$

Accordingly, 1 h after the alteration of PEEP the APV is determined again ($APV_{(2)\mathrm{measured}}$) and the measured volume difference ($\Delta APV_{\mathrm{measured}} = APV_{(2)\mathrm{measured}} - APV_{(1)\mathrm{measured}}$) is compared with the predicted volume difference [$\Delta APV_{\mathrm{predicted}} = C \times (\mathrm{PEEP}_2 - \mathrm{PEEP}_1)$]. $\Delta APV_{\mathrm{measured}}$ is 1.5 times larger than $\Delta APV_{\mathrm{predicted}}$ (Fig. 5). The quotient $\Delta APV_{\mathrm{measured}}/\Delta PEEP$ is the difference in volume divided by the change in pressure and therefore describes a distensibility of the lung. Obviously, for the same situation there are two almost totally different elasticities; what are their differences?

The C we are familiar with is analyzed within one breath; it fixes the relationship between volume and pressure which can be examined within one breath cycle, that is within a few seconds; so C quantifies a "rapid distensibility." In contrast to this, the quotient $\Delta APV_{\mathrm{measured}}/\Delta PEEP$ covers the relationship between a variation of pressure ($\Delta PEEP$) and the consecutive alteration of volume ($\Delta APV_{\mathrm{measured}}$) and therefore quantifies a "slow distensibility." So the "slow distensibility" observed over an hour is considerably larger than the "rapid distensibility" observed within the space of one breath. Our investigation of $\Delta APV_{\mathrm{measured}}/\Delta\mathrm{PEEP}$ shows that the lung has several mechanical features and that their time constants are broadly distributed; they may partially lie within the range of the breath cycle but some time constants can also be much larger.

A Cycle of PEEP Steps

The goal of the following investigation was to estimate the upper limit of these time constants. Every hour the PEEP was altered a step: from an initial value of

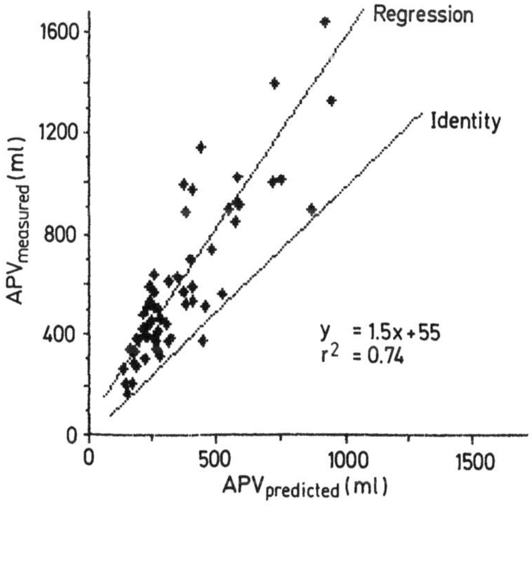

Fig. 5. Measured pulmonary volume ($APV_{measured}$) vs predicted pulmonary volume ($APV_{predicted}$) in 14 patients with acute respiratory insufficiency, in which PEEP is increased in steps of 6 mbar from 0 to 24 mbar. The actual measured APV is 1.5 times larger than predicted on the basis of the actually measured compliance. See text

12 mbar (reference situation 1) to 18 mbar, then to 24 mbar, back to 18 mbar, then back again to the initial value (reference situation 2), then to 6 mbar, to 0 mbar, to 6 mbar, and finally returned to the initial value of 12 mbar (reference situation 3). Each hour after a change in PEEP the patient was monitored while in the new steady state; the entire PEEP step cycle lasted 9 h (Fig. 6). We found that after high PEEP (reference situation 2) the APV rises above the initial value (reference situation 1) and after low PEEP (reference situation 3) the APV falls below it, i.e, a change in the pulmonary volume, brought about by a change in PEEP, does not level out after an hour.

We may draw the following three conclusions: (1) Certain mechanical properties of the lung can only be described with time constants which last considerably longer than the breath cycle time of the given respiratory frequency; the length of individual time constants can lie in the region of hours. (2) Long and short time constants are both effective at the same time. (3) Very long time constants cannot be detected during a mechanical ventilation which repeats breaths with identical flow patterns in monotone.

A variety of mechanisms could be responsible for the slow distensibility, for example, slow viscous changes in the pulmonary tissues or a slow displacement of the intrapulmonary blood volume. Our measurements do not allow any assertions to be made regarding the responsible mechanisms.

The Time Course of Passive Expiration

Theory of Passive Emptying

If we allow the simplification that the respiratory system is one compartment, its expiratory behaviour is sufficiently identified with a C and a flow resistance (R)

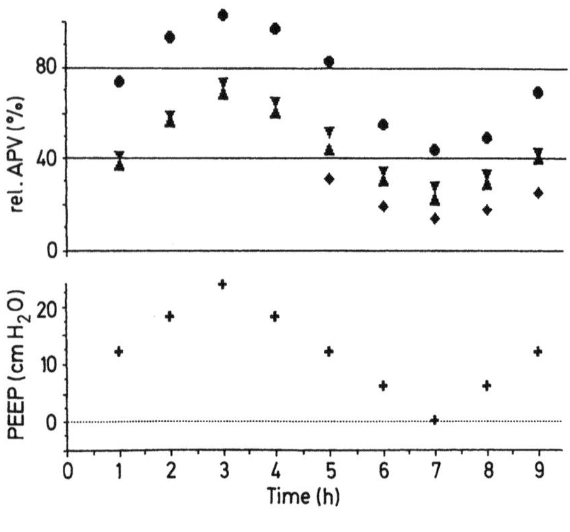

Fig. 6. Changes of pulmonary volume in four patients when a PEEP cycle is applied. *Above*, lung volume assessed with the N_2 washout (*APV*, accessible pulmonary volume) is given in % of the expected pulmonary volume in the sitting position estimated on the basis of anthropometric data (*rel. APV*). *Below*, PEEP ± time when PEEP was changed (e.g., PEEP started with 12 cm H_2O at 0 h and was increased to 18 cmH_2O at 1 h, etc.). See text

and thus can be comprehensively described with the time constant ($\tau = C \times R$). In this simplified monocompartmental model the expiratory flow ($\dot{V}$) decreases exponentially over the course of expiration in accordance with Eq. 4, in which $\dot{V}_0$ is the initial flow (peak expiratory flow in our simplified monocompartmental model); t the time; TE the expiratory time; and τ the time constant. Thus:

$$\dot{V} = \dot{V}_0 \times \mathrm{e}^{-t/\tau} \tag{4}$$

The expired volume (V) at a specified time starting from the beginning of expiration can be calculated with the integral:

$$V_{TE} = \int_0^{TE} \dot{V} \mathrm{d}t = \dot{V}_0 \times \tau \times (1 - \mathrm{e}^{-TE/\tau}) \tag{5}$$

Compartments with a long τ thus need more time for expiration. If there is no extended breathing time (TE) available, the slow compartments do not exhale completely during expiration (Fig. 7), so that the following inspiration begins before the expiratory flow has fallen to zero. Therefore, at the time this expiratory exhalation has been terminated by the onset of the following inspiration, pulmonary gas volume has not yet come down to functional residual capacity (FRC) and the tidal volume of the following inspiration is grafted onto an enlarged lung volume. Therefore, if TE gets shortened, the lung volume rises from breath to breath until a new equilibrium state is reached and the lung volume remains constant at a larger level; the new state is characterized by a higher end-inspiratory airway pressure and, consequently, by a higher level expiratory flow pattern.

Accordingly, with constant PEEP the completeness of expiration is determined by two factors which act independent of each other:

1. The pathological alterations in the respiratory system which slow down the expiratory flow pattern. The functional weight of these pathological alterations can be quantitatively described with the expiratory time constant (τ).
2. The expiratory time (TE) which the ventilatory pattern – chosen by the medical team – de facto allows for expiration.

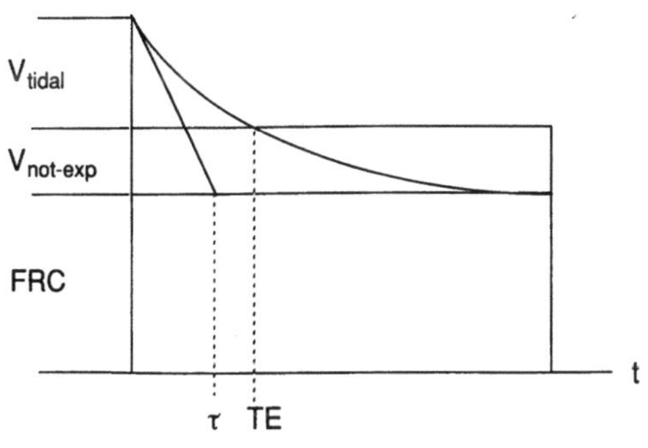

Fig. 7. A passively emptying volume model. The emptying process is fully described by the time constant (τ). An unlimited expiratory time (TE) allows an equilibrium of the model and atmospheric pressures to be reached so that gas flow becomes zero. This volume corresponds to the functional residual capacity (FRC). When TE is shorter emptying is incomplete, and a certain volume is not expired ($V_{not-exp}$). The volume which can be expired during TE is the actual tidal volume (V_{tidal}). See text

If we describe passive expiration with the physical interrelations of Eq. 5, it is obvious that the expired volume is determined predominantly by TE/τ. Consequently, the actual *TE* setting at the ventilator and the patient's momentary pathology, quantified by τ, together form the expiratory quotient TE/τ, which tells how much of the volume inspired, in addition to the FRC, is exhaled. If *TE* is three times longer than τ, 95% of tidal volume is expired. With either a larger *R* and/or a larger *C* τ increases proportionally, and a proportionally longer *TE* is needed for complete expiration.

Indeed, the *I/E* ratio (inspiration time/expiration time or inspiration time/breath cycle time) has been used for many years to describe the respiration pattern and so TE has obviously long been taken into consideration. However, the duration of inspiration does not influence the expiratory exhalation, and thus the piece of information, that *TE* alone holds throughout, is unfortunately lost by the formation of the quotient *TI*/*TE*. Inspiratory gas flow and inspiratory time define tidal volume, and all three together determine the intrapulmonary gas distribution. Nevertheless, during expiration it is not a specific ratio of *TI* to *TE* that determines the process of exhalation, but a specific duration of *TE*, i.e, so and so many ms. With the quotient of TE/τ the *TE* is normalized with the individual momentary expiration pathology, τ. After these theoretical considerations we were interested in discovering how the expiratory quotient, TE/τ, is manifested in practice.

The Effect of a Change in TE

In the last paragraph it was demonstrated that, in the theoretical monocompartmental model, incomplete expiration can be created by forcing the following inspiration to begin before the expiratory gas flow has fallen to zero. This can be the case for normal *TE* if the expiratory flow resistance is increased, as for example in obstructive lung disease. It can also hold true for normal flow resistance if *TE* is altered to an especially short time, as for example with inverted ratio ventilation. This poses the questions whether these theoretical findings hold in patients ventilated for ARI and whether TE/τ is clinically important as a quantitative measure of the incompleteness of expiration.

We therefore measured, in patients mechanically ventilated for ARI, the *C* of the total respiratory system (C_{trs}), the *R* of the total respiratory system, which includes the resistance of the endotracheal tube (R_{trs}), and the external expiratory resistance (R_{ext}) localized in the expiratory valve. Expiratory τ was calculated according to:

$$\tau = C \times (R_{trs} + R_{ext}) \qquad (6)$$

The three respiration variables inspiratory flow ($\dot{V}$), tidal volume (VT), and end-inspiratory pause (EIP) clearly specify the inspiratory flow pattern. The supplementary variable *TE* then specifies the breathing frequency. The changes in the respiration pattern and their bearing on the pulmonary function indices (function values) are given in Tables 1–6 as mean values and as paired

Table 1. Ventilatory setting I

Pattern	PEEP cm H_2O	Δ	VT (ml)	Δ	AF b/min	Δ
Flow +	11.3	+ 0.1	1034	− 7	14.5	0.0
Flow −	11.3	− 0.4	1032	− 41	14.5	− 0.1
EIP	11.3	− 0.5	1028	− 10	14.3	− 0.5
Flow +, EIP	11.3	+ 0.1	1025	+ 14	14.3	− 0.7

b/min, breaths per minute

Table 2. Ventilatory setting II

Pattern	$\dot{V}$Im ml/s	Δ	EIP ms	Δ	TE ms	Δ
Flow +	529	+ 502	49	− 36	2034	+ 1012
Flow −	538	− 182	53	+ 74	2080	− 871
EIP	534	− 7	52	+ 942	2113	− 764
Flow +, EIP	536	+ 493	57	+ 992	2129	+ 170

Table 3. Usual observations

Pattern	VdS CO_2 ml	Δ	$\dot{V}CO_2$ ml/min	Δ	C.I. L/min/m²	Δ	$\dot{Q}S/\dot{Q}T$ %	Δ
Flow +	299	+ 13	236	− 20	3.25	− 0.26	22.0	+ 1.5
Flow −	298	+ 20	238	− 9	3.25	− 0.48	21.5	− 3.4
EIP	293	− 32	239	+ 2	3.13	− 0.16	20.8	− 2.8
Flow +, EIP	294	− 51	232	− 2	3.29	− 0.18	22.2	− 0.6

Table 4. Additional observations I

	TE ms	Δ	$\dot{V}$Ee ml/s	Δ	APV ml	Δ	IPEEP Cm H_2O	Δ
Flow +	2034	+ 1012	102	− 83	2043	− 279	12.9	− 0.9
Flow −	2080	− 871	111	+ 308	2232	+ 496	12.9	+ 4.5
EIP	2113	− 764	102	+ 252	2151	+ 484	12.8	+ 3.3
Flow +, EIP	2129	+ 170	92	− 27	2197	− 28	12.8	+ 0.1

Table 5. Additional observations II

Pattern	Paw (mean) cm H_2O	Δ	$\dot{V}E_{max}$ ml/s	Δ	V_{rest} ml	Δ
Flow +	21.4	− 3.1	1643	− 36	85	− 57
Flow −	20.9	+ 7.1	1648	+ 192	95	+ 204
EIP	21.1	+ 8.5	1614	+ 55	88	+ 165
Flow +, EIP	20.7	+ 2.7	1657	− 75	81	+ 10

Table 6. Additional observations III

	C_{trs}		τ		TE/τ		PEEP – IPEEP	
Pattern	ml/cm H_2O	Δ	ms	Δ	—	Δ	cm H_2O	Δ
Flow +	45	0	636	+ 48	3.6	+ 1.6	1.7	– 0.9
Flow –	48	– 13	682	– 127	3.5	– 1.2	1.6	+ 4.9
EIP	46	– 10	676	– 67	3.5	– 1.2	1.5	+ 3.8
Flow +, EIP	47	– 1	652	+ 40	3.9	0.0	1.5	0.0

differences. Still, a change in any one of the three respiration variables is not without further consequences for the patient (Fig. 8). For example, if only $\dot{V}$ were lowered the *TI* and the breath cycle time (*Tc*) would be lengthened, the respiratory frequency (*RF*) would thus be lowered, and CO_2 would be retained. In our investigation, $PaCO_2$ and thus RF are kept constant by means of an additional adaptation of the *TE*. The initial respiration setting and the alterations of the individual ventilatory variables are described in Tables 1 and 2. The general observations are given in Table 3 and the additional observations in Tables 4, 5, and 6.

A surprising finding in the measurement of the initial situation was that the end-expiratory gas flow ($\dot{V}$Ee) did not fall to zero but (on average) only reached about 100 ml/s; the process of passive expiration was therefore not completed when the following inspiration started. If – at the end of expiration – gas is still flowing, a driving pressure must be available at that time, i.e., at the end of expiration there must still be available an intrapulmonary pressure which is higher than PEEP. Pepe and Marini (1982) called this intrapulmonary pressure "intrinsic PEEP." We therefore measured the intrinsic PEEP (IPEEP); the maneuver to assess IPEEP is shown in Figs. 9 and 10.

Table 5 shows that in the reference situation IPEEP was up to 1.3 mbar higher than PEEP; *TE* was at 2000 ms and *APV* at 2100 ml. Starting from this reference pattern (*VT*, 11 ml/kg; $\dot{V}$, 500 ml/s; EIP, 50 ms; RF, 14 b/min; PEEP, 11 mbar), we varied *TE*: (a) by raising $\dot{V}$ by 100%; (b) by lowering $\dot{V}$ by 40%; (c) by administering an EIP of 1 s, and (d) by raising $\dot{V}$ by 100% together with administration of an EIP of 1 s (see Fig. 8). PEEP was kept constant; $PaCO_2$ and RF did not change. We now looked for a correlation between $\dot{V}Ee$, TE/τ, IPEEP, and APV and the interdependence of the changes in the respiratory pattern already described.

IPEEP is scarcely altered by a rise in flow, shows a clear rise during a reduction of flow and during EIP, and does not change during the combination of a rise in flow and EIP. The incompleteness of expiration thus increases with inverted ratio ventilation and increases clearly during respiration with an EIP. As expected, APV is larger in both of these situations by about 500 ml. Conversely, during the increase in flow, *TE* is prolonged by about 1000 ms and APV falls by about 300 ml. Thus, lung volume is not only dependent on PEEP,

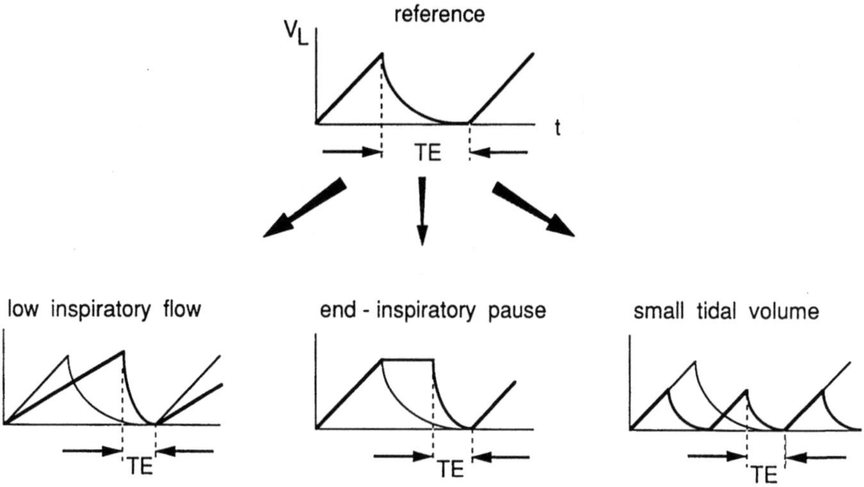

Fig. 8. In order to decrease expiratory time (*TE*) in the volume controlled ventilated patient there are three possible ways to change the ventilatory setting: (1) reduction of inspiratory flow (*below, left*); (2) application of an end-inspiratory pause (*below, center*), and (3) reduction of the tidal volume forces (*below, right*) to increase respiratory frequency and avoid CO_2 retention due to the reduction in alveolar minute volume. The reduction in respiratory frequency shortens respiratory cycle time and consequently also TE. In the three *lower* diagrams, the reference pattern from the upper *diagram* is drawn as a *thin line*; the new pattern is superimposed as a *thick line*

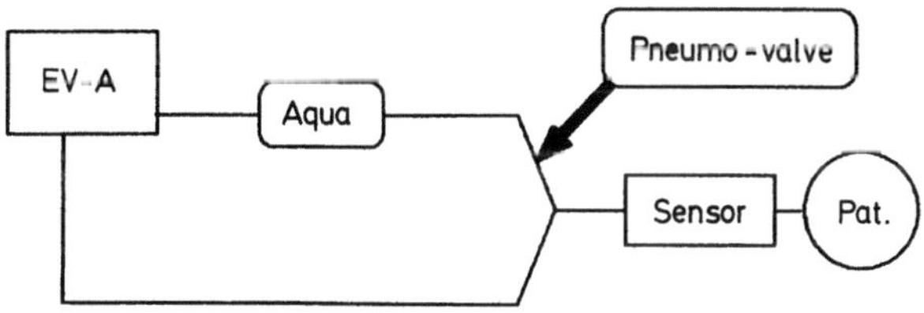

Fig. 9. Tubings in a ventilated patient which allow the performance of an intrinsic PEEP maneuver. A valve is inserted in the inspiratory tube (between nebulizer and Y-piece). This valve can close off the inspiratory line directly at the patient

but also on the completeness of expiration, which was manipulated in this study by inspiratory flow and the EIP.

The difference between IPEEP and external PEEP (PEEP) is called auto-PEEP (auto-PEEP = IPEEP − PEEP). Figure 11 presents auto-PEEP vs TE/τ; an impressive correlation is apparent. Auto-PEEP is directly dependent on TE/τ and this dependence is clearly demonstrated within a range of $TE/\tau = 1$ to $TE/\tau = 9$. When $\dot{V}Ee$ is plotted against auto-PEEP a clear dependency is shown as well (Fig. 12). The plot of $\dot{V}Ee$ vs TE/τ likewise shows an exponential dependence (Figs. 13 and 14). The expiration is practically complete if the expiratory quotient has a value greater than 3. These observations were condensed

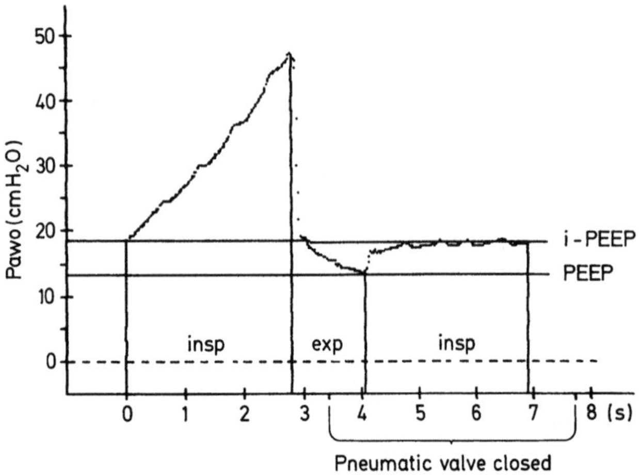

Fig. 10. Recording of airway pressure (*Pawo*) during normal inspiration (*insp*) and expiration (*exp*). During expiration (at 3.4 s) the pneumatic valve (see Fig. 9) is closed by the investigator. Then, as soon as the next inspiration starts, the expiratory valve in the ventilator closes automatically. The ventilator delivers inspiratory gas against the closed pneumatic valve; the inspiratory pressure limit is thus exceeded and the inspiratory gas flow stops. For the total duration of an inspiration (from 4.1 s to 6.8 s) the patient is totally shut off from the ventilator and no volume change is possible at the endotracheal tube. Within this time a redistribution of intrapulmonary gas will occur and intrapulmonary pressure differences will equilibrate. If the equilibrated intrapulmonary pressure – as measured at the endotracheal tube – is higher than the external PEEP, this intrapulmonary pressure is called intrinsic PEEP (IPEEP)

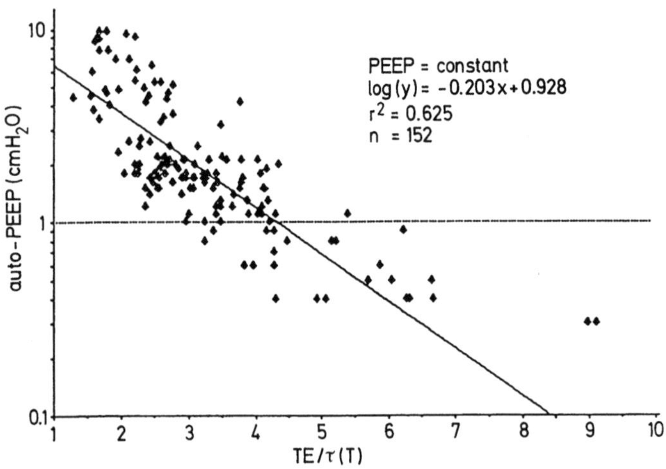

Fig. 11. Semi logarithmic plot of auto-PEEP against TE/τ (T). The relation between auto-PEEP and TE/τ is obviously an exponential one. See text

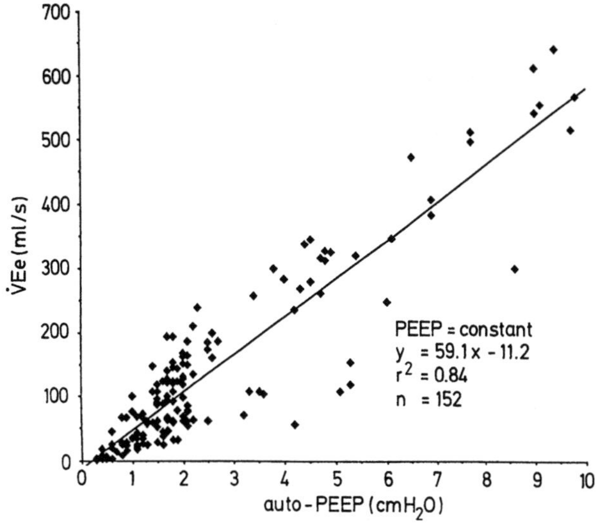

Fig. 12. End-expiratory flow (V̇Ee) vs auto-PEEP. The higher the auto-PEEP the higher V̇Ee; 152 measurements in 14 patients with acute respiratory insufficiency demonstrate a good correlation. See text

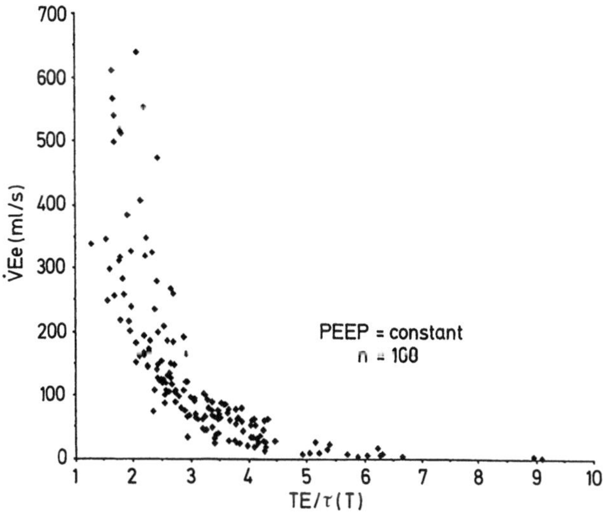

Fig. 13. End-expiratory flow (V̇Ee) vs TE/τ in 168 measurements. The data suggest an exponential relation. See Fig. 14

in Fig. 15, in which the plot of $\Delta\dot{V}Ee$ against ΔAPV shows that an increase in $\dot{V}Ee$ caused an enlargement of APV.

In ventilated patients, C and R should therefore be measured so that τ can be calculated. Following this, the TE necessary for a complete expiration – which is

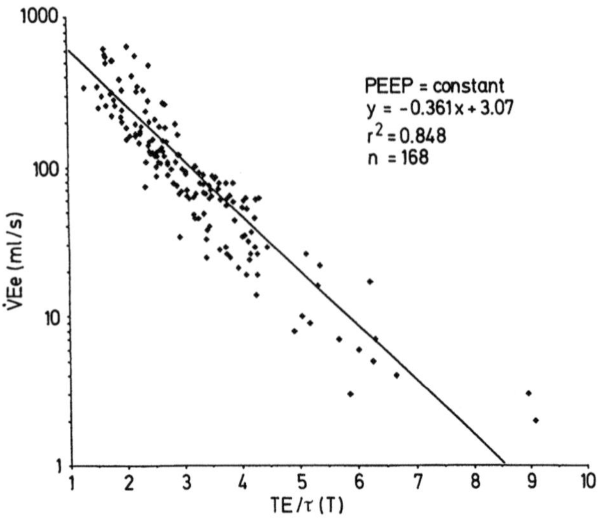

Fig. 14. Semi logarithmic plot of end-expiratory flow (V̇Ee) vs TE/τ demonstrates an exponentional dependency with a surprisingly good correlation ($r^2 = 0.848$). See text

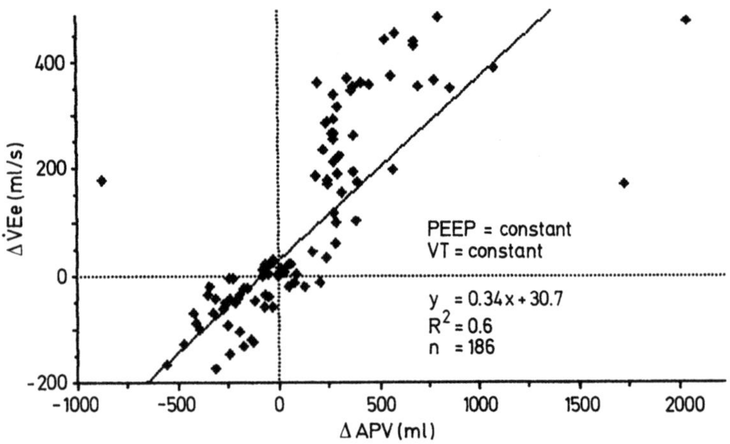

Fig. 15. Paired differences (result after the change of the setting minus result before the change of the setting) of end-expiratory flow (ΔV̇Ee) vs paired differences of accessible pulmonary volume (ΔAPV); 186 pairs with a change in inspiratory flow, end-inspiratory pause, or both with PEEP and tidal volume kept constant. An increase in end-expiratory flow always corresponds to an increase in pulmonary volume. See text

three to four times larger than τ – can be calculated and employed at the bedside by adjusting the ventilatory pattern at the respirator. On the other hand, if the medical team decides to deliberately create an auto-PEEP by using the inverted ratio ventilation mode, a TE/τ smaller than 2.5 can be chosen by assessing τ and setting the appropriate TE at the ventilator.

Concluding Remarks

We have established that time constants of different lengths are present in the lungs at the same time and that very long time constants appear. We have also determined that one does not necessarily have to reach all the goals of mechanical ventilation in each breath simultaneously; they can also be reached one after another, i.e., in consecutive breaths. Finally, we ask whether we can use these findings to outline a new form of ventilation. We believe that, in the future, mechanical respiration will no longer be carried out with the constant repetition of breaths with identical flow patterns, i.e., it will no longer be monotone as it is today, but very different breaths will be strung together to define a sequence. Such a sequence (consisting of a number of breaths with different flow patterns) will be employed again and again. The sequences of different flow patterns would then be pre-programmed on a proven pattern and the different flow patterns would then be adapted to the patient with an automatic control system, using actual measurements as feedback. We are presently concerned with the development of such a ventilatory mode. In contrast to the current monotone ventilation, we call it polymorphous ventilation.

Acknowledgement. The participating investigators were, in Basel, J.X. Brunner[1], and E. Grädel[1]; in Augsburg, J. Eckart[2], J. Birle[2], Ch. Knothe[2], and in Lübeck, E. Hecker[3], W. Beissert[3], D. Fiebelkorn[3], H.J. Kohl[3], D. Weismann[3], and H.J. Friedrich[4].

References

Beecher HK (1933a) Measured effect of laparotomy on respiration. J Clin Invest 12:639–650
Beecher HK (1933b) Effect of laparotomy on lung volume. Demonstration of a new type of pulmonary collapse. J Clin Invest 12:651–658
Beecher HK, Bradshaw HH, Lindskog G (1933) Effect of laparotomy and abdominal distention on lung volume. J Thorac Surg 2:444–450
Bendixen HH (1964) Atelectasis and shunting. Anesthesiology 25:595–596
Bendixen HH, Laver MB (1965) Hypoxia in anesthesia. A review. Clin Pharmacol Ther 6:510–539
Bendixen HH, Hedley-Whyte J, Laver MB (1963) Impaired oxygenation in surgical patients during general anesthesia with controlled ventilation. A concept of atelectasis. N Engl J Med 269:991–996
Berggren SM (1942) The oxygen deficit of arterial blood caused by non-ventilating parts of the lung. Acta Physiol Scand [Suppl] 11:1–92
Brunner JX, Wolff G (1988) Pulmonary function indices in critical care patients. Springer, Berlin Heidelberg New York
Clemens JA, Hustead RF, Johnson RP, Gribetz I (1961) Pulmonary surface tension and alveolar stability. J Appl Physiol 16:444–450

---

[1] Clinical Physiology, Clinic for Cardiac and Thoracic Surgery, University of Basel, Kantonsspital, Basel, Switzerland
[2] Division for Anesthesiology and Operative Intensive Care Medicine, Central Clinics, Augsburg, FRG
[3] Drägerwerk AG, Lübeck, FRG
[4] Institut für Med. Statistik und Dokumentation der Med. Universität, Lübeck, FRG

Dantzker DR, Brook CJ, Dehart P. Lynch P, Wef JG (1979) Ventilation-perfusion distributions in the adult respiratory distress syndrome. Am Rev Respir Dis 120:1039–1052

Froese AB, Bryan C (1974) Effects of anesthesia and paralysis on diaphragmatic mechanics in man. Anesthesiology 41:242–255

Hedenstierna G, Strandberg A, Brismar B, Lundquist H, Svensson L, Tokics L (1985a) Functional residual capacity, thoracoabdominal dimensions, and central blood volume during general anesthesia with muscle paralysis and mechanical ventilation. Anesthesiology 62:247–254

Hedenstierna G, Strandberg A, Brismar B, Lundquist H, Tokics L (1985b) What causes the lowered FRC during anaesthesia? Clin Physiol 5:133–141

Hedenstierna G, Lundquist H, Lundh B, Tokics L, Strandberg A, Brismar B, Frostell C (1989) Pulmonary densities during anaesthesia. An experimental study on lung morphology and gas exchange. Eur Respir J 2(6):528–535

Pepe E, Marini J (1982) Occult positive end-expiratory pressure in mechanically ventilated patients. Am Rev Respir Dis 126:166–170

Ralph DD, Robertson HT, Weaver LJ, Hlastala MP, Carric CJ, Hudson LD (1985) Distribution of ventilation and perfusion during positive end-expiratory pressure in the adult respiratory distress syndrome. Am Rev Respir Dis 131:54–60

Rehder K, Sessler AD, Marsh HM (1975) General anesthesia and the lung. Am Rev Respir Dis 112:541–563

Rehder K, Cameron PD, Krayer S (1985) New dimensions of the respiratory system (editorial). Anesthesiology 62:230–233

Tokics L, Hedenstierna G, Strandberg A, Brismar B, Lundquist H (1987) Lung collapse and gas exchange during general anesthesia: effects of spontaneous breathing, muscle paralysis, and positive end-expiratory pressure. Anesthesiology 66:157–167

Westbrook PR, Stubbs SE, Sessler AD, Rehder K, Hyatt RE (1973) Effects of anesthesia and muscle paralysis on respiratory mechanics in normal man. J Appl Physiol 34:81–86

Wolff G et al. (1979) Beatmung mit intermittierend ansteigendem PEEP. Annual assembly of the Swiss Society for Intensive Care Medicine, 16–17 Nov 1979, Geneva

Wolff G. Brunner JX, Grädel E (1986) Gas exchange during mechanical ventilation and spontaneous breathing. Intermittent mandatory ventilation after open heart surgery. Chest 89:11–17

Success of Pressure Support Ventilation and Combined High Frequency Ventilation with respect to Extravascular Lung Water

J. Zeravik, J. Eckart, G. Blümel and U.J. Pfeiffer

Introduction

The goals of mechanical ventilatory support in patients with acute respiratory insufficiency (ARI) are to supply adequate ventilation and oxygenation with minimal cardiocirculatory embarrassment. The most common mode for providing this support is continuous positive pressure ventilation (CPPV). Recently, inspiratory pressure support ventilation (PSV) has been made available in several ventilators. This kind of ventilation, which augments spontaneous inspiration with an adjustable amount of inspiratory pressure, is of particular interest as a weaning method. Compared to Synchronized intermittent mandatory ventilation (SIMV) a reduced oxygen breathing cost has been reported [1]. Another alternative to CPPV for treatment of ARI is high frequency ventilation (HFV), [2], which has been used with varying results. A new method of HFV was introduced in 1983, in which a combination of conventional ventilation and HFV was used; this was referred to as combined HFV (CHFV) [3].

It would be of interest to determine if there was a specific indication to ventilate patients suffering from ARI, who are currently being managed with CPPV, with PSV or CHFV as long-term method of ventilation. Subsequently, the question arises what variables should be used in order to define a clear-cut indication for PSV or CHFV? With the clinical introduction of extravascular lung water (EVLW) measurement (estimated by extravascular lung thermal volume, ETV) [4, 5] a new lung related quantity became available. In order to ascertain advantages or disadvantages of PSV or CHFV, oxygenation indices and parameters related to lung mechanics have been measured. ETV seems to be a parameter which is more related to the severity of the insult to the lung than are oxygenation indices or lung mechanics. The objective of this study was to assess: (a) the short-term changes in hemodynamics and oxygenation in patients transferred from CPPV to PSV or CHFV and (b) if the degree of lung water accumulation prior to PSV or CHFV would influence the patients response to PSV or CHFV.

Materials and Methods

The study was performed in 56 patients, 29 of them randomly assigned to the PSV group and 27 patients to the CHFV group. Additionally, for each group there was a control group ($n = 27$ for the PSV control group; $n = 20$ for the CHFV control group). All patients were admitted to and managed in the surgical intensive care unit. The patients had the following injuries or diagnosis: road accidents with blunt chest trauma, multiple fractures, neurologic trauma, complications after abdominal or orthopedic surgery.

The patients had to meet the following entry criteria:

1. Densities on the chest X-ray
2. Managed by volume cycled ventilation (Servo Ventilator 900 C, Siemens Elema, Solna, Sweden) with a tidal volume (Vt) of 12–18 ml/kg body weight
3. Inspiration/expiration (I/E) ratio of 1/1 or less
4. PEEP of 5 cm H_2O or higher
5. Respiratory rate (RR) 12–18 breaths/min to achieve a $PaCO_2$ of 45 ± 10 mmHg
6. FiO_2 of 0.4 or more in order to achieve a PaO_2 of 90 ± 15 mmHg with no improvement during the preceeding 24 h

Hemodynamics had to be stable; changes in the supply of vasoactive drugs and diuretics or measures which would influence the circulating blood volume were not allowed.

Catheterization and Measurements

A 7.5 F5 lumen Swan-Ganz pulmonary artery thermodilution catheter (Edwards Laboratories, Santa Ana, CA) and a 5 F femoral artery catheter equipped with fiber-optic and thermistor (Pulsion Medizintechnik, München, FRG) were placed in each patient for monitoring of central venous (CVP), mean pulmonary artery (MPAP), pulmonary capillary wedge (PCWP), and mean arterial (MAP) pressure, for withdrawal of blood samples, and for thermal dye dilution. Both the pulmonary artery and arterial catheters were connected to an integrated fiberoptic monitoring system (COLD Z-02, Pulsion Medizintechnik, Munich, FRG) [6]. A 10 ml bolus of 5% glucose containing 0.75 mg/ml indocyanine green dye at 0°–4 °C was injected into the right atrium at a rate of 10 ml/s with a temperature controlled pneumatic injector (Pulsion, Munich, FRG). The injection was started at beginning of expiration. The dye and the thermal curve recorded in the femoral artery were used for the calculation of cardiac output (C.O.), intrathoracic blood volume (ITBV), and ETV (normal range: 6–9 ml/kg). The coefficient of variation of five repeated estimations of ETV with this system in another group of intensive care patients ($n = 12$) was determined to be 7.6%.

Calculated Hemodynamic and Respiratory Variables

Arterial (CaO_2) and mixed venous oxygen contents (CvO_2), stroke volume index (SVI), oxygen delivery index (DO_2I), oxygen consumption index (VO_2I), and the percentage of intrapulmonary shunt (Qs/Qt) were calculated using standard formulas.

Study Protocol

When assigned to the PSV group, the patients sedation was reduced and/or substituted by analgesics. Hemodynamic and gas exchange variables were measured before the mode of ventilation was changed from CPPV to PSV. PSV was then applied with the Servo 900C. The level of pressure support during inspiration was chosen in order to achieve a $PaCO_2$ of 45 $\pm$ 10 mmHg. A negative pressure of 0.5–1.5 cmH_2O on the expiratory limb of the patient circuit triggered inspiratory flow to provide the set level of the inspiratory pressure. PEEP was adjusted in order to achieve the same mean airway pressure (MPaw) as during CPPV. The hemodynamic and gas exchange variables were determined again 6 h after switching to PSV.

When assigned to the CHFV group the patients were intubated transorally with a Hi-Lo-Jet tube (Mallinckrodt Inc., Argyle, NY). CPPV was continued through the larger lumen. Mpaw was measured through the smallest lumen of this tube, while the third lumen was closed during CPPV. Hemodynamic and gas exchange variables were measured before the mode of ventilation was changed from CPPV to CHFV. CHFV was then applied with the Servo Ventilator 900C and the high frequency unit (Siemens Elema, Solna, Sweden). The conventional CPPV was reduced to a Vt of 4–5 ml/kg; the RR was kept unchanged as was the I/E ratio. The HFV component was applied through the unused third lumen of the endotracheal tube. The frequency was set to 10 Hz; the duty cycle was 50%; the Vt of HFV was 9–11 ml/kg during CPPV inspiration and was reduced to 4–5 ml/kg during CPPV expiration in order to obtain a $PaCO_2$ of 45 $\pm$ 10 mmHg. In order to reduce the inadvertent PEEP, during the last 5% of CPPV expiration time HFV was not applied. PEEP was adjusted in order to achieve the same MPaw as during CPPV. The hemodynamic and gas exchange variables were determined again 6 h after switching to CHFV. In the 27 patients of the PSV control group and the 20 patients of the CHFV control group CPPV was continued with unaltered ventilation patterns. The hemodynamic and gas exchange variables were determined twice with an interval of 6 h according to the PSV and CHFV group.

Statistical Analysis

The change in oxygenation index PaO_2/FiO_2 was used to quantify the effect of the alternative ventilation mode. In order to find out if there is an initial lung-related parameter indicating the efficacy of PSV or CHFV, linear regression analysis was performed between ETV (during CPPV) and the change in

PaO_2/FiO_2. The Wilcoxon matched pairs signed ranks analysis was applied for evaluation of significant differences of the measured variables between CPPV and 6 h PSV or CHFV.

Results

PSV Group

According to regression analysis of ETV (during CPPV) and the change of PaO_2/FiO_2 ($r = 0.7$) we estimated that the x-intercept for this variable was around 12 ml/kg (Fig. 1), meaning that below an ETV value (during CPPV) of 12 ml/kg an improvement of oxygenation due to PSV occurred; above this value an impairment was found. In patients with an ETV > 12 ml/kg ($n = 12$) the mean ETV value was 16.7 (± 1.10) ml/kg. The inspiratory pressure support was 24.3 (± 2.20) cm H_2O. There was a significant decrease of PaO_2/FiO_2 and an increase of SVI (Table 1). In patients with an ETV < 12 ml/kg ($n = 17$) the mean ETV value was 7.91 (± 0.60) ml/kg. The inspiratory pressure support was 22.3 (± 1.42) cmH_2O. There was a significant increase of PaO_2/FiO_2 of 15% with a simultaneous increase of CI and SVI of more than 20%. Therefore, as a result, DO_2I increase of around 25% (Fig. 2) occurred. VO_2I did not change significantly, but there was a good correlation between VO_2I and DO_2I when the mode of ventilation was changed from CPPV to PSV at the same MPaw (Fig. 3).

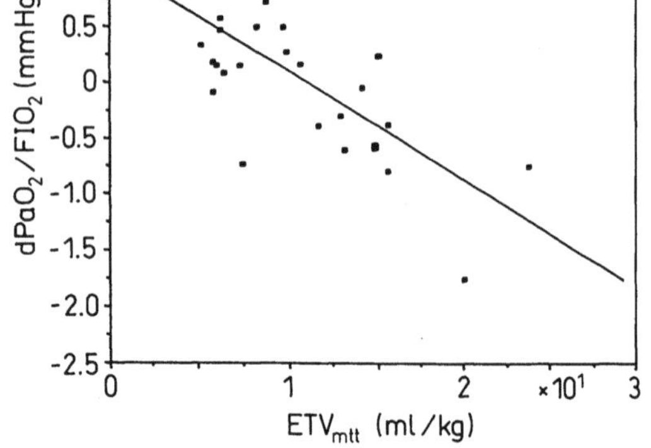

Fig. 1. Relationship between the extravascular lung thermal volume (*ETV*) and the change (*d*) of the oxygenation index (*PaO₂/FIO₂*) after 6 h PSV ($n = 29$)

Table 1. Selection of the hemodynamic and respiratory variables in the PSV group with ETV < 12 ml/kg and ETV > 12 ml/kg

	ETV < 12		ETV > 12	
Parameter (mean ± SE)	CPPV	PSV	CPPV	PSV
n	17		12	
CI ($1/min \times m^2$)	4.10 ± 0.35	4.73 ± 0.29**	5.01 ± 0.52	5.32 ± 0.57
SVI (ml/m^2)	40.5 ± 3.88	46.8 ± 3.42*	45.7 ± 4.57	52.4 ± 6.16
ITBVI (ml/m^2)	801 ± 49.1	888 ± 54.6	943 ± 51.5	968 ± 61.5
ETV (ml/kg)	7.91 ± 0.60	7.78 ± 0.55	16.7 ± 1.10	16.3 ± 1.17
Q_s/Q_t (%)	20.7 ± 1.55	20.4 ± 1.67	24.2 ± 2.10	26.9 ± 3.18
PaO_2/FiO_2 (mm Hg)	239 ± 16.3	271 ± 17.4**	232 ± 25.8	201 ± 26.6**
VO_2I ($ml/min \times m^2$)	177 ± 10.6	193 ± 12.0	206 ± 16.0	226 ± 20.9
DO_2/I ($ml/min \times m^2$)	694 ± 61.4	826 ± 56.7**	844 ± 81.0	888 ± 92.3

Values are means ± standard error.
*, $p < 0.05$; **, $p < 0.01$

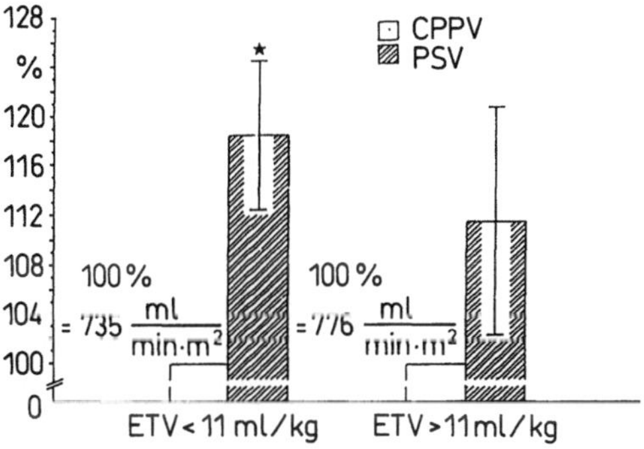

Fig. 2. Change of the percentage oxygen delivery index (DO_2I) induced by PSV in dependency of ETV

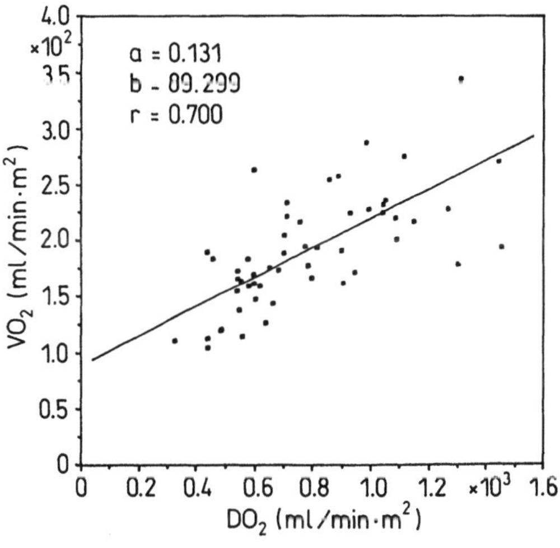

Fig. 3. Relationship between oxygen delivery index (DO_2I) and oxygen consumption index (VO_2I) induced by PSV ($n = 29$)

CHFV Group

Regression analysis performed in the same way as in the PSV group showed an ETV value (during CPPV) of around 15 ml/kg. Above this value, with a mean ETV of 22.3 ($\pm$ 1.60) ml/kg ($n = 17$) and the same MPaw, an improvement of oxygenation with an increase of PaO_2/FiO_2 of more than 40% occurred (Fig. 4) during CHFV. Qs/Qt was reduced by 25%, and there was a slight decrease of CI by 10% with a nearly unaltered DO_2I (Table 2). In patients with an ETV < 15 ml/kg, with a mean ETV of 10.8 ($\pm$ 0.89) ml/kg ($n = 10$), no changes could be detected between CPPV and CHFV. Figure 5 and 6 show the regression analysis dITBV/dCI for the CHFV subgroups with ETV < 15 ml/kg and ETV > 15 ml/kg. A significant correlation between dITBV and dCI exist for both groups ($r = 0.90$ and $r = 0.60$).

In the PSV and CHFV control groups, in which CPPV remained unchanged, no significant change of any variable was detected.

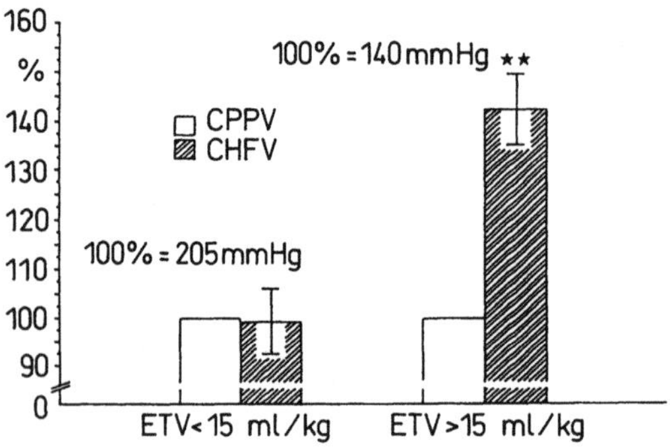

Fig. 4. Change of the PaO_2/FiO_2 in percent induced by CHFV in dependency of ETV;**, $p < 0.01$

Table 2. Selection of the hemodynamic and respiratory variables in the CHFV group with ETV < 15 ml/kg and ETV > 15 ml/kg

	ETV < 15		ETV > 15	
Parameter (mean $\pm$ SE)	CPPV	CHFV	CPPV	CHFV
n	10		17	
CI ($1/min \times m^2$)	4.36 $\pm$ 0.51	3.71 $\pm$ 0.21	4.45 $\pm$ 0.28	3.92 $\pm$ 0.24**
SVI (ml/m^2)	42.7 $\pm$ 6.24	36.2 $\pm$ 2.54	40.7 $\pm$ 2.16	36.4 $\pm$ 1.91*
ITBVI (ml/m^2)	900 $\pm$ 64.8	834 $\pm$ 39.2	834 $\pm$ 50.5	796 $\pm$ 45.2
ETV (ml/kg)	10.8 $\pm$ 0.89	10.5 $\pm$ 0.64	22.3 $\pm$ 1.60	21.9 $\pm$ 1.50
Q_s/Q_t (%)	26.3 $\pm$ 2.51	27.0 $\pm$ 2.83	33.5 $\pm$ 2.71	25.7 $\pm$ 2.87**
PaO_2/FiO_2 (mm Hg)	205 $\pm$ 18.8	202 $\pm$ 21.2	141 $\pm$ 17.1	198 $\pm$ 22.7
VO_2I ($ml/min \times m^2$)	173 $\pm$ 12.4	164 $\pm$ 14.9	203 $\pm$ 13.7	199 $\pm$ 12.6
DO_2/I ($ml/min \times m^2$)	699 $\pm$ 75.3	600 $\pm$ 47.7	764 $\pm$ 41.5	697 $\pm$ 33.9

Values are means $\pm$ standard error.
*, $p < 0.05$; **, $p < 0.01$

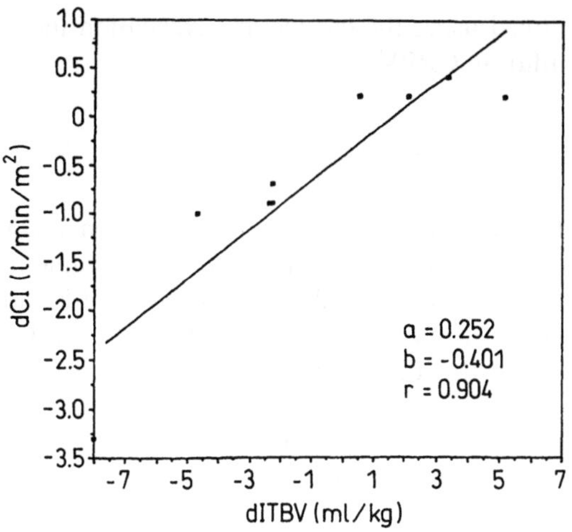

Fig. 5. Relationship between the change of intrathoracic blood volume (*dITBV*) and the subsequent change of cardiac index (*dCI*) induced by CHFV in the CHFV subgroup with ETV < 15 ml/kg ($n = 10$)

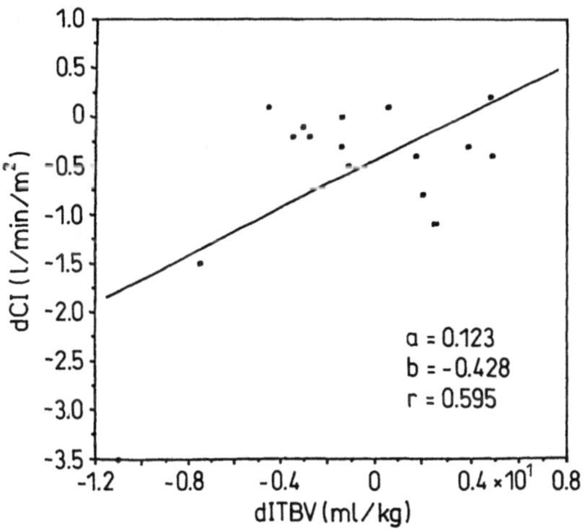

Fig. 6. Relationship between the change of intrathoracic blood volume (*dITBV*) and the subsequent change of cardiac index (*dCI*) induced by CHFV in the CHFV subgroup with ETV > 15 ml/kg ($n = 17$)

Discussion

The goal of this study was to determine if there is a lung related parameter which would clearly define the efficacy of PSV or CHFV in patients with ARI, thus eliminating the need for trial and error. Therefore we investigated the relationship between the success of ventilation and several lung-related parameters. The change in oxygenation was quantified using the change in oxygenation index $dPaO_2/FiO_2$ based on the ETV (during CPPV).

PSV Group

The correlation between ETV (CPPV) and the change in oxygenation index PaO_2/FIO_2 after 6 h PSV revealed an x-intercept of an ETV(CPPV) value of around 12 ml/kg, indicating that below an ETV(CPPV) value of 12 ml/kg an improvement of oxygenation may be achieved with PSV; above this value deterioration is more likely. Based on this the patients were divided into two groups, one with ETV(CPPV) < 12 ml/kg and one with ETV(CPPV) > 12 ml/kg. Hedenstierena et al. [7] reported an ETV value of 8 ml/kg in healthy volunteers using the Pulsion COLD equipment; our normal ETV range is between 6–9 ml/kg.

PSV in Patients with ETV < 12ml/kg

The mean ETV (CPPV) of the subgroup with ETV < 12 ml/kg was 7.91 ± 0.6 ml/kg and thus can be considered as normal. However, this subgroup had a remarkably impaired oxygenation as judged from the mean PaO_2/FIO_2 (239 ± 16.3 mm Hg) during CPPV. Shunt was obviously impaired ($Qs/Qt = 20.7 \pm 1.55$) as well. The densities in the lung X-ray indicated a moderate lung injury.

The thoracic cavity consists of two rapidly changing compartments, the blood volume and the gas compartments, and the rather slowly changing extravascular lung water compartment and the almost invariable compartments represented by the tissues of the heart, the lung, and the vessels. For the evaluation of effects of changes in ventilation not only the gas volume compartment, but also the ITBV and EVLW (accurately estimated by ETV) compartments are of utmost importance. In a study of the changes in thoracic compartments and dimensions induced by general anesthesia leading to subsequent muscle paralysis and mechanical ventilation, Hedenstierna et al. [7], utilizing multiple breath nitrogen washout to measure FRC and thermal-dye dilution to quantify ITBV and ETV, showed that ITBV and FRC were significantly decreased during CPPV compared to spontaneous ventilation and that ETV was not influenced.

During a CPPV inspiration the driving pressure for an increase of the thoracic dimensions is transmitted through the lung and to the intrathoracic structures: gas volume increases and ITBV decreases. By contrast, during a spontaneous inspiration the activation of the respiratory muscles increases both the thoracic dimensions and the volume of intrathoracic structures: ITBV increases in parallel to the increasing gas volume.

PSV is a combined form with an initial phase of spontaneous breathing followed by a phase of positive pressure ventilation with spontaneous timing of start and duration of inspiration. At the beginning of inspiration pleural pressure is lowered with the patient's effort to initiate a breath. Simultaneously, the volume of the thoracic cage and the volume of the intrathoracic structures start to increase: gas volume and ITBV increase. Inspiratory pressure support is provided as soon as the airway pressure falls below the preset trigger level. Thus, the thoracic volume continues to increase similar to CPPV. That is, gas volume increases further and ITBV decreases from the elevated level. As a net effect mean ITBV should be higher than during CPPV. This is confirmed by the significantly increased ITBV during PSV in the subgroup with ETV < 12 ml/kg.

The reason for the improvement of oxygenation during PSV may be an increase in FRC. Comparing PSV with an inspiratory pressure support of 10 cm H_2O to spontaneous breathing (SB) in patients with almost healthy lungs, Brochard et al. [8] did not find any differences of end-expiratory transpulmonary pressure. They concluded that FRC was the same during SB as during this form of PSV. CPPV with muscle paralysis has been shown to lower FRC and ITBV significantly if compared to spontaneous breathing [7]. The latter changes were caused by both a reduction of the cross-sectional chest area and by a cranial shift of the diaphragm. The patients in our investigation did not receive paralytic drugs, but they were well sedated during CPPV; during PSV sedation was reduced. Thus, it is likely that heavy sedation during CPPV decreased FRC via a reduction of the thoracic volume due to the reduced or abolished respiratory muscle activity and that FRC increased towards normal during PSV. Consequently oxygenation improved during PSV even in the presence of an increased CI.

During PSV SI and CI increased significantly in this group of patients with normal ETV but impaired oxygenation. The increase in CI and SI can be explained by the increase in preload. As we have shown recently in critically ill surgical patients, ITBV accurately reflects cardiac preload [9] and ITBV was significantly increased during PSV in the group with ETV < 12 ml/kg.

Due to the increased CI, DO_2I was increased significantly, while VO_2I remained unchanged. Therefore, the oxygen cost of breathing during PSV in the group with the low ETV value does not constitute an important factor. This is in accordance with Viale et al. [10].

PSV in Patients with ETV > 12 ml/kg

It should be pointed out that the most significant difference between the two ETV groups was the more then doubled ETV value in this group (16.7 $\pm$ 1.17). PSV at the same MPaw as during CPPV caused a significant impairment of oxygenation and Q_s/Q_t, whereas the hemodynamic pattern remained nearly unchanged. A higher ETV implies a more severe condition; patients in this group are obviously unable to adequately accommodate the mechanical expansion of the lungs by the ventilator and thus the preset level of pressure support is reached at a lower tidal volume. This could be explained by a reduced compliance or by reduced efficiency of the respiratory muscles due to the illness itself.

CHFV Group

The main findings in this group were that, below an ETV value of 15 ml/kg, CHFV did not influence hemodynamics or oxygenation significantly. CHFV markedly improved oxygenation and slightly depressed CI above an ETV value of 15 ml/kg, though CHFV was compared with CPPV at the same MPaw. In the clinical management of CHFV we did not observe barotrauma or a relevant cardiocirculatory embarrassment. In addition, there never were problems with CO_2 removal, probably because CHFV with the HFV component given in expiration reduced $PaCO_2$. This effect on $PaCO_2$ was most likely due to an increased washout of dead space. CHFV increased PaO_2/FIO_2 more than 40% in the CHFV group with ETV > 15 ml/kg. This marked improvement of oxygenation cannot be ascribed to the slight reduction of CI of around 10% only. The reduction of percent shunt in this group may have contribute both to the reduction of CI and to the ventilatory recruitment of previously perfused but underventilated areas of the lung. Enhanced gas mixing and convection of oxygen in the conducting airways [11] with the aid of high frequency pulses seems to increase the efficiency of the conventional breaths. Another reason for this improvement could be explained by the better opening of terminal airways and fluid-filled alveoli in this group with high pulmonary edema. This mechanism can be caused or at least amplified by an additional PEEP, as it was reported that HFV produces a certain amount of auto-PEEP [12, 13]. In a recent investigation, the dissociation of MPaw and lung volume during HFV was clearly shown [14].

As mentioned above, Hedenstierna et al. [7] have demonstrated that the thermal dye technique is useful in characterizing the variable intrathoracic volumes, as there are also extravascular lung parenchymal volume (estimated by ETV) and ITBV in addition to the measurement of FRC. We did not measure FRC, but ITBV and ETV. ETV changes slowly and does not seem to be susceptible to intrathoracic volume changes [7], whereas a compression of intrathoracic structures containing blood (estimated by ITBV) seems to be reasonable if lung volume or, more precisely, FRC increases during CHFV. ITBV reflects global preload for the heart [15] and, consequently, a reduction of ITBV would cause a decrease of C.O. This mechanism is demonstrated in the regression analysis between dITBV and dCI in both CHFV subgroups yielding correlation coefficients of $r = 0.90$ and 0.60 (Figs. 5, 6).

ITBV was not influenced significantly by CHFV. Therefore, a change in preload is not responsible for the significant decrease of CI in the CHFV subgroup with ETV > 15 ml/kg. Based on the position of the y-intercept this CI reduction occurs, independent of changes in preload, by the onset of CHFV. This kind of CI reduction can only be interpreted as a slight impairment of cardiac function. However, looking at cardiopulmonary function as a whole, the reduction of CI is outweighed by better oxygenation as CHFV does not affect DO_2 significantly. As there is a dissociation of MPaw and lung volume with the onset of CHFV, however, it is not recommended to maintain the same MPaw as during CPPV. An increased lung volume with CHFV probably provokes reduction of the pulmonary vascular bed thereby decreasing C.O.

Conclusions

Many ventilatory modes have recently been made available even though criteria regarding their application are meager. This is mainly because the evaluation parameters used seem to be too insensitive and/or nonspecific. These results demonstrate that ETV may help to distinguish patient populations with moderate and severe ARI which can benefit significantly from either PSV or CHFV. PSV improves oxygenation, hemodynamics, and re-establishment of patient control of ventilation in the moderate form of ARI. CHFV remarkably improves oxygenation without clinically relevant embarrassment of hemodynamics in the severe form of ARI. However, further investigations are necessary to evaluate if such a PSV or CHFV protocol reduces the overall need for mechanical ventilation and improves patient outcome.

References

1. McIntyre NR (1986) Respiratory function during pressure support ventilation. Chest 89:677–683
2. Hurst JM, Branson RD, DeHaven CB (1987) The role of high frequency ventilation in posttraumatic respiratory insufficiency. J Trauma 27:236–242
3. El-Baz N, El Ganzouri A, Invahovich A (1983) combined high frequency ventilation for treatment of severe respiratory failure. In: Scheck PAE, Sjostrand UH, Smith RBP (eds) Perspectives in high frequency ventilation. Hoff, The Hague
4. Lewis FR, Ellings VB (1978) Microprocessor determination of lung water using thermal green dye double indicator dilution. Surg Forum 29:182–184
5. Peiffer U, Zimmermann G (1984) Fehlermöglichkeiten und Grenzen der Lungenwasserbestimmung mit der Thermo-dye-Technik. Maudrich, Vienna. Beitr Anästhesiol Intensivmed 6:81–104
6. Pfeifer U, Birk M, Aschenbrenner H, Blümel G (1982) The system for quantitating thermal dye extravascular lung water. In: Prakash O (ed) Computers in critical care and pulmonary medicine, vol 2. Plenum, London, pp 123–125
7. Hedenstierna G, Strandberg A, Brismar B, Lundquist H, Svensson L, Tokics L (1985) Functional residual capacity, thoracoabdominal dimensions, and central blood volume during general anesthesia with muscle paralysis and mechanical ventilation. Anesthesiology 62: 247–254
8. Brochard L, Pluskwa F, Lemaire F (1987) Improved efficacy of spontaneous breathing with inspiratory pressure support. Am Rev Respir Dis 136:411–415
9. Peiffer UJ, Zeravik J, Eckart J, Blümel G (1989) Intrathoracic blood volume accurately reflects circulating volume status. Crit Care Med 17 412):522
10. Viale JP, Annat GJ, Bouffard YM, Delafosse BX, Bertrand OM, Motin JP (1988) Oxygen cost of breathing in postoperative patients. Chest 93:506–509
11. Ericsson I (1982) The role of conducting airways in gas exchange during high frequency ventilation – a clinical and theoretical analysis. Anesth Analg 61:483–489
12. Beamer WC, Prough DS, Royster R, Johnston WE, Johnson JC (1984) High frequency ventilation produces auto-PEEP. Crit Care Med 12:734–737
13. Lazarus G, Rothhammer A, Lazarus W, Weis KH (1986) Hämodynamische Nebenwirkungen der high-frequency jet ventilation (HFJV) als Funktion des Lungenvolumens. Anaesthesist 35:24–29

14. Smith DW, Frankel L, Ariagno RL (1988) Dissociation of mean airway pressure and lung volume during high-frequency oscillatory ventilation. Crit Care Med 16:531–535
15. Pfeiffer U, Aschenbrenner G, Kolb E, Blümel G, Peiffer HG (1986) Die Messung des intrathorakalen Blutvolumens als sensitiver Parameter zur Steuerung der Volumensubstitution bei Intensivpatienten. Chir Forum 86:203–207

Biphasic Positive Airway Pressure (BIPAP)

H. Benzer, M. Baum, C. Hörmann, Ch. Huber, W. Koller, T. Luger, C. Putensen, and G. Putz

During the past few years, research in the field of ventilatory support [1] has mainly focused on the development of modes combining mechanical ventilation with spontaneous breathing (augmented ventilation). Mechanical ventilation can be combined with spontaneous breathing either by intermittent administration (mechanical breath – spontaneous breath) or by providing continuous ventilatory support during every breath. The first of these two principles is utilized by all modes of intermittent mandatory ventilation (IMV); the second principle is the basis of the large variety of inspiratory assists (IA). Both strategies aim at mechanically assisting patients with insufficient spontaneous ventilation by using an artificial ventilation system which provides part of the ventilatory work. In order to improve the gas exchange for oxygen, an appropriate amount of lung volume at end-expiration must be maintained by positive end-expiratory pressure (PEEP, CPAP). Biphasic positive airway pressure (BIPAP), which is described in the following, is an attempt at providing ventilatory support with the CPAP function of the respirator.

BIPAP may best be described as a combination of spontaneous breathing and time-cycled, pressure-controlled mechanical ventilation (Fig. 1). According to an adjustable sequence, the pressure is cyclically switched between high and

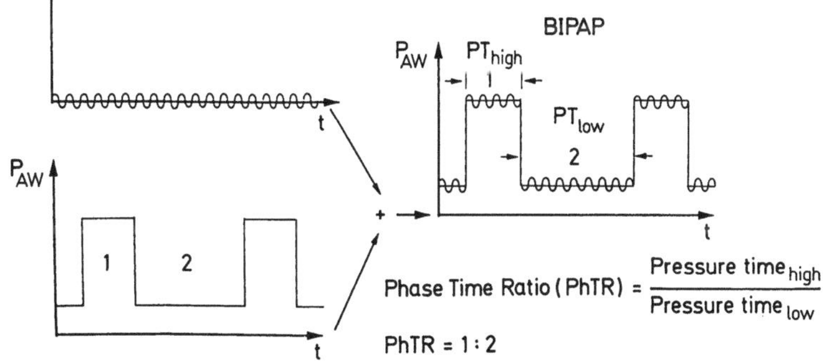

Fig. 1. The combination of spontaneous breathing (*above*) and pressure-controlled, time-cycled ventilation (PC ventilation) (*below*) in the BIPAP system depicted schematically. The inspiration-expiration ratio (I:E) of 1:2 during controlled ventilation corresponds with the phase-time ratio (PhTR) of 1:2 in the BIPAP mode. Time pressure high (TP_{hi}) is duration of the phase at the upper pressure level; time pressure low (TP_{lo}) is duration of the phase at the lower pressure level

low (pressure high, P_{hi}; pressure low, P_{lo}). At both pressure levels, which can be independently adjusted, spontaneous breathing (CPAP) is possible. The contribution of mechanical ventilation consists in the volume displacement caused by switching between the two pressure levels.

On principle, any duration of the two pressure phases (time pressure high, TP_{hi}, and time pressure low, TP_{lo}) is possible. In analogy to the inspiration-expiration ratio of controlled ventilation, the phase-time ratio (PhTR) is calculated as the ratio between the durations of the two pressure phases. A PhTR of 2:1 corresponds to inversed ratio ventilation (IRV) transferred to the BIPAP mode (Fig. 2) and is called IR-BIPAP. This setting is comparable to the airway pressure release ventilation (APRV) [8] described recently.

The varying degrees of ventilatory assistance administered makes it difficult to integrate the BIPAP system in a conventional classification system. When spontaneous ventilation is completely absent, BIPAP provides time-cycled, pressure-controlled controlled ventilation. When the patients starts spontaneous breathing at the low pressure level, BIPAP corresponds with constant pressure IMV. The new concept of ventilation BIPAP is realized as soon as the patient shows spontaneous ventilation at both pressure levels.

The technical realization of BIPAP was based on a simple version of a continuous flow CPAP system which was modified for the weaning phase (Fig. 3). While the inspiratory limb of the CPAP system remains unchanged, the conventional expiratory/PEEP valve is replaced by a pneumatically controlled membrane valve (ex valve). A magnetic valve switches between P_{hi} and P_{lo}, controlling the pop-off pressures of the expiratory valve. The two CPAP pressure levels can be adjusted via special controllers; the magnetic valve is

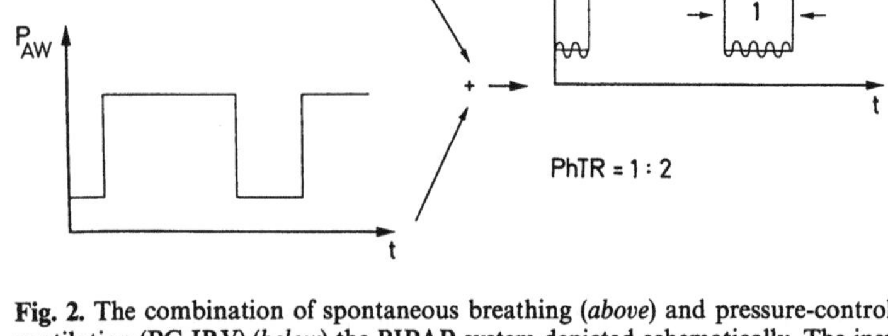

Fig. 2. The combination of spontaneous breathing (*above*) and pressure-controlled, inversed ratio ventilation (PC-IRV) (*below*) the BIPAP system depicted schematically. The inspiration-expiration ratio (I:E) of 2:1 during controlled ventilation corresponds with the phase-time ratio (PhTR) of 2:1 in the BIPAP mode

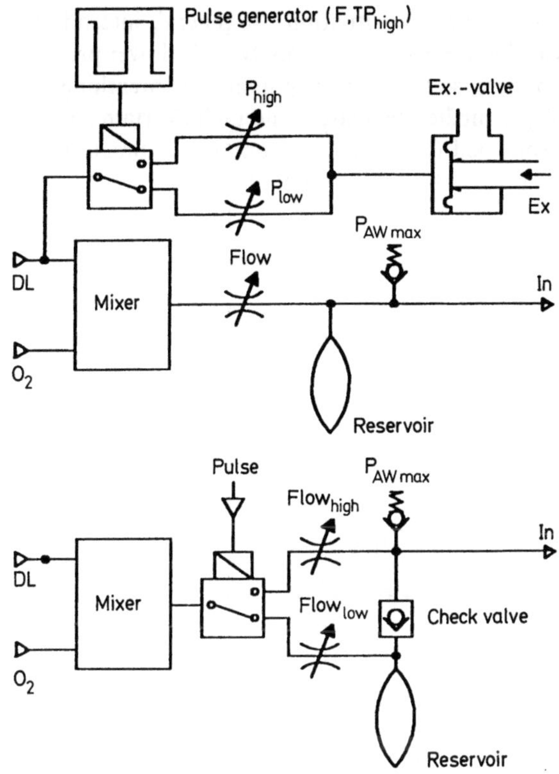

Fig. 3. Continuous flow BIPAP system (*above*) and modified inspiratory limb to avoid large volume displacements of the reservoir bag (*below*). The expiratory/PEEP valve is controlled by a magnetic valve switching between two independently adjustable pressures (P_{hi}, P_{lo}) at BIPAP frequency (F). *DL*, air; O_2, oxygen; TP_{hi}, time pressure high; TP_{lo}, time pressure low; PAW_{max}, check valve; *IN*, inspiratory limb; *EX*, expiratory limb

operated by an impulse generator, controlling the frequency (F) and duration of the P_{hi} phase (TP_{hi}). With adequate sizing of the reservoir bag (compliance) and correct setting of the expiratory/PEEP valve (resistance), this ventilatory system allows the unrestricted spontaneous breathing of a high-flow CPAP system.

To avoid large volume displacements of the reservoir bag as a result of the difference in BIPAP pressure, an additional magnetic valve and a check valve permit access to the reservoir bag only during the P_{lo} phase. This system demands a higher flow during the P_{hi} phase to keep the pressure constant during spontaneous breathing at this pressure level.

An alternative to the continuous flow system described above is the demand valve system which was realized as the Dräger-EVITA respirator.

Clinical work has shown that the BIPAP system is particularly useful in the phase of weaning. During the initial phase of weaning, constant-volume mechanical ventilation is replaced by the BIPAP mode using the same settings. This means that BIPAP is started as a mode of constant-pressure, time-cycled ventilation with the same frequency and I:E ratio as before, with the P_{lo} corresponding to the PEEP and the P_{hi} corresponding to the CMV end-inspiratory pressure. If a similar gas exchange is achieved by the new setting, the mechanical ventilatory support is slightly reduced by a minor reduction in P_{hi}

and analgosedation is adapted to the new situation. In general, intermittent spontaneous breathing starts at that time, most commonly at the lower pressure level (Fig. 4). In an attempt to increase the part of spontaneous breathing, the difference in pressure ($P_{hi} - P_{lo}$) is further decreased, and under certain circumstances the level times are prolonged (F). Regular spontaneous breathing at both pressure levels indicates successful weaning (Fig. 5).

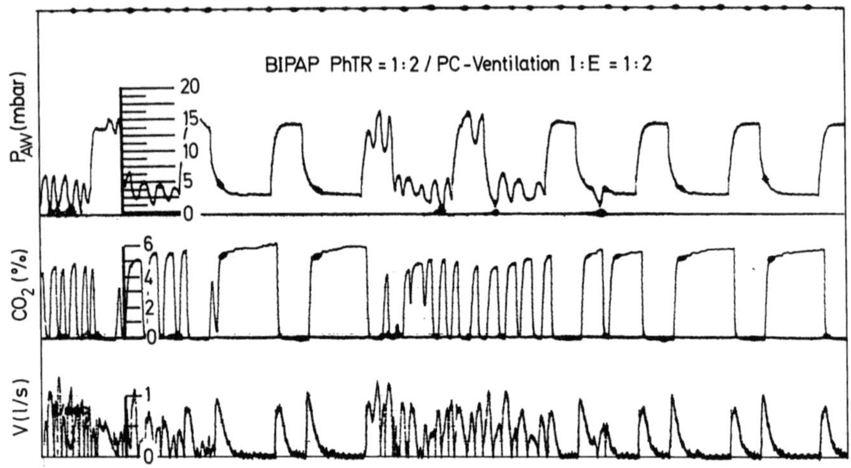

Fig. 4. Original registration of airway pressure (PAW) and expiratory CO_2 (% CO_2) under pressure-controlled, time-cycled ventilation (PC ventilation) with the continuous flow system set to a I:E ratio of 1:2. BIPAP takes effect with the patient's onset of spontaneous breathing. The flow ($\dot{V}$) (l/sec) measured by a hot wire anemometer near the tube shows the attempt to distinguish between spontaneous and mechanical ventilation. Upper pressure level (P_{hi}) = 15 mbar, lower pressure level (P_{lo}) = 4 mbar, phase-time ratio (PhTR) = 1:2, BIPAP frequency (F) = 12/min

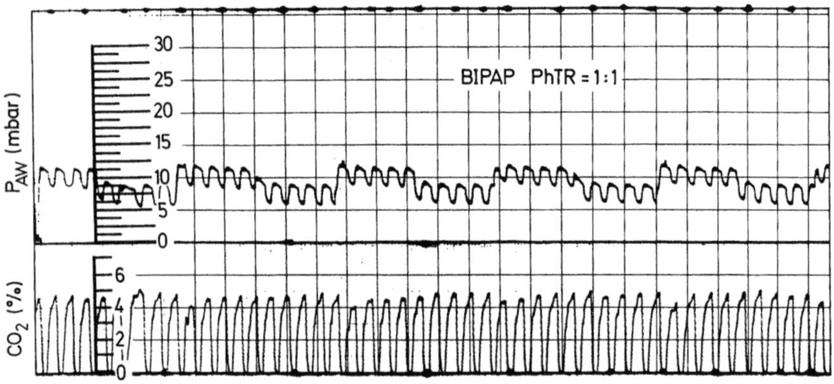

Fig. 5. Original registration of airway pressure (PAW) and expiratory CO_2 (% CO_2) under BIPAP. Spontaneous breathing at both pressure levels. Upper pressure level (P_{hi}) = 9 mbar, lower pressure level (P_{lo}) = 6 mbar, phase-time ratio (PhTR) = 1:1, BIPAP frequency (F) = 4/min. CPAP frequency = 30/min

Our present considerations regarding the setting of BIPAP parameters can be simplified as follows: The low pressure level determines the gas exchanging surface. Pressure difference ($P_{hi} - P_{lo}$) and level durations (times) determine the proportion of mechanical ventilation. The pressure levels should be long enough to allow spontaneous breathing.

This can also be achieved with an IR-BIPAP setting, as shown in Fig. 6 at a frequency of 5/minute and a PhTR = 2:1. In the same patient, a setting providing the same mean airway pressure (P_{aw}) and a PhTR = 1:2 did not change gas exchange (Fig. 6). If P_{lo} periods are considerably shorter, as suggested for APRV, spontaneous breathing is possible only at the high pressure level (P_{hi}) (Fig. 7).

Discussion

The application of the BIPAP system was originally aimed to provide ventilatory support in a CPAP system; clinical experience has demonstrated its technical feasibility and clinical applicability. Moreover, this mode of ventilation has proved to be a useful tool for assisting spontaneous breathing during many stages of illness. The unrestricted possibility of spontaneous breathing is helpful in realizing early weaning [1]. Since the BIPAP system eliminates the voluntary act of volume replacing constant mechanical ventilation by augmented ventilation, the choice of the appropriate moment to start the process of weaning is no longer of importance.

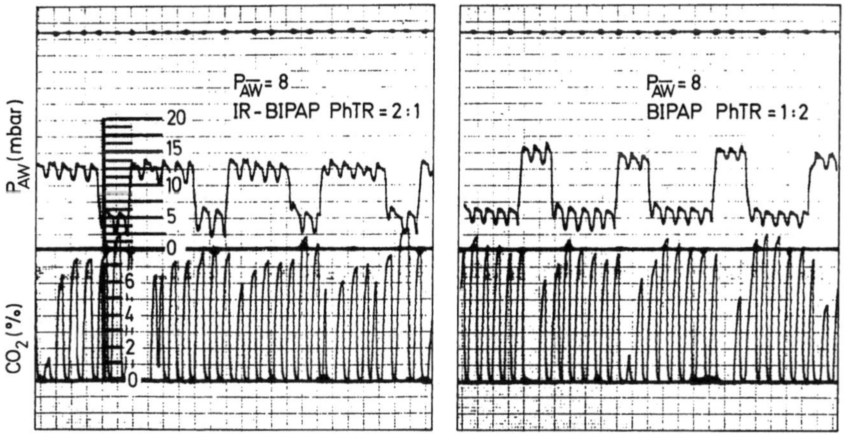

Fig. 6. Original registration of airway pressure (PAW) and expiratory CO_2 (% CO_2) under IR-BIPAP (left) and BIPAP (right) in a patient with a constant airway pressure (P_{aw}) = 8 mbar. IR-BIPAP: Upper pressure level (P_{hi}) = 12 mbar, lower pressure level (P_{lo}) = 4 mbar, phase-time ratio (PhTR) = 2:1, BIPAP frequency (F) = 5/min. CPAP frequency = 30/min. BIPAP: Upper pressure level (P_{hi}) = 14 mbar, lower pressure level (P_{lo}) = 6 mbar, phase-time ratio (PhTR) = 1:2, BIPAP frequency (F) = 5/min. CPAP frequency = 30/min.

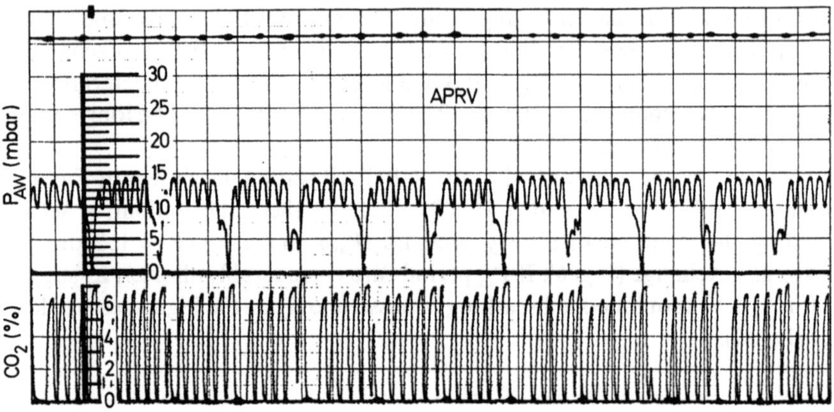

Fig. 7. Original registration of airway pressure (PAW) and expiratory CO_2 (% CO_2) under airway pressure release ventilation (ARPV). Upper pressure level (P_{hi}) = 12 mbar, lower pressure level (P_{lo}) = 2 mbar, phase-time ratio (PhTR) = 3.5:1, BIPAP frequency (F) = 7/min. CPAP frequency = 35/min.

In most cases a time-cycled, pressure-controlled mode for controlled ventilation will also be sufficient in severely injured lungs, e.g., by using pressure-controlled IRV (PC-IRV) [3, 4]. We would not like to claim, however, that the BIPAP mode is a "universal mode" of ventilation. In patients under controlled mechanical ventilation requiring higher pressure we still prefer a time-cycled, volume constant mode of ventilation.

The procedure described above has proved useful in clinical practice. However, since some of the BIPAP mechanisms are not yet completely clear, it may require some modifications. The significance of the phase-time ratio, for example, is still obscure. At present, we use a ratio < 1, which means that TP_{lo} is longer than TP_{hi}. In contrast, APRV uses extremely short phases of P_{lo} that do not allow spontaneous breathing at the lower level. In order to achieve better mechanical support of ventilation in the APRV mode, P_{hi} must be set relatively high (approx. 25–30 mbar), sometimes higher than seems to be reasonable for optimal oxygenation.

Study of intensive care patients has shown that the BIPAP mode is superior to CPAP with regard to oxygenation. This observation has not been confirmed by systematic examinations so far, which is partly due to the difficulties involved in setting up this kind of study. Results of other studies (fluctuating PEEP) [9], however, still leave this possibility open.

It is highly probable that lung mechanics are optimized by a more even distribution of the mechanically administered proportion of the tidal volume through spontaneous breathing. PEEP wave examinations [5] in patients under controlled mechanical ventilation have confirmed this assumption. In this study we observed by stepwise increase in PEEP that, after three breaths at the new PEEP level, the FRC increased significantly more than it could be expected from the so-called static compliance [3]. This mechanism probably contributes to the effect of the BIPAP system, particularly if the duration of the two phases is relatively long.

Although questions are still open, we think that even today the BIPAP system is a very promising aid in the process of early weaning, because it is very easy to administer and less invasive than other modes of ventilation.

References

1. Benzer H, Koller W, Putensen C (1987) Beatmung: Logik der Verfahren. In: Just OH, Krier C (eds) Aktuelle Anaesthesie und Intensivmedizin, Vol 147. Thieme, Stuttgart, pp 148–157
2. Gabriele G, Rosenfeld CR, Fixler DE (1977) Continuous airway pressure breathing with the head box in the newborn lamb: effect on regional blood flows. Pediatrics 59:858
3. Gattinoni L, Pesenti A, Caspani ML, Pelizzola A, Mascheroni D, Marcolin R, lapichino G, Langer M, Agostini A, Kolobow T, Melrose DG, Damia G (1984) The role of total static lung compliance in the management of severe ARDS unresponsive to conventional treatment. Intensive Care Med 10:121–126
4. Lachmann B, Haendly B, Schulz H, Jonson B (1980) Improved arterial oxygenation, CO_2 elimination, compliance and decreased barotrauma following chances of volume-generated PEEP ventilation with inspiratory/expiratory I/E ratio of 4:1 in patients with severe adult respiratory distress syndrome (ARDS). Intensive Care Med 10:121–126
5. Putensen C, Baum M, Koller W, Putz G (1989) PEEP-Welle: ein automatisiertes Verfahren zur bettseitigen Bestimmung der Volumen/Druck-Beziehung beatmeter Patienten. Anaesthesist 38:214–219
6. Simonneau G, Lemaire F, Harf A, Carlet J, Teisseire B (1982) A comparative study of the cardiorespiratory effects of continuous positive pressure ventilation in acute respiratory failure. Intensive Care Med 8:61–67
7. Steinhoff H, Falke K, Schwarzhoff W (1982) Enhanced renal function with intermittent mandatory ventilation in acute respiratory failure. Intensive Care Med 8:74–96
8. Stock MC, Downs JB, Frolicher DA (1987) Airway pressure release ventilation. Crit Care Med 15:62–66
9. Uchida H, Inaba H, Sato J, Sakurada M, Mizuguchi T (1988) Fluctuating PEEP versus conventional PEEP in diffuse and unilateral lung injury induced by oleic acid. Acta Anaesthesiol Scand 32:420–426

Technical Aspects of Patient-Ventilator Interactions

R.M. Kacmarek, H. Cohen, and R.L. Goulet

It has become increasingly clear that during patient-initiated volume-limited mechanical ventilatory assistance numerous factors can affect patient synchrony with the mechanical ventilator, the two most important being inspiratory trigger sensitivity and peak inspiratory flow. Decreasing inspiratory trigger sensitivity requires a greater system pressure change resulting in greater patient effort to initiate a mechanical breath [1, 2]. This greater effort reflects an increase in ventilatory drive, for there is good correlation between mouth occlusion pressure ($P_{0.1}$) and the pressure required to trigger a mechanical breath [3]. In addition, Gurevitch and Gelmont [4] recently noted an increased delay in establishing system pressure during mechanical volume-limited breaths as trigger sensitivity is decreased.

The matching of machine peak inspiratory flow rates to patient demands is also essential to the establishment of synchrony during mechanical ventilation [2, 5, 6]. In fact, if matching is poor, the patient's work of breathing during the mechanical breath may rival that during unassisted spontaneous ventilation [5]. That is, the energy cost of mechanical ventilation can equal that of spontaneous ventilation. This problem has been reviewed in detail by Marini et al. [5] and is depicted in Fig. 1. Essentially, if system peak flow is incapable of matching

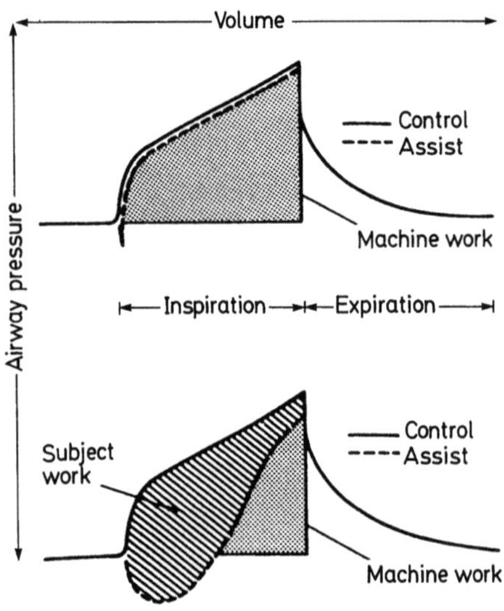

Fig. 1. Pressure-volume loops (pressure at airway opening) developed during volume-limited mechanical ventilation. *Top*, Control and idealized assisted volume ventilation. No difference in loops. *Bottom*, Control and actual assisted volume ventilation. The differences in area (*hatched*) represent work performed by the subject or patient during delivery of a mechanical breath. (From Marini et al. [5])

patient demands, a large percentage of the work of breathing would be performed by the patient in spite of the mechanical ventilator. It may be true that gas exchange or efficiency of ventilation is improved but the load on the ventilatory muscles may remain essentially unchanged. Any difference in the pressure-volume loop developed during assisted ventilation, when compared to controlled ventilation, represents work performed by the patient. To minimize this discrepancy, peak inspiratory flow must be kept high (60–90 liters/min) and inspiratory times kept short (0.8 – 1.2 s).

It has been well recognized since the early 1980s [7–10] that improperly designed continuous-flow continuous positive airway pressure (CPAP) systems and demand-flow ventilator CPAP systems increase patients' work of breathing. Problems with CPAP systems were primarily due to inadequate system flow and were easily remedied by adjustment of delivered flow. The major concerns of demand systems were their sensitivity [9] and the capability of demand flow to match patients' demand [8] during the initial phase of inspiration. The newest generation of mechanical ventilators has markedly improved upon the function of demand systems [11, 12]. However, many demand-flow ventilators still impose additional work when compared to continuous-flow systems [12]. This, coupled with the potential of artificial airways to markedly elevate imposed work of breathing [13, 14], particularly in patients with enhanced ventilatory drives, small-sized artificial airways, and nasal intubation, has raised concerns about all patients breathing spontaneously via ventilator systems.

The heightened awareness of these problems has led to the increasing use of inspiratory pressure support (IPS) during CPAP, the spontaneous breathing phase of synchronized intermittent mandatory ventilation (SIMV), or as an independent mode of ventilation. IPS, because of its inherent flow delivery capabilities, appears to be able to match the spontaneously breathing patient's ventilatory demand as well as or better than any of the other modes of ventilation currently available. With IPS, the maximum gas flow delivery is based on the inherent design of the ventilator and the patient's ventilatory demand. All ventilators providing IPS are capable of exceeding peak inspiratory flows of patients by 50% or more [15]. Each is capable of producing a unique inspiratory pressure waveform (Fig. 2). The termination of inspiration is based on delivered gas flow. When flow diminishes to a predetermined level the unit cycles to exhalation. Some terminate the IPS breath when peak flow is 25% of maximum flow (Servo 900C) [15]; others terminate IPS at a flow as low as 2 liters/min (Ohmeda CPU-1) [15].

Clinically, we have noticed a large variation in patient tolerance of various ventilators with IPS at similar levels and postulated that alterations in peak inspiratory flow and expiratory trigger flow would affect the ventilatory pattern, established with a given ventilator, as well as affect the ventilatory drive of patients receiving pressure support.

To study the effects of these two variables, we used a prototype Bear 3 ventilator and a Drager IRISA ventilator. During inspiratory pressure support, the expiratory trigger setting on the Bear 3 could be varied from 25% to

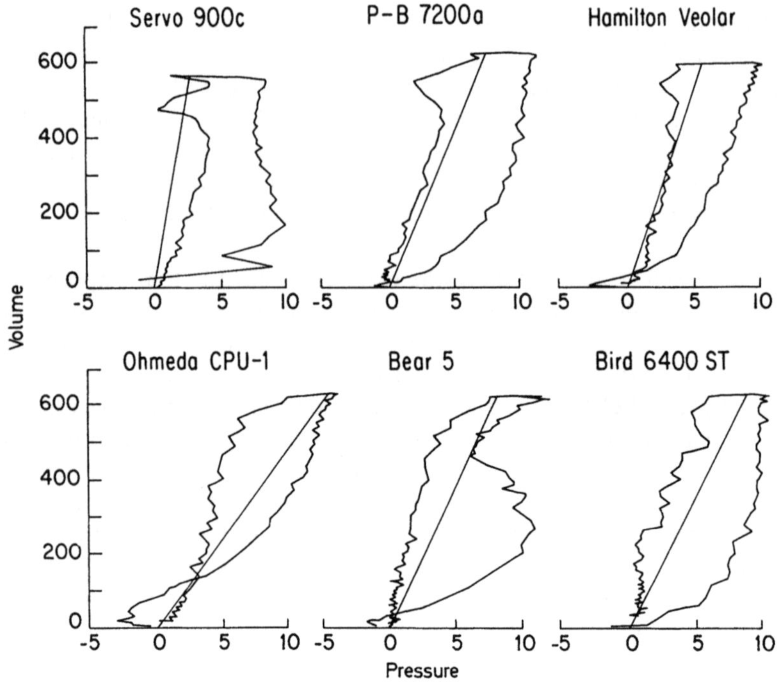

Fig. 2. Representative pressure-volume loops during spontaneous breathing via a lung model at an IPS level of 10 cmH_2O. (From Kacmarek [15])

35% to 50% of peak inspiratory flow. The IRISA ventilator has the capability of varying the configuration of the inspiratory pressure curve, which results in an alteration in the maximum inspiratory flow initially established during IPS. Measured on a lung model, the full range of alterations in the inspiratory pressure curve at a peak inspiratory flow of 40 liters/min caused peak flow delivery to vary from 71 to 53 liters/min [11].

The preliminary results we present here were determined in eight patients with the Bear 3 and in four different patients with the IRISA. During each application we adjusted the IPS level to at least overcome the work imposed by the ventilator-endotracheal tube system, establishing an acceptable ventilatory pattern for each patient. This resulted in applied IPS levels between 10 and 20 cmH_2O. In addition to changes in respiratory rate, tidal volume, pulse, and blood pressure, we analyzed the inspiratory pressure waveform produced by each alteration.

Figure 3 illustrates the approach used during airway pressure waveform analysis. The inspiratory phase was divided in three time frames: 1) A to B represents the time between patient initiation of inspiration and the ventilator providing sufficient gas flow to begin to pressurize the system (trigger time, T_T); 2) B to C represents the time from initial pressurization of the system to the

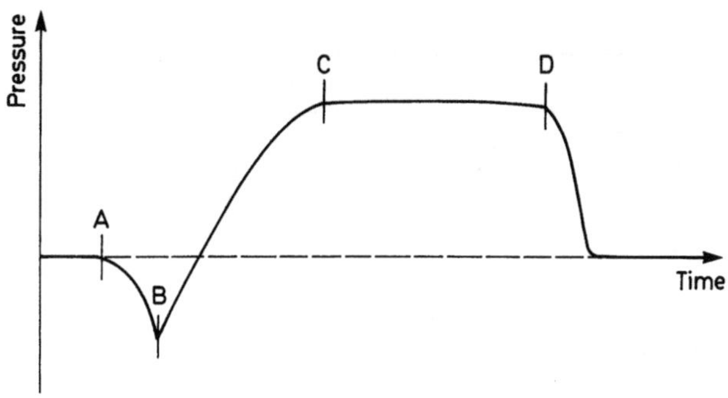

Fig. 3. Method used to analyze the inspiratory pressure waveform produced during IPS with Bear 3 and Drager IRISA ventilators. *A-B*, time of trigger; *B-C*, time from trigger to plateau pressure; *C-D*, time of plateau; *A-D*, total inspiratory time. The vertical distance *A-B* represents trigger pressure. See text for details

attainment of the plateau pressure (IPS level, T_{Tp}); 3) C to D represents the time that IPS (plateau pressure) was maintained (T_p), while A to D is the total patient inspiratory time (T_{TOT}). The vertical distance (pressure axis) on Fig. 3 between A and B represents the amount of pressure generated by the patient during triggering of the ventilator to inspiration (trigger pressure, P_T). In addition, we calculated the product of P_T and T_T, the pressure time product (P–T product), as an index of ventilatory drive [6].

The results of the Bear 3 trial are listed in Table 1. Note that no statistically significant differences existed for any of the directly measured variables. Although respiratory rate (RR) tended to be higher at the 50% trigger setting, as did P_T, tidal volume (V_T) tended to be lower. The T_P and T_{TOT} tended to be longer at the 25% setting. When the P–T product was determined, the 35% and 50% settings differed from the 25% setting. In spite of the overall consistency in waveform, we considered the P-T product increase as a reflection of changing ventilatory drive. Since the unit triggered to exhalation sooner at the 50% setting, patients were required to perform additional effort to ventilate, establishing a trend toward higher RRs and lower V_Ts.

Similar findings have been recently reported by Braschi et al. [16]. Using a prototype Hamilton Veolar ventilator on a series of nine patients, the expiratory trigger setting was varied between 3% and 56% of peak inspiratory flow rate. They noted a reduction in RR with an increase in V_T as the trigger sensitivity was decreased (near 3% setting). However, they noted, as we, that the optimal expiratory trigger setting varied across the whole spectrum of trigger settings. Optimal level seemed to be based on the therapeutic endpoint and patient ventilatory drive but tended to cluster more at low trigger settings than high.

The results of the IRISA trial are listed in Table 2. As you will note, statistically significant differences were present for RR, T_T, P_T, P–T product, T_{TP}, T_P, and T_{TOT}. From this data the number two setting, the pressure waveform

Table 1. Bear 3 trial ($n = 8$)

Expiratory trigger[a]	25%	35%	50%
RR (per min)	20 ± 7	21 ± 8	23 ± 7
V_T (ml)	616 ± 286	603 ± 324	577 ± 333
T_T (s)	0.25 ± 0.11	0.22 ± 0.06	0.21 ± 0.06
P_T (cmH_2O)	3.2 ± 1.0	3.3 ± 2.0	3.4 ± 1.4
P-T (cmH_2O–s)	0.48 ± 0.15	0.69 ± 0.21*	0.75 ± 0.31*
T_{TP} (s)	0.37 ± 0.06	0.32 ± 0.14	0.34 ± 0.08
T_p (s)	0.41 ± 0.21	0.38 ± 0.27	0.35 ± 0.23
T_{TOT} (s)	1.03 ± 0.28	0.97 ± 0.25	0.91 ± 0.22

All values: mean ± SD.
*$p < 0.05$ ANOVA
[a] See text for definition of variables.

Table 2. IRISA trial ($n = 4$)

Pressure wave[a]-form setting	One	Two	Three	Four
RR (per min)	21.0 ± 7.1	15.8 ± 3.9*	22.7 ± 9.1	20.1 ± 5.3
V_T (ml)	356 ± 126	364 ± 182	248 ± 32	323 ± 81
T_T (s)	0.18 ± 0.09	0.18 ± 0.01	0.11 ± 0.05*	0.22 ± 0.11
P_T (cmH_2O)	1.27 ± 0.49	0.94 ± 0.22*	1.28 ± 0.38	1.53 ± 0.27
P-T (cmH_2O)	0.23 ± 0.09*	0.18 ± 0.06*	0.14 ± 0.04*	0.33 ± 0.18
T_{TP} (s)	0.34 ± 0.19*	0.81 ± 0.16	0.84 ± 0.26	0.93 ± 0.21
T_p (s)	0.38 ± 0.21	0.54 ± 0.47	0.19 ± 0.20*	0.20 ± 0.17*
T_{TOT} (s)	0.89 ± 0.25*	1.53 ± 0.43	1.14 ± 0.28*	1.35 ± 0.28

All values: mean ± SD.
* $p < 0.05$ ANOVA
[a] Setting one resulted in the highest peak flow which decreased progressively at the two, three, and four settings (see text for definition of variables).

resulting in the second-highest maximum inspiratory flow, produced the most acceptable overall ventilatory pattern. Alterations in available peak inspiratory flow resulted in profound variation in patient inspiratory effort (P_T), ventilatory drive (*P–T*), and overall ventilatory pattern. As with the expiratory trigger setting, large individual variations existed. Those patients with the highest ventilatory drive required the highest setting (one in Table 2) for the establishment of the most acceptable ventilatory pattern, while those with lower drives tolerated the lower flow capability settings better (two and three in Table 2). Similar findings were reported by Li-Ing and MacIntyre [17]. They used the IRISA to establish IPS_{max} (V_T of 10–12 ml/kg) and found that a lower IPS level was required to establish V_T at lower available peak flow setting capabilities.

Pressure support has been considered by many as a mode of ventilation best tolerated by the spontaneously breathing patient because of the mechanical ventilator's ability to independently contour delivery of gas to the patient's demands. Our preliminary data, along with that of others [16, 17], suggest that there may be a need for more clinician control over IPS delivery characteristic to ensure maximizing the synchrony of the patient-ventilator system. Based on these data, we believe patient tolerance of IPS would be improved if the capability to vary peak inspiratory flow during IPS was available on ventilator systems.

References

1. Christopher KL, Neff TA, Bowman JL et al. (1985) Demand and continuous flow intermittent mandatory ventilation systems. Chest 87:625–630
2. Marini JJ, Capps JS, Culver BH (1985) The inspiratory work of breathing during assisted mechanical ventilation. Chest 87:612–618
3. Fernandez R, Benito S, Sanchis J, Milie-Emili J, Net A (1988) Inspiratory effort and occlusion pressure in triggered mechanical ventilation. Intensive Care Med 14:650–653
4. Gurevitch MJ, Gelmont D (1989) Importance of trigger sensitivity to ventilator response delay in advanced COPD with respiratory failure. Crit Care Med 17:354–359
5. Marini JJ, Rodriguez RM, Lamb V (1986) The inspiratory workload of patient-initiated mechanical ventilation. Am Rev Respir Dis 134:902–909
6. Marini JJ, Smith TC, Lamb VJ (1988) External work output and force generation during synchronized intermittent mechanical ventilation. Am Rev Respir Dis 138:1169–1179
7. Gibney RTN, Wilson RS, Pontoppidan H (1982) Comparison of work of breathing on high gas flow and demand valve. Chest 82:692–695
8. Viale JP, Annat G, Bertrand O (1985) Additional inspiratory work in intubated patients breathing with continuous positive airway pressure systems. Anesthesiology 63:536–539
9. Henry WC, West GA, Wilson RA (1983) A comparison of the oxygen cost of breathing between a continuous-flow CPAP system and a demand-flow CPAP system. Respir Care 28:1273–1281
10. Katz JA, Kraemer RW,. Gjerde GE (1985) Inspiratory work and airway pressure with continuous positive pressure delivery systems. Chest 88:519–526
11. Hirsch CA, Kacmarek RM, Stanek K (1988) Mechanical ventilator demand-valve function with and without continuous positive airway pressure (CPAP) and pressure support (PS) (abstract). Respir Care 33:908
12. Samodelov LF, Falke KJ (1988) Total inspiratory work with modern demand valve devices compared to continuous flow CPAP. Intensive Care Med 14:632–639
13. Bolder PM, Healy TEJ, Bolder AR et al. (1986) The extra work of breathing through adult endotracheal tubes. Anesth Analg 65:853–859
14. Shapiro M, Wilson RK, Casar G et al. (1986) Work of breathing through different sized endotracheal tubes. Crit Care Med 14:1028–1031
15. Kacmarek RM (1988) The role of pressure support ventilation in reducing work of breathing. Respir Care 33:99–120
16. Braschi A, Sala Gallini G, Rodi G et al. (1989) Relationship between sensitivity of the expiratory trigger and breathing pattern during pressure support ventilation (abstract). Am Rev Respir Dis 139:A361
17. Li-Ing H, MacIntyre NR (1989) Pressure supported breaths: ventilatory effects of breath initiation and breath termination design characteristics. Crit Care Med 17:S26

Learnt Ventilation Processes

E. Hecker, P. Gebhardt, and D. Weismann

The title "Learnt Ventilation Processes" presents a particular challenge in view of the fact that learnt processes have not, as yet, been applied in practice. It is difficult to report on something which at best is still at the research stage. In addition, two questions present themselves: what are learnt ventilation processes used for and why the processes developed to date are not entirely adequate?

It will be helpful to approach this challenge by first looking at ventilation patterns. If we look at the changes of airway pressure and flow during controlled ventilation, spontaneous breathing, and the processes which support spontaneous breathing we find several completely different typical patterns. The distinguishing characteristics of these patterns will be woven into the main theme of this lecture which explores the terms "controlling", "regulating", and "learning".

Controlling

Controlling is a process in which an input variable influences an output variable. The characteristic of control is an open loop system.

In controlled ventilation the machine controls the breathing of the patient by regularly applying a pre-set volume. The action sequence runs from the machine to the patient. It is therefore necessary to relax the patient in order to eliminate the "disruptive variable" of the patient's spontaneous breathing. In spontaneous breathing, on the other hand, the supply of gas by a continuous positive airway pressure (CPAP) appliance is controlled by the spontaneous breathing of the patient. Here, the machine should play a passive role.

When both ventilator and spontaneous breathing by the patient provide the control, the result will be opposed sequences of action with interaction between the patient and machine, which leads to "fighting" by the patient (Fig. 1).

When the patient is breathing spontaneously, controlled ventilation is not the best solution. The dominance of aggressive ventilation therapy, with sedation and controlled ventilation, now appears to have had its day.

For a long time it was thought that using controlled ventilation could help the patient to overcome temporary breathing problems. Then it was realised that, although controlled ventilation did provide temporary alleviation, there were side effects on the lungs and other organs. Consequently, today the tendency is to use spontaneous breathing – or processes supporting spontaneous

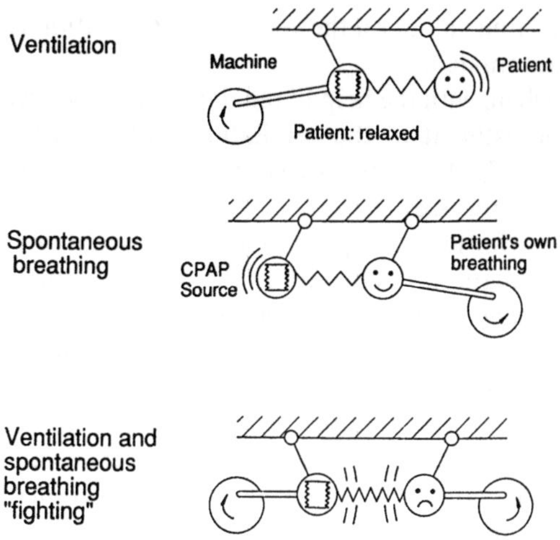

Fig. 1. Different modes of ventilation

breathing – as early and for as long as possible both to prevent the "unphysiological" phase of controlled ventilation and to make use of the positive effects of spontaneous breathing on the circulation and other organs. Today we understand ventilation therapy as "weaning from day one". It was, therefore, necessary for the ventilator to adapt to the patient's spontaneous breathing rather than for the patient to have to adapt to the ventilator.

The first step in this direction was to extend the concept of controlled ventilation so that it became assisted ventilation with the help of a trigger function. Here the ventilation frequency was adjusted to the patient's own rhythm and deviations. Then a controlled mechanism with intermittent mandatory ventilation (IMV) was developed for weaning which consisted of a chronological sequence of controlled ventilation interspersed with timed windows of spontaneous breathing. In this process the concept of control with its open loop system is still dominant. For IMV, an adequate IMV frequency has to be pre-set to safeguard minimum ventilation for the patient. Changes in patient status are not automatically recorded and corrections must be made manually on the IMV. This manual correction can be regarded as a first step towards regulation.

Regulating

Regulating is a process involving the continuous recording of regulated variables, comparison with desired values, and correction by adjustment to desired values. The characteristic of regulation is the closed loop system.

The advantage of regulation is that changes in a regulated function caused by disruptive variables can be recorded in the control loop and corrected. In this way, regulated ventilation processes can be adapted to changes in patient status. However, regulation involves extra expense because these systems require a doctor's continual attention to adjusting values on the ventilator. Regulation is, therefore, becoming increasingly automated.

We live in an age of regulating when, with the help of regulated processes, we try to achieve the best possible adjustment to the ventilation pattern of the patient with spontaneous breathing. To illustrate this point we would like to consider a few regulated ventilation processes.

To improve the weaning process Hewlett et al. [1] proposed the mandatory minute volume (MMV) process. Regulation is achieved by the desired value of minute volume being set. The spontaneously breathed minute volume is continuously compared as the actual value with the desired value. When the difference between the desired value and the actual value reaches the volume of a respiratory stroke the machine issues a mandatory stroke to make up the difference. In contrast to IMV, the result, i.e. the frequency of mechanically applied respiratory strokes, is dependent on the spontaneous breathing action of the individual patient rather than on a pre-set machine frequency.

The augmented processes, known as "pressure support", "inspiratory help system" and "assisted spontaneous breathing" (ASB) can also be regulated to improve adjustment to a patient with spontaneous breathing.

We would now like to discuss the process of weaning by means of a MMV with variation of ASB level. A minute volume is given as the desired value. Where the minute volume spontaneously breathed by the patient with ASB does not reach the MMV desired value, the assistance to spontaneous breathing (ASB level) is increased in steps. This deepens the stroke volume breathed by the patient and also the minute volume. Where the desired value of minute ventilation is reached or exceeded, the amount of spontaneous assistance is automatically reduced.

Such MMV, regulated by the process of ASB, avoids the use of machine-controlled respiratory strokes necessary in other MMV concepts with all the physiological disadvantages for the patient.

A further example of regulation is normoventilation with regulation of breathing minute volume by measurements of end-tidal CO_2 partial pressure. This ventilation pattern may, for example, be used in anaesthesia in order to reduce the tendency to hyperventilation. The application of such an algorithm is subjected to the patient being stable, i.e. that the end-tidal CO_2 partial pressure is correlated with the arterial CO_2 partial pressure and that the alveolar arterial difference remains constant.

A desired value of the endtidal partial pressure to be reached is set and then continuously compared breath by breath with the CO_2 values emitted by the patient. When the desired value and the actual value differ, the frequency or stroke volume of controlled ventilation is adjusted.

Weaning by means of "carbon dioxide mandatory ventilation" (CO_2MV) according to Chopin et al. [2] is yet another example.

In the case of a chronic destructive pulmonary disease (COPD) patient there is an individual correlation between the arterial and the end-tidal CO_2 partial pressure. In the steady state, the arterial end-tidal CO_2 partial pressure remains constant, even during changes of CO_2 production. Under these conditions, the ventilator can control the weaning of the patient. This is done by a change-over, controlled by the end-tidal CO_2 partial pressure, between controlled ventilation and CPAP. The end-expiratory CO_2 partial pressures are, therefore, compared breath by breath with two threshold values, P_{ETint} and P_{ETmax}. When the end-tidal CO_2 exceeds the P_{ETmax} threshold for a period T1 the CPAP ventilator is changed over to controlled ventilation.

The CO_2 flushing process is improved by controlled ventilation and the CO_2 concentration will fall below the P_{ETint} threshold. After a period T2 has passed, the ventilator is again changed over to the CPAP operating mode. In this way an individual patient weaning pattern is achieved. Figure 2 shows the development of the weaning pattern, published by Chopin. It compares the transcutaneously measured $P_{TC}CO_2$ and the end-expiratory PCO_2.

Weaning patients is the crucial element in the processes we have considered, since the co-ordination of the ventilator and the patient's spontaneous breathing requires special adjustment. When the regulated ventilation processes become too complex in their algorithms, the operator is unable to understand clearly what is happening. He is no longer able to distinguish where the ventilation dynamics come – from changes in the patient or from adjustments made by the resulting algorithm.

At this point, the limits of regulated ventilation processes become apparent. These lie in the complexity of the algorithms and the resulting loss of understanding by the operator. Moreover, regulation which has the essential purpose of eliminating short-term deviations has inherent limits. Longer-term ventilation changes cannot, as yet, be controlled in the same way. However, there is

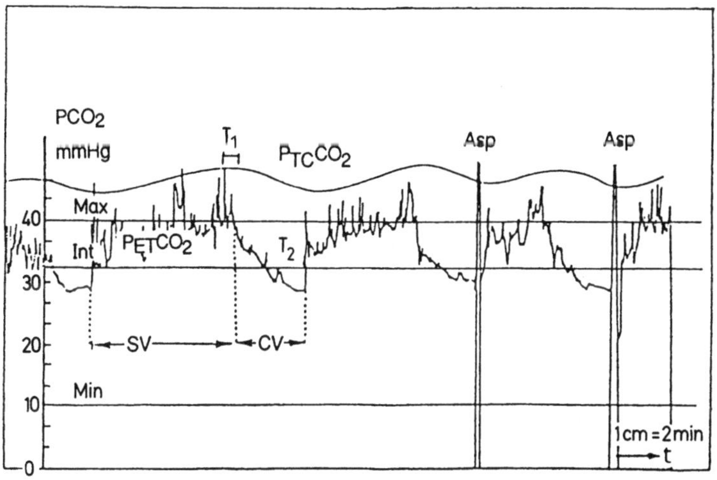

Fig. 2. Weaning: CO_2 mandatory ventilation. Simultaneous recording of transcutaneous and expired partial pressure of CO_2($P_{TC}CO_2$ and $P_{ET}CO_2$). (According to Chopin et al. [23])

a need for "long-term adjustment" to influence continuously the entire course of ventilation therapy for individual patients. Today, doctors work to both control and regulate ventilation processes on ventilators. They use several different approaches to adjust ventilation patterns independently of patient status. These approaches may be applied to the working out of learnt processes. Two examples of different ventilation strategies are:

1. The differential ventilation approach, according to Wolff [3], with basic setting and initial adjustment of the pattern as well as a seven step programme with a gradual increase in the "aggressiveness" of ventilation. It is shown here in a simplified form on the parameter-ventilation mechanics (Table 1).
2. The Benzer strategy during ventilation and weaning [4]. Here the aggressiveness of ventilation is increased in a four-stage step-by-step approach, or reduced for weaning. The target parameter in this strategy is peak inspiratory flow (PIF). It is the product of positive end expiratory pressure (PEEP), inspiration to expiration time ratio (I:E) and inspiratory oxygen fraction. Benzer calls for comprehensive monitoring to carry out this strategy (Table 2) [6–8].

Table 1. Ventilation mechanics according to Wolff [3]

Step 1	Increase TV to 1700 as long as Paw(t) < ca. 30–40
Step 2	Prolong inspiration, that is reduce flow and shorten expiration (up to 2:1)
Step 3	PEEP 5
Step 4	PEEP 10
Step 5	PEEP 10 and Inflation hold 0.6
Step 6	PEEP 10 to 20 and Inflation hold to 1.2
Step 7	PEEP 10 to 20 and Inflation hold 0.6–1.2 physical cooling

Table 2. Step by step approach to ventilation and weaning according to Benzer and Koller [4]

PIF ↑↑			
Ventilation ↓	Step I	CPAP	Weaning ↑
	Step II	IMV, HFP	
	Step III	Continuous positive pressure ventilation (PEEP) I:E ratio 1:2 PEEP 5–10 cmH_2O	
	Step IV	Inversed ratio ventilation (IRV) I:E ratio 1:1–3:1 PEEP 5–10 cmH_2O	
	Alternatives	HFV, extracorporeal CO_2 elimination	
	Wet lung	CAVH	
			PIF ↓↓

Learning

Learning how then can the strategies we have discussed be put into practice in a technical system for learnt ventilation processes? First we must define the term "learning" as follows: 'Acquiring certain patterns of reaction based on certain patterns of stimulation.' A child learns, for example, that touching a hot cooker top hurts. Based on the learnt stimulation pattern "hot", it will in future not carry out the reaction "touch".

In the context of our discussions, the term "learnt processes" needs to be simplified and limited so that it does not concern itself with the process of "acquiring" but rather with the process of reaction based on a certain stimulation. Learnt, recognised consequences influence future action.

A learnt process means, therefore, recognising "stimulation patterns" from measured values and then changing the desired values in regulated systems. What is crucial in defining learnt ventilation processes is the analysis of the stimulation patterns that will have to be recognised.

The automated application of the ventilation strategies discussed earlier is difficult when the basis for decision making is poorly defined. The scientific literature describes the processes which can, with the help of "standard basic decision making", can be used for pattern recognition to produce proposals for the adjustment of ventilation parameters. We are referring here to a paper by Holtzman and Seiver [5] which described the process of determining adjustments by decision-making processes.

Decision-making analysis has a key role in this process. It differs from both descriptive sciences and engineering sciences in its normative character and is used to work out guidelines for correct action.

How do experts reach a proper understanding of the decision-making process? The answer to this question is that they serve their apprenticeship in real decision-making situations where they can gain insight and progressively build up and refine a model of decision-taking. The consequences which flow from these decisions must then be documented in an appropriate manner.

An effective way of doing this is to use influence diagrams. Influence diagrams are easy to understand, can be defined mathematically, are general in nature and allow decision-making rules to be stated concisely. By using an influence diagram, mathematically different descriptive relationships can be shown simultaneously. For example, the input variable fractional inspiratory oxygen (FIO_2) can be assigned a range of values, the deterministic variable DO_2 can be assigned a function and the stochastic variable survival can be assigned a probability of survival dependent on oxygen toxicity (Fig. 3).

With the assistance of specialists the full relationship between inspiratory oxygen concentration and survival probability can be shown in a decision diagram. Input variables, which have to be determined on the patient at regular intervals, are required in order to be able to adjust the statement of relationships for each individual patient status. When this is done a decision diagram is

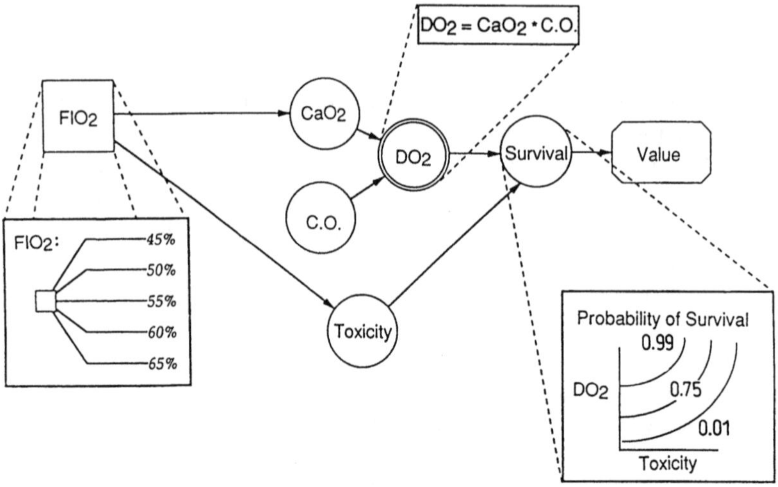

Fig. 3. Influence diagram: presentation patterns. The decision variable is the fractional inspiratory oxygen (FIO_2), the deterministic variable (DO_2) is assigned a function, and the stochastic variable *survival* is assigned a probability

created which is mathematically and structurally defined and which contains the influence parameters for individual patients (Fig. 4).

The decision analysis method now allows us to reduce the complexity of the influence diagram by using suitable algorithms. The result is a simple relationship between inspiratory oxygen concentration and survival probability.

We can now use the decision diagram. For example, when the data are entered we can find the optimum inspiratory oxygen concentration which the patient requires at that precise time. If the input values are updated a few hours later we will then find the optimum inspiratory oxygen concentration for the patient at that moment (Fig. 5).

All other essential parameters can be entered in the influence diagram in analogous fashion. The drawing up of influence diagrams from decision-making situations may be compared with the drawing up of maps in geography. Whereas maps facilitate future orientation, influence diagrams facilitate the carrying-out of therapy decisions.

If we now attempt to reply to our earlier question on the need for learnt ventilation processes, we will find the answer in the need for a longer-term ventilation regime. The benefit to the patient lies in the continuous monitoring of patient status which can then be carried out and in the possibility of reacting continuously using an adequate ventilation pattern for the individual patient. A further benefit lies in the existence of a uniform basis for regulation for all members of the therapy team.

Before a therapy proposal system, such as the one outlined here, can be applied, ventilation strategies must be translated into appropriate influence diagrams. Also essential are regulated ventilation processes, which desired

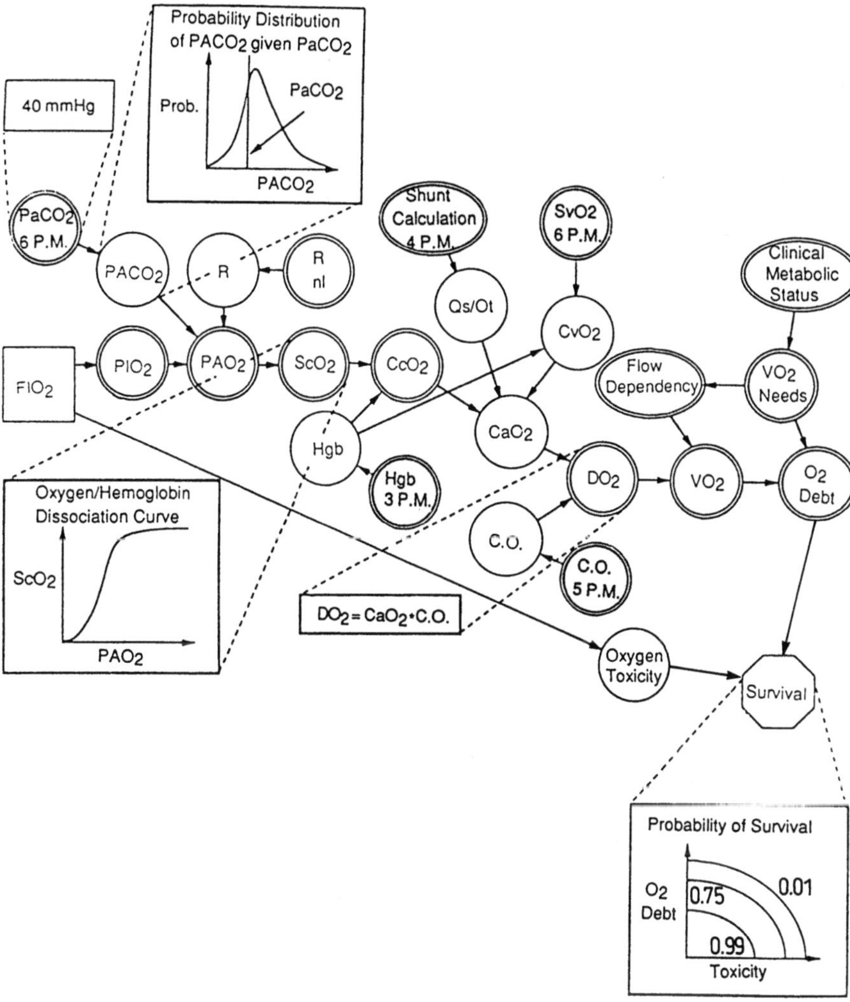

Fig. 4. Influence diagram: total relationship between inspiratory oxygen concentration and survival probability

values can be changed in accordance with the learnt and recognised parameter patterns derived from the influence diagram.

A further essential is thorough monitoring of the measured parameters used in the influence diagrams. These must be derived from valid measurements and should, therefore, be validated.

Given these factors we could expect therapy-supporting processes in the future. At present, the main difficulty is the transfer of expert knowledge into influence diagrams, and consequently this is now the subject of intensive research.

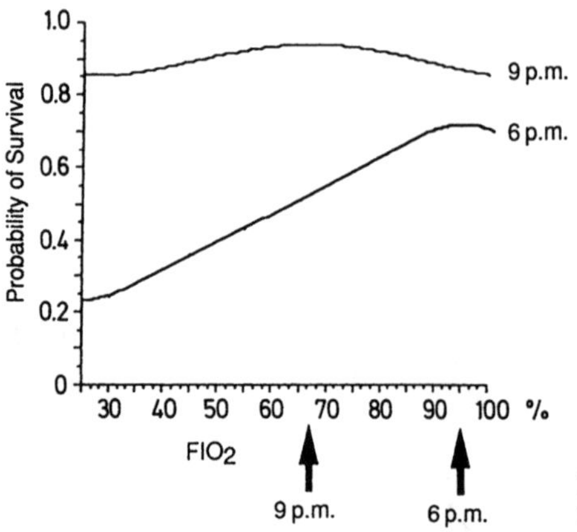

Fig. 5. Different optimum oxygen concentrations (*arrows*) at two different times

References

1. Hewlett AM, Platt AS, Terry VG (1977) Mandatory minute volume: a new concept in weaning from mechanical ventilation. Anaesthesia 32:163–169
2. Chopin C, Chambrin MC, Mangalaboyi J, Lestarel P, Fourrier F (1989) Carbon dioxide mandatory ventilation (CO_2MV): a new method for weaning from mechanical ventilation. Int Clin Monit Comput 6:11
3. Wolff G (1983) Die Künstliche Beatmung auf Intensivstationen, 3rd edn. Springer, Berlin Heidelberg New York, p 166
4. Benzer M, Koller W (1987) Die Strategie der Beatmung. Intensivmedizin 24:214
5. Seiver A, Holtzman S (1988) Decision analysis: a framework for critical care decision assistance. International symposium on computer-assisted decision support and data base management in anaesthesia, intensive care and cardio-pulmonary medicine (1988), Rotterdam
6. Putensen C, Baum M, Koller W, Putz G (1989) PEEP-Welle: ein automatisiertes Verfahren zur bettseitigen Bestimmung der Volumen/Druck-Beziehung der Lunge beatmeter Patienten. Anaesthesist 38:214
7. Stock C, Downs J, Frohlicher D (1987) Airway pressure release ventilation. Crit Care Med 15:462
8. Lemaire F (1984) L'aide inspiratoire: progräs decisif ou mode passagüre? Räan Soins Intens Mäd Urg 4 (5)

Part 9:

Tissue Oxygenation and Organ Metabolism

Diagnostic and Therapeutic Possibilities of a Computer-Based Hemodynamic Multisensor System

K. Stangl, M. Laule, A. Wirtzfeld, and R. Heinze

Introduction

In recent years advances in sensor technology and microelectronics have opened the way to new dimensions in monitoring and treatment, and growing attendance has been focussed on the development of multifunctional catheters. This approach, however, sets high demands on technology to achieve long-term stability of the sensors and on operational complexity and memory capacity of the processing units.

For diagnostic and therapeutic reasons we developed a computer-based multisensor system.

Design of the Multisensor System

For performing the tests we have developed a multisensor catheter and a computerized measuring and evaluating system connected thereto.

The Multisensor Catheter

The multisensor catheter is shown in Fig. 1. The 7F catheter has the tip electrode in the ventricle, an electrode 4 cm behind the tip, and an electrode 8 cm behind the tip, which is positioned in the atrium. Two piezoresistive pressure sensors are implemented in the ventricle and in the atrium; the catheter also disposes of an

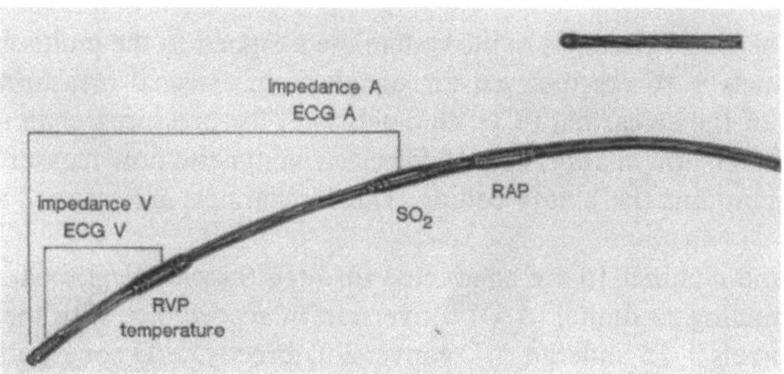

Fig. 1. Design of the multisensor catheter. *A*, atrium, *V*, ventricle

optoelectric sensor we have developed for reflection-oximetric determination of the oxygen saturation. This sensor is placed 8 cm behind the tip and comes to lie in the atrium; a thermistor is also integrated into the sensor for measuring temperature in the ventricle.

The following measuring methods are used:

- The intracardiac ECG is measured between the tip and the lower indifferent electrode of the catheter. The amplification factor is 200.
- The atrial ECG is taken between the lower atrial and tip electrodes; it is also amplified by a factor of 200. Both ECGs are measured at half the repeating cycle, namely at 0.5 ms.
- The impedance measurement is performed using a bipolar rectangular pulse with a frequency of 16 kHz. The ventricular impedance is measured between the indifferent electrode and the tip electrode; the atrial impedance is determined between the lower atrial electrode and the tip. The repeating cycle for both impedances is 1 ms. To determine the right ventricular stroke volume one utilizes the frequency parts above 1 Hz, to determine the respiratory rate the frequency parts below 1 Hz.
- The pressure measurement is performed via piezoresistive pressure sensors which sensitivity is 20 μV/mmHg. The frequency is 2 kHz, the amplitude 1.2 mA.
- The temperature measurement is performed via a thermistor having a direct current of 100 μA; the sensitivity is 1/100°C/ohm.

The oxygen saturation sensor comprises a phototransistor, a light-emitting diode with 630 nm in the red light range, and a light-emitting diode of 910 nm that works in the infrared range. For both light-emitting diodes the supplied alternating current is 1.6 mA. The reflected light is measured by the phototransistor; the photocurrent is amplified by a factor of 20.

Data Processing

The measuring system connected to the catheter is shown with its components in Fig. 2. The system is used in a hemodynamic animal model (pigs) shown in Fig. 3.

The first seven of the 16 channels of the system are assigned to the multisensor catheter. Channels 8–16 are reserved for signals from external measuring devices: channel 8 for the epicardial ECG, channels 9–11 for pressures, channel 12 for the surface ECG, and channels 13–15 for electromagnetic flow measurements; channel 16 contains the binary coding. The 16 channels are scanned at 400 Hz.

Channels 1–8 and channel 16 are conducted through the electrical separation and undergo analog to digital (A/D) conversion in accordance with their scanning rate. Channels 9–15 undergo A/D conversion directly. A/D conversion is performed using a 16-channel A/D converter board. The electrical separation

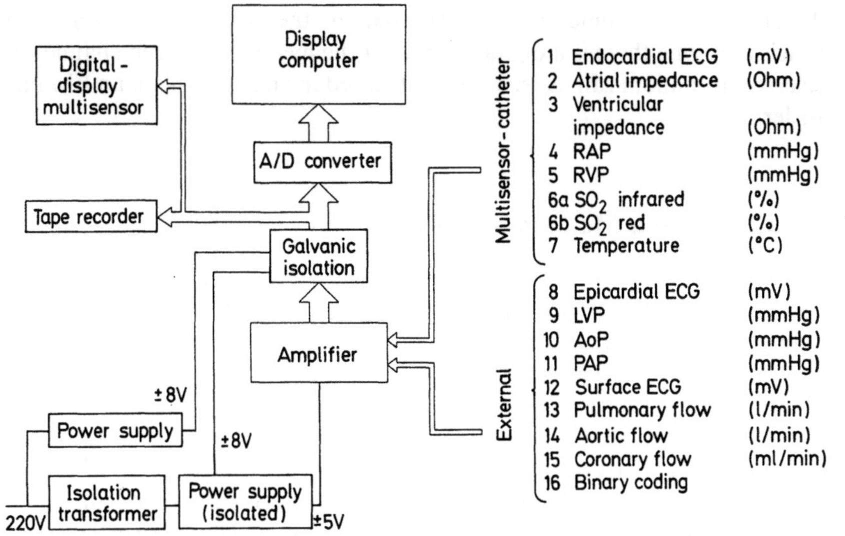

Fig. 2. Block diagram of the multisensor system

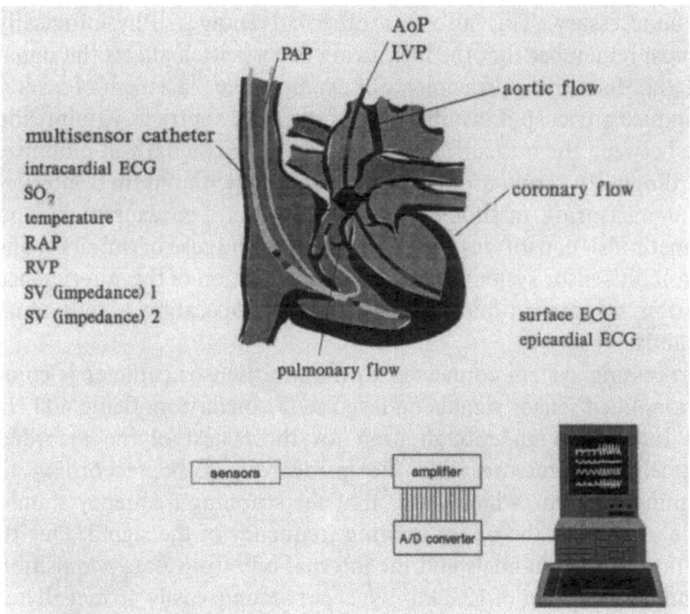

Fig. 3. Hemodynamic animal model (pigs)

between the mains and the patient is performed at the output of the measuring amplifier.

The incoming data are stored on a computer (Compaq Deskpro 386) on a 130-megabyte hard disk. A scroller board is used for the data throughput.

Eight channels at a time can be displayed on the screen online; for seven channels at a time there is a digital display of the mean values. Ten channels to be selected at random can be recorded and stored in analog form on an FM tape recorder.

The Rationale of a Multisensor System

The multisensor catheter developed by us allows for simultaneous detection and for comparison of different parameters under identical physiological and experimental conditions using a reference model of a healthy heart. By registering the intracardiac ECG, central venous blood temperature, the oxygen saturation, the stroke volume, and the pressures of the right heart, it allows for detection of an essential part of the stress-induced adaptation processes of the body which can be detected with measuring technology implemented in cardiac pacemakers.

A very essential advantage of such a multisensor catheter is that the simultaneous measurement of several parameters minimizes the invasiveness of the examination for patients and test persons, since a multisensor catheter makes further access unnecessary. This also has other advantages. Physiologically speaking, one must remember that the measuring process itself affects the signal to be measured (the Heisenberg principle). For example, the placement of several catheters may induce a tricuspid insufficiency of the right ventricle. Minimizing the interference between the measuring process and the biosignal will minimize this error accordingly. In terms of measuring technology, the mutual interference of different measuring methods – such as impedance measurement and polarographic methods – constitutes a great problem in the case of simultaneous measurement. A multisensor system allows for compensation of this interference by synchronization, staggered timing, or pulse interval operation of individual measuring methods.

The data processing system connected to the multisensor catheter is computerized. The amplified sensor signals undergo A/D conversion. Being 400 Hz these scanning rates are high enough even for the fastest of the recorded parameters, namely the pressures and the intracardiac ECG, according to Shannon's scanning theorem, which states that the scanning frequency should be at least twice as high as the upper-limiting frequency of the signal. Due to these scanning rates on 16 channels and the internal offsetting, data acquisition results in the immense data set of 12.8 kilobytes per second, easily 46 megabytes per hour. This data set becomes clearer when one realizes that one megabyte of information will cover about 250 single-spaced standard-size pages. In animal experiments lasting between 5 and 8 h, about 300 megabytes of raw data must thus be processed and stored per test, a task that can currently only be accomplished by the most powerful computers.

The reasons for implementing a computerized measuring system in spite of these technical difficulties lie in the enormous possibilities offered by a digital system. Unlike the measuring systems commonly used in medicine, using recorders as the output medium for the analog data, this data concept allows for both analog and digital storage of the raw data and for access after any time intervals. Furthermore, the digital data format ensures high data security, since falsification during transmission, component drift, distortion by nonlinear components, and the coupling-in of interference signals are virtually ruled out. One of the major reasons for digital systems is that this data format is the basic precondition for all further microprocessor-controlled processing. While analog signal processing necessitates elaborate hardware implementation even for simple signal processing steps, such as maxima formation, and makes it very difficult to perform complex computing operations, the digital data format allows for any kind of further processing by the computer through the use of appropriate software. Data reducing methods such as the formation of minima, maxima, and means, differential and integral formation, and filtering methods such as frequency analyses can be performed automatically by the computer. Furthermore, complex mathematical operations to be performed on the data are virtually impossible without this computer technology.

It is clear from all this that the adequate processing of large numbers of biological signals with a reasonable amount of effort presupposes such a measuring system while, conversely, digital systems open up new dimensions for setting off biological signals.

Intrathoracic Blood Volume Accurately Reflects Circulating Volume Status in Critically Ill Patients

U.J. Pfeiffer, J. Zeravik, M. Lichtwarck-Aschoff and J. Obermaier

Introduction

In general, central venous pressure (CVP) and pulmonary capillary wedge pressure (PCWP) are used for control and management of circulating blood volume. It has been demonstrated that there is a good correlation between left atrial pressure and PCWP during spontaneous breathing and intermittent positive pressure ventilation [1, 2, 7]. However, the introduction of continuous pressure ventilation (CPPV) has complicated the use of, e.g., PCWP as the indicator of left ventricle (LV) preload greatly; more than 10 years ago it was shown that PCWP poorly reflects circulating volume status during CPPV in subjects with normal lungs [13, 16]. In an investigation by Shippy et al. [12] of over 1500 occasions of clinical indication or suspicion of either hypovolemia or hypervolemia during periods of critical illness in patients admitted to the surgical ICU or during early resuscitation from hypotensive shock with administration of a fluid load, blood volume and values of the commonly monitored variables, including CVP, PCWP, and cardiac output (C.O.), improved appropriately. However, the correlation coefficients, in general, were not good. The authors concluded that the commonly monitored variables in and of themselves do not reflect adequately the blood volume status in critically ill patients.

In mechanically ventilated dogs we have already demonstrated that intrathoracic blood volume (ITBV) is more sensitive to hemorrhage than CVP or PCWP (Fig. 1) [10] and that ITBV accurately reflects the intravascular volume status during mechanical ventilation with PEEP [14]. In addition, a retrospective analysis of two groups of patients subjected to different infusion regimens has revealed that ITBV was the only variable reflecting volume status [8]. The aim of this prospective study in critically ill patients was to compare ITBV to the commonly monitored variables with regard to ability to indicate the circulating volume status and without regard to the mode of mechanical ventilation.

Patients and Methods

The study was performed in 26 patients (mean age 39.4 years) with acute respiratory failure. They had the following primary diagnoses at the time of admission to the ICU: multiple trauma ($n = 11$), pneumonia ($n = 4$), neurological

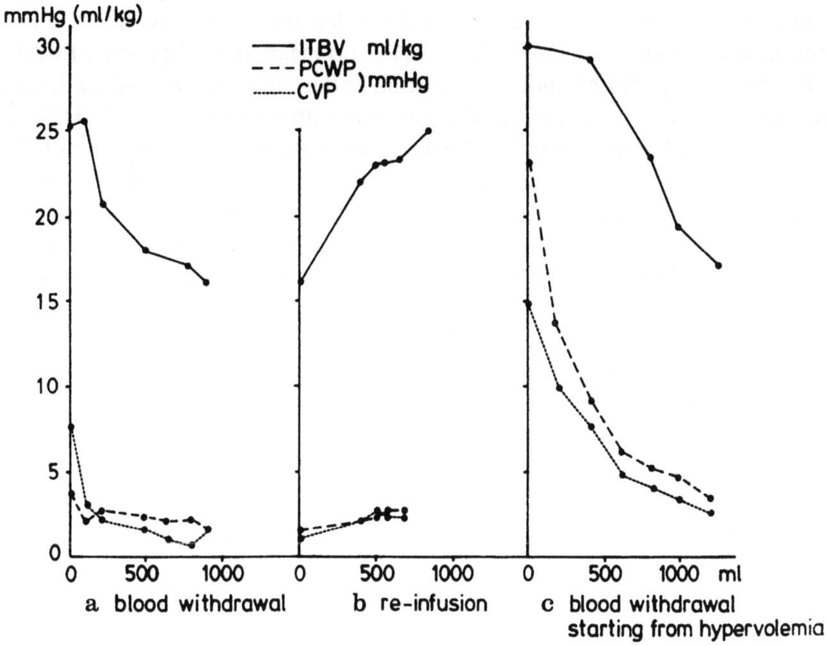

Fig. 1. Typical course of central venous pressure (*CVP*), pulmonary capillary wedge pressure (*PCWP*), and intrathoracic blood volume (*ITBV*) during blood withdrawal and reinfusion in an anesthetized, paralyzed, and mechanically ventilated dog

trauma ($n = 5$), blunt chest trauma ($n = 2$), peritonitis after abdominal surgery ($n = 4$). All patients were admitted to and managed in the surgical ICU and required mechanical ventilation. They were either on CPPV or on combined high frequency ventilation (CHFV) or on pressure support ventilation (PSV). The ventilation patterns and PEEP were adjusted as frequently as necessary. During PSV the patients received less sedatives than during CPPV or CHFV. Volume or diuretics were given according to the circulating volume patterns, which were estimated from CVP, PCWP, C.O., and urine output. Patients with a history of cardiac insufficiency and those requiring positive inotropic or vasoactive drugs were excluded. The study protocol was approved by the institutional ethics committee and informed consent was obtained from the patients or their next of kin.

Catheterization and Measurements

A 7.5 F5 lumen Swan Ganz pulmonary artery thermodilution catheter (Edwards Laboratories, Santa Ana, CA) and a 5.0 F femoral artery catheter equipped with fiber-optics and thermistor (5F Pulsiocath FTL, Pulsion Medizintechnik,

Munich, FRG) were placed in each patient for monitoring of CVP, mean pulmonary artery pressure (MPAP), PCWP, and mean arterial pressure (MAP) and for thermal dye double indicator dilution as described below. Both catheters were connected to an integrated fiber-optic monitoring system (COLD Z-02 System, Pulsion Medizintechnik, Munich, FRG). Figure 2 is a drawing of the thermal dye measuring system. A 10–20 ml bolus of 5% glucose containing 0.75 mg/ml of indocyanine green dye at 0°–4°C was injected into the right atrium at a rate of 10 ml/s with a temperature controlled pneumatic injector (ZI-03 Injector, Pulsion). The dye and the thermal curve recorded in the femoral artery were used for the calculation of C.O., ITBV, and extravascular thermal volume (ETV), as previously described [16]. Figure 3 explains the size and the calculation of ITBV. The COLD system rejects thermal dye measurements if the C.O. measured simultaneously in the pulmonary artery deviates more than $\pm$ 15% from the femoral artery C.O. or if ETV calculated with the slope volume method deviates more than $\pm$ 15% from the ETV value calculated with the mean transit time method [16]. The coefficient of variation of five successive ITBV determinations in these patients was determined to be 8.3% (single measurements).

Calculated Variables

Systemic (SVRI) and pulmonary vascular resistance index (PVRI), the arteriovenous O_2 content difference ($C(a-v)O_2$), the oxygenation index

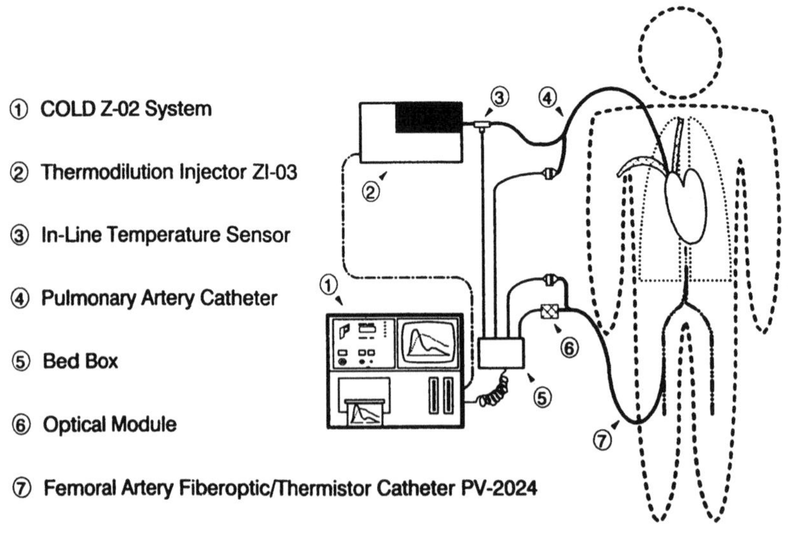

Fig. 2. The COLD Z-O_2 Femoral-pulmonary artery

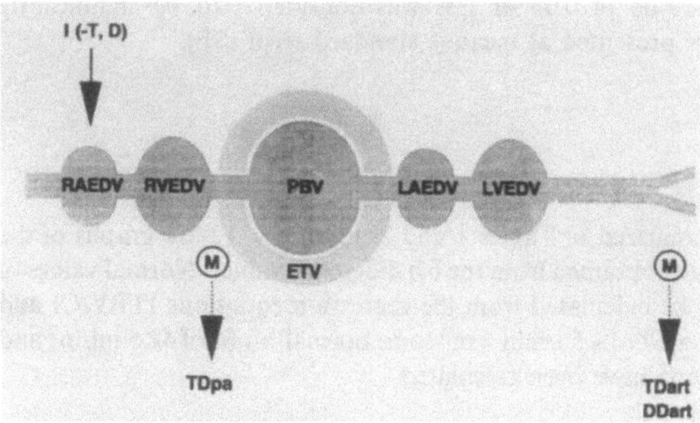

Fig. 3. The size and the calculation of intrathoracic blood volume (ITBV). *RAEDV*, right artial end-diastolic volume; *RVEDV*, right ventricular end-dialstolic volume; *PBV*, pulmonary blood volume; *LAEDV*, left atrial end-diastolic volume; *LVEDV*, left venticular end-diastolic volume; *ETV*, extravascular thermal volume; *I(-T,D)*, injection with negativ heat and dye; *M*, measuring point; *TDpa*, thermodilution in the pulmonary artery; *TDart*, thermodilution in femoral artery; *DDart*, dyedilution in the femoral artery. ITBV = MTTD C.O.TDart, where MTTD is the mean transit time o dye and C.O.TDart is the cardiac output measured by thermodilution in the femoral artery

(PaO_2/FiO_2), the percentage of intrapulmonary shunt (Q_s/Q_t), the oxygen delivery (DO_2I) and the oxygen consumption index (VO_2I) were calculated using standard formulas.

Study Protocol

The patients were placed in a supine position at least 15 min before data collection was started. All pressure measurements were performed at end expiration without removal of PEEP. Indocyanine injection was started at the beginning of expiration. Thermal dye dilution derived variables were determined as a mean of three successive measurements. Data were collected in intervals of 6 h for a maximum period of 4 days.

Statistical Analysis

It was assumed that relevant changes in myocardial inotropic state or changes in afterload did not occur in these patients during the time of the investigation. Validity of this assumption given, a change of a preload-dependent variable would indicate a change of cardiac preload. Therefore, linear regression analyses were performed between the preload-indicating variables, CVP, PCWP, and ITBVI, and the preload-dependent variables, stroke index (SI), Cardiac index (CI), DO_2I, SvO_2, and SVRI, for absolute values as well as for 6 h differences in the variables. A p-value of 0.05 or less was considered to be significantly different. Results are presented as mean ± standard error (SE).

Results

The results are summarized in Tables 1 and 2. Figures 4–12 are graphs of the most important results obtained from the 6 h difference values. Normal values of ITBV and SI could be calculated from the regression equations ITBV/CI and ITBV/SI. Assuming a CI of 4.5 $l/min \times m^2$ to be normal, an SI of 42.5 ml/m^2 and an ITBV of 847 ml/m^2 have been calculated.

Discussion

The validity and accuracy of the measurement of ITBV may be derived from the accuracy of the measurement of extravascular lung water (EVLW), accurately estimated by ETV. ETV is calculated from the difference of total thoracic thermal volume and ITBV. In several experimental investigations ETV has been

Table 1. Correlation coefficients of the regression analyses between absolute values

	CVP	*PCWP*	*ITBVI*
CVP	—	0.54**	– 0.39*
PCWP	0.54**	—	– 0.18
ITBV	– 0.39*	– 0.18	—
CI	– 0.05	– 0.09	0.53**
SI	– 0.09	– 0.14	0.56**

*, $p < 0.05$; **, $p < 0.01$; $n = 256$

Table 2. Correlation coefficients of the regression analyses between 6-h differences in measured values

	dCVP	*dPCWP*	*dITBVI*
dCVP	—	0.27	– 0.15
dPCWP	0.27	—	0.09
dITBV	– 0.15	0.09	—
dCI	– 0.18	– 0.04	0.75**
dSI	– 0.14	– 0.02	0.69**
dSVRI	0.01	– 0.01	– 0.48**
dDO_2I	– 0.1	– 0.06	0.71**
dVO_2I	– 0.1	– 0.05	0.37*
$dSvO_2$	– 0.07	– 0.04	0.33*

*, $p < 0.05$; **, $p < 0.01$; $n = 229$

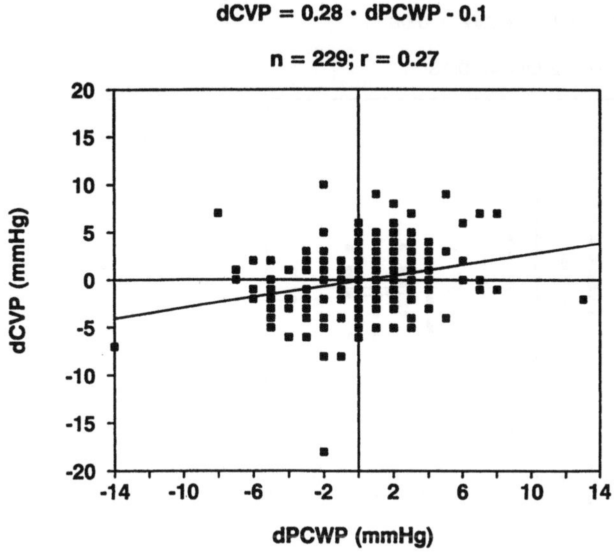

Fig 4. Relationship between the change in central venous pressure (*dCVP*) and the change in pulmonary capillary wedge presure (*dPCWP*) ($n = 229$, $r = 0.27$)

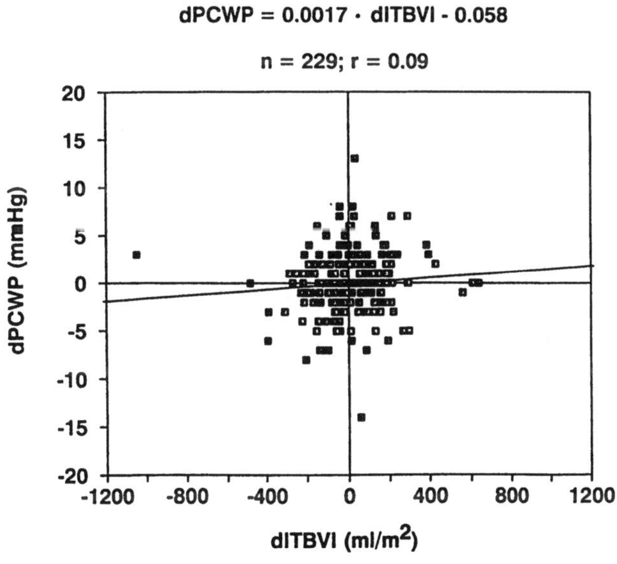

Fig. 5. Relationship between the change in pulmonary capillary wedge pressure (*dPCWP*) and the change in intrathoracic blood volume (*dITBV*) ($n = 229$, $r = 0.09$)

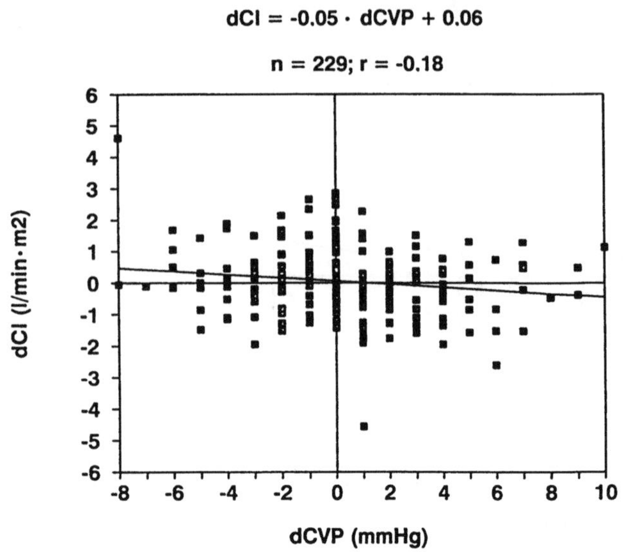

Fig. 6. Relationship between the change in cardiac index (*dCI*) and the change in central venous pressure (*dCVP*) ($n = 229$, $r = -0.18$)

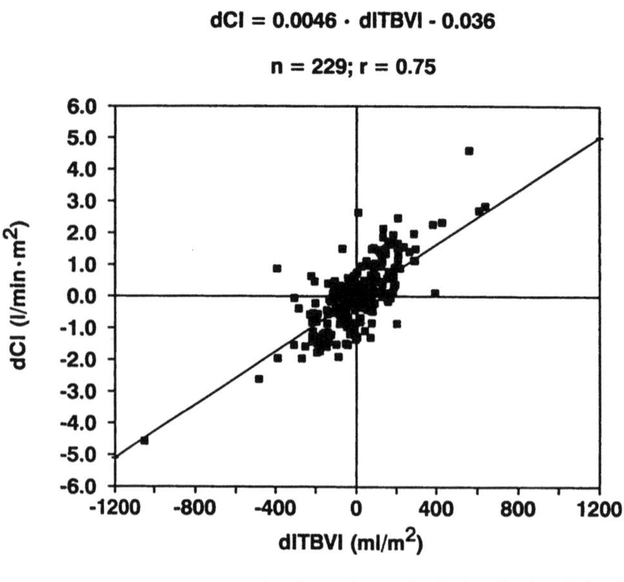

Fig. 7. Relationship between the change in cardiac index (*dCI*) and the change in intrathoracic blood volume (*dITBV*) ($n = 229$, $r = 0.75$)

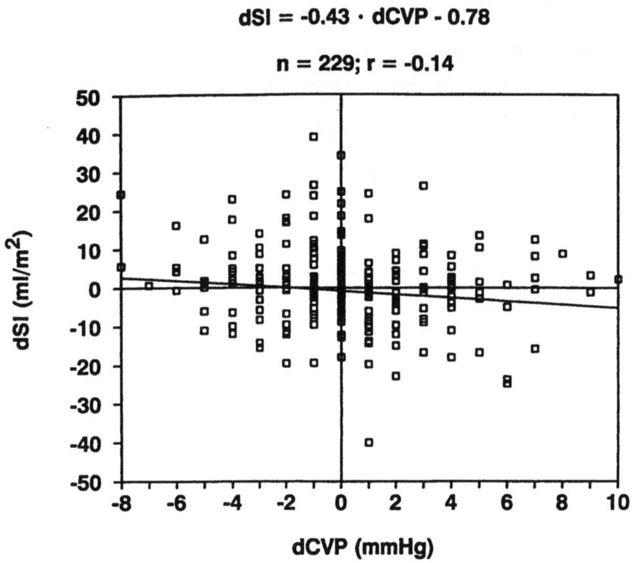

Fig. 8. Relationship between the change in stroke index (*dSI*) and the change in central venous pressure (*dCVP*) ($n = 229$, $r = -0.14$)

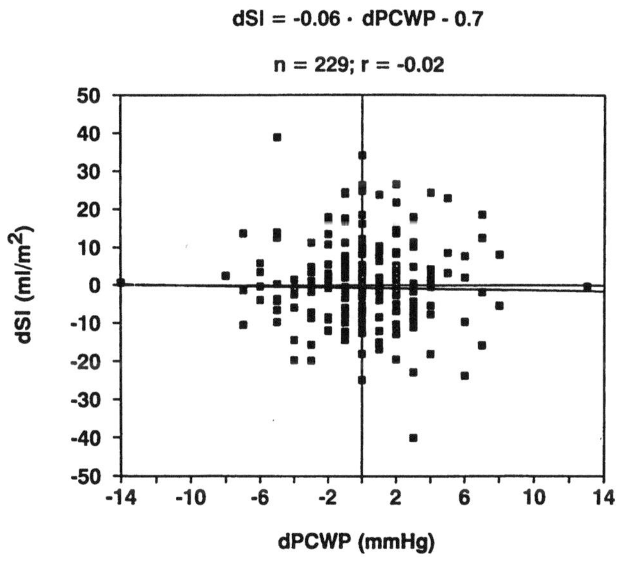

Fig. 9. Relationship between the change in stroke index (*dSI*) and the change in pulmonary capillary wedge pressure (*dPCWP*) ($n = 229$, $r = -0.02$)

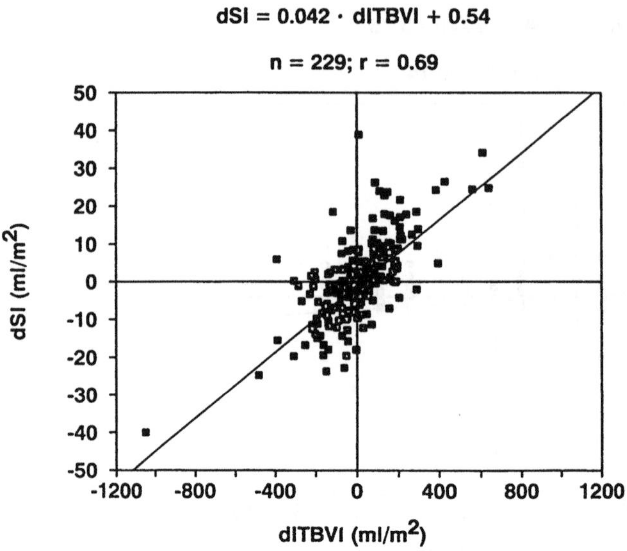

Fig. 10. Relationship between the change in stroke index (*dCI*) and the change in intrathoracic blood volume (*dITBV*) ($n = 229$, $r = 0.69$)

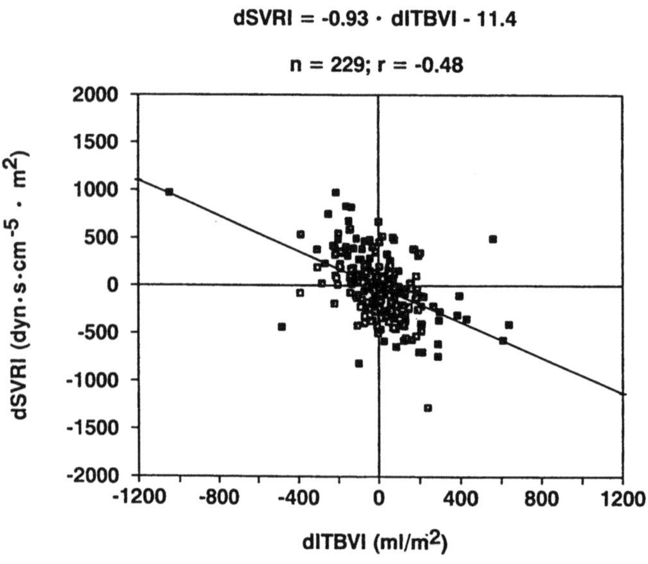

Fig. 11. Relationship between the change in systemic vascular resistance index (*dSVRI*) and the change in intrathoracic blood volume (*dITBV*) ($n = 229$, $r = -0.48$)

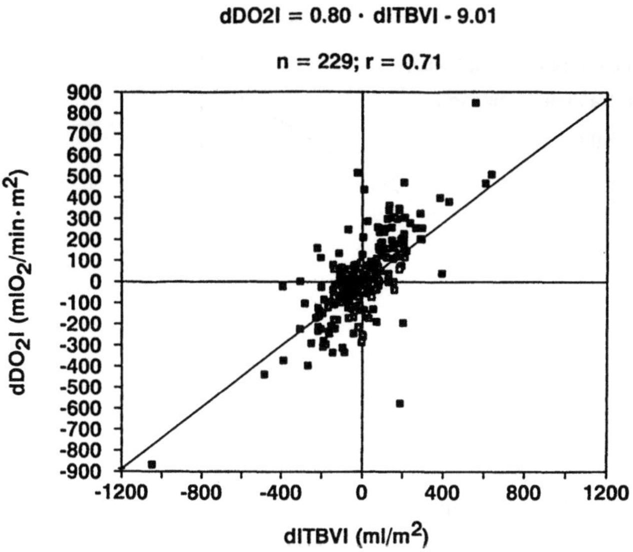

Fig. 12. Relationship between the change in oxygen delivery index (*dDO_2I*) and the change in intrathoracic blood volume (*dITBV*) ($n = 229$, $r = 0.71$)

compared to postmortem determined EVLW and an excellent correlation has been found between EVLW and ETV. Figure 13 shows the results of two studies with different methods of producing pulmonary edema. Moreover, we [9] and others [15] have shown that the measurement of ETV with the Pulsion COLD system was not dependent on flow. On the contrary, a flow dependency of the method has been shown for the Edwards lung water computer [4, 9, 15]. From this we conclude that the determination of ITBV, as a side product of the calculation of ETV, must be as accurate as the ETV measurement.

ITBV reflects the volume of the following six partial volumes: right atrial end-diastolic volume (RAEDV), right ventricular end-diastolic volume (RVEDV), pulmonary blood volume (PBV), left atrial end-diastolic volume (LAEDV), left ventricular end-diastolic volume (LVEDV), and aortic blood volume (AoV). The aorta does not have significant volume-capacitive properties which have to be regarded here; hence, AoV, with a normal value of about 100 ml/m^2, can be regarded as a constant and may be subtracted from the normal value of ITBV yielding a capacitive intrathoracic volume of about 750 ml/m^2. PBV, with a normal value of about 250 ml/m^2, does not account for more than 33% of the normal capacitive intrathoracic volume. Thus, at least two-thirds of ITBV is cardiac preload.

CVP and PCWP both represent the intravascular pressure at a certain point in the circulation. In surgical critical care medicine both pressures are used as indicators of circulating volume status and statements like "wedge pressure was well maintained" or "wedge pressure was kept above 15 mm Hg" are familiar descriptions of volume supply. On the other hand, in cardiology PCWP in

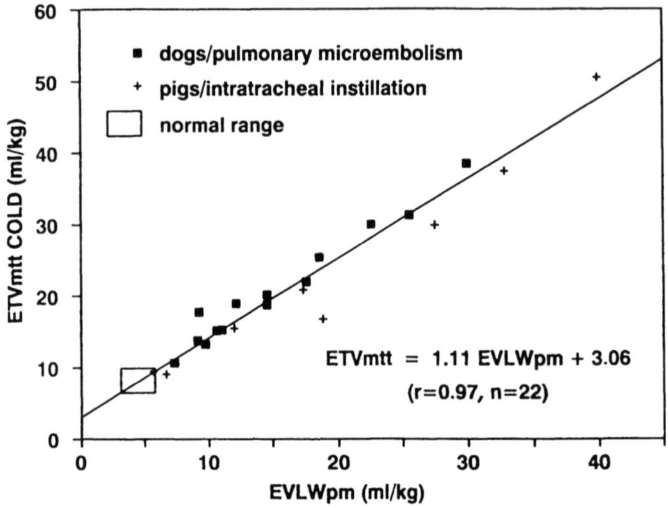

Fig. 13. The results of two studies with different methods of producing pulmonary edema

particular is used as an indicator of left heart function. This obvious discrepancy hallmarks the trivial and inadmissible assumptions made by therapists. In fact, any pressure measured in the low pressure capacitance system is the result of four different mechanisms: (1) function of the cardiac ventricle downstream, (2) circulatory filling volume, (3) intrathoracic pressure or, more precisely, extramural pressure, and (4) venomotor tone [11]. Thus it becomes clear that changes in CVP or PCWP cannot be easily interpreted as changes of cardiac preload or myocardial function. Moreover, technical difficulties add to the overinterpretation of the "filling" pressures. Keeping in mind that a 5 cm error in the height of the zero reference of the pressure transducer causes an error of almost 4 mm Hg, the value of CVP and PCWP measurements, in light of their wide normal ranges of about 8 mm Hg, are questionable [11]. Even in a standardized experimental setting with CPPV, the sensitivity of CVP to blood withdrawal was almost nil; the sensitivity of PCWP, with a value of 16 ml/kg blood withdrawal/mm Hg PCWP decrease, was not much better. Some authors try to get an impression of circulatory filling with CVP and/or PCWP measurements during removal of PEEP ventilation [3, 5, 6]. What is the sense, however, of such a maneuver when the critically ill patient has to survive and the therapist needs to quantify circulatory filling status with PEEP installed?

In conclusion, CVP and PCWP measurements cannot reliably indicate circulating volume status in a ventilated critically ill patient, whereas ITBV quantifies total cardiac preload without removal of PEEP, without cessation of ventilation, and without regard to patient position. The thermal dye technique measures ITBV and ETV simultaneously and thus quantifies two of the three variable volumes in the chest (Fig. 14). Therefore, this technique can provide proper management of the ventilated critically ill patient.

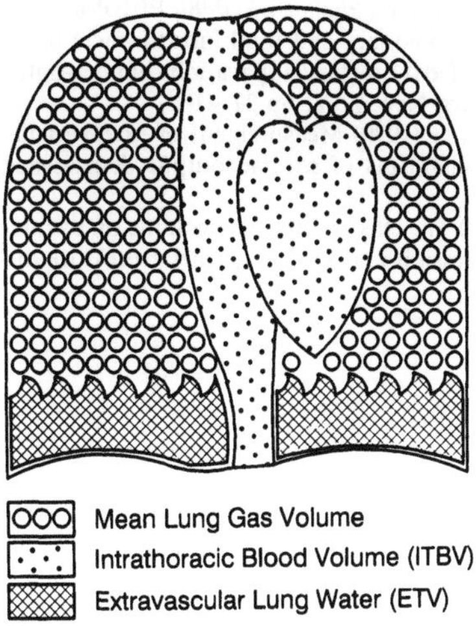

Fig. 14. The three variable volumes in the chest

References

1. Batson GA, Chandrashekar KP, Payas Y, Rickards DF (1972) Measurement of pulmonary capillary wedge pressure by flow directed Swan-Ganz catheter. Cardiovasc Res 6:748–752
2. Buchbinder N, Ganz W (1976) Hemodynamic monitoring: invasive techniques. Anesthesiology 45:146–155
3. De Campo T, Civetta JM (1979) The effect of short-term discontinuation of high-level PEEP in patients with respiratory failure. Crit Care Med 7:47–49
4. Fallon KD, Drake RE, Laine GA, Gabel JC (1985) Effect of cardiac output on extravascular lung water estimates made with the Edwards lung water computer. Anesthesiology 62:505–508
5. Gershan JA (1983) Effect of positive end-expiratory pressure on pulmonary capillary wedge pressure. Heart Lung 12:143–148
6. Hardy JD, Garcia JB, Hardy JA (1974) Fluid replacement monitoring: effect of dextran overload, norepinephrine drip and positive pressure ventilation on systemic arterial, right atrial, pulmonary wedge and left atrial pressure in dogs. Ann Surg 180:162–166
7. Humphrey CB, Oury JH, Virgilio RW, Gibbons JA, Folkerth TL, Shapiro AR, Fosburg RG (1976) An analysis of direct and indirect measurement of left atrial filling pressure. J Thorac Cardiovasc Surg 71:643–647
8. Pfeiffer H-G, Pfeiffer UJ, Aschenbrenner G, Kolb E, Blümel G (1990) Intrathoracic blood volume is a useful guide for volume substitution in intensive care patients. In: Lewis FR, Pfeiffer UJ (eds) Practical applications of fiberoptics in critical care monitoring. Springer, Berlin Heidelberg New York, pp 42–44
9. Pfeiffer UJ, Zimmermann G (1984) Fehlermöglichkeiten und Grenzen der Lungenwasserbestimmung mit der Thermo-Dye Technik. Beitr Anaesthesiol Intensivmed 6:81–104
10. Pfeiffer UJ, Perker M, Zeravik J, Zimmermann G (1990) Sensitivity of central venous pressure, pulmonary capillary wedge pressure, and intrathoracic blood volume as indicators of acute and chronic hypovolemia. In: Lewis FR, Pfeiffer UJ (eds) Practical applications of fiberoptics in critical care monitoring. Springer, Berlin Heidelberg New York, pp 25–31
11. Sampliner JE, Piluk HC (1986) Hämodynamische und respiratorische Überwachung. In: Berk JL, Sampliner JE (eds) Handbuch der Intensivmedizin. Karger, Basel, pp 61–92
12. Shippy CR, Appel PL, Shoemaker WC (1984) Reliability of clinical monitoring to assess blood volume in critically ill patients. Crit Care Med 12:107–112
13. Tooker J, Huseby J, Butler J (1978) The effect of Swan-Ganz catheter height on the wedge pressure-left atrial pressure relationship in edema during positive pressure ventilation. Am Rev Respir Dis 117:721–725

14. Wellhöfer H, Zeravik J, Perker M, Blümel G, Zimmermann G, Pfeiffer UJ (1990) PEEP-induced changes of pulmonary capillary wedge pressure, prepulmonary and total intrathoracic blood volume in anesthetized dogs. In: Lewis FR, Pfeiffer UJ (eds) Practical applications of fiber-optics in critical care monitoring. Springer, Berlin Heidelberg New York, pp 32–41
15. Wickerts C-J, Jakobsson J, Frostell C, Hedenstierna G (1990) Measurement of extravascular lung water by thermal-dye dilution technique: mechanisms of cardiac output dependence. Intensive Care Med 16: 115–120
16. Zarins CK, Virgilio RW, Smith DE, Peters RM (1977) The effect of vascular volume on positive endexpiratory pressure induced cardiac output depression and wedge-left atrial pressure discrepancy. J Surg Res 23:348–360.

Adult Respiratory Distress Syndrome and Metabolic Organ Dysfunction

M. Georgieff and K. Tschaikowsky

The adult respiratory distress syndrome (ARDS) is a group of disease states seen in the posttraumatic or septic patient that have a relatively constant pathologic presentation. A distant focus of tissue trauma or infection usually initiates the ARDS response by generating a systemic inflammatory reaction. The systemic response can be the result of intense local inflammation (e.g., pancreatitis) or a circulating factor (e.g., endotoxin, bacteria, or microemboli). Two major components of the ensuing systemic response can be distinguished. First, the release of mediator precursors from cell membranes, in particular arachidonic acid and platelet-activating factor. The precursor source can be pulmonary or systemic. Second, the activation of a number of cascades including complement with generated C5a along with activation of the coagulation, fibrinolysis, and kinin cascades. The basic defect as a result of all the above described changes is an acute alteration in microvascular membrane integrity. This leads to alterations in regional blood flow and subsequent inadequate oxygen supply.

In normal subjects oxygen consumption (VO_2) is protected in the face of dropping oxygen delivery (DO_2) levels by increased tissue oxygen extraction. Widened arteriovenous oxygen content difference ($DAVO_2$) and reduced mixed venous oxygen saturation (SVO_2) are seen. VO_2 and DO_2 become directly dependent below a critical DO_2 which has been found to occur at an oxygen extraction ratio (OER) of approximately 0.7–0.8 or oxygen delivery of less than 7–9 ml/kg per min. Anaerobic metabolism and lactic acid production occur, even though a simple relationship with derangements of VO_2 cannot be documented. Tissue OER seems to be impaired in sepsis and ARDS. Pathologic supply dependency of oxygen uptake occurs. In sepsis the OER is close to 0.5 at DO_2 of more than 50% compared to control [1]. Patients with ARDS have an OER as low as 0.3 in association with low $DAVO_2$ and high SVO_2; supply dependency of VO_2 on oxygen delivery shows a plateau 2.5–3 times greater than in non-ARDS patients and that it occurs at DO_2 levels around 21 ml/kg per min [2]. For any given level of DO_2, the VO_2 is less than in patients without ARDS and remains supply-dependent at much higher levels. The abnormal pattern of peripheral oxygen metabolism termed "pathological supply dependency" [3] is characterized by the following: (1) a linear relationship of VO_2 and DO_2 above the normal threshold, (2) a relatively fixed oxygen extraction ratio ($VO_2:DO_2$) at varying levels of DO_2 (3) the tendency for VO_2 to increase to supranormal levels as supply is increased, and (4) a possible limitation in the maximal OER achieved when oxygen delivery is severely reduced [3–5]. This pattern may be due to loss of autoregulation, peripheral microembolization, or other mechanisms resulting in increased diffusion pathway and maldistribution of oxygen delivery. Bihari [6] speaks of a covert oxygen deficit which occurs under these circumstances and rates this phenomenon as one of the key initiators of multiple organ failure (MOF).

The incidence of MOF in critically ill patients is 5%–10% [7], with a mortality rate of 60%–80% depending on the number of organs involved and the control of infection [7, 8]. Failure occurs simultaneously or sequentially in different organs, suggesting a common etiology. Although the sequence of organs involved is variable and unpredictable, the lungs are often the first to be damaged, or at least to manifest functional disturbances before renal, hepatic, hematologic, and gastrointestinal (GI) impairment [8]. However, the damaging process also involves the GI tract and the liver very early, resulting in important morphologic and functional changes. But because of the paucity of specific GI symptoms, the GI dysfunction is not recognized immediately unless particular attention is given to the problem. Up to 100% of critically ill patients show evidence of stress lesions in the upper GI tract [9].

The relationship between shock and pancreatitis suggests that ischemia is one of the causes of pancreatitis. It has also been shown that low flow state can aggravate the severity of pancreatitis with progression of pancreatic edema to necrosis [10].

Jaundice with sepsis is associated with mortality approaching 90% [11]. The liver blood flow usually reaches 800–1200 ml/min and is determined by three parameters: the hepatic arterial vascular resistance, the portal vein flow determined by the vascular resistance of the intestine and the spleen, and the hepatic portal vascular resistance [12]. Central venous pressure elevation creates distension of the intrahepatic vessels and decrease of the liver blood flow. This situation is seen during positive pressure mechanical ventilation, right cardiac failure, or pancreatitis.

As far as hormones are concerned, cholecystokinin increases intestinal and, thereby, portal blood flow. Insulin is without effect on the liver perfusion, but glucagon increases total liver blood flow. This hormone [13] has several actions: it causes intestinal vasodilation leading to an increased portal flow and increased portal resistance; but the most important action of glucagon is its antagonistic effect of vasoconstriction in the hepatic arterial vasculature, neutralizing the effect of anoxia and increasing the hepatic blood flow [12]. Norepinephrine decreases the liver blood flow by inducing vasoconstriction in the hepatic artery and the portal vein, and by decreasing the splanchnic flow. At the same time, systemic artery pressure is increased. Hypocapnia reduces arterial and portal venous blood flow [12]. Hypoxemia is one of the main factors of severe impaired hepatic function. It induces an excretory defect, according to the majority of authors [14, 15]. Portal venous blood flow contributes to 70% of the liver blood flow and supplies 70% of its oxygen requirements in human beings. The portal venous saturation is 35%. In shock and sepsis, the portal venous flow decreases significantly and its saturation can decrease to as low as 10%. The use of vasopressors will further decrease the liver blood flow [16]. It seems so that adequate oxygenation is more important than the supply of the required blood flow [17]. When PO_2 is reduced to a value below 50 mmHg, the lactate/pyruvate ratio increases in the hepatocytes [18]. Hypoperfusion can also induce the formation of oxygen-derived free radicals; the liver cell, very rich in xanthine oxidase, will be injured through lipid peroxidation and membrane dysfunction [19, 20].

The reticuloendothelial system (RES) is at the center of hepatic dysfunction and pathogenesis in MOF. The RES is able to clear endotoxins, microorganisms, activated immune complexes, inert colloids, and clotting factors [21]. Bacteria coming from the GI tract are filtered by the liver, preventing their passage to the systemic circulation; a blockade of the RES is thus associated with an increased risk of bacteremia [22]. Its capacity is limited by the magnitude of hepatic blood flow. In obstructive jaundice, the RES is reduced to 15% of its function and bacteria are found in the lung trapped, but not killed [23]. It is argued that the stage of immunodeficiency predisposes to infectious complications [24].

The hepatic oxygen consumption decreases with low systolic pressure (below 60 mmHg) [25]. Concomitantly, cellular AMP and ATP levels decrease, showing mitochondrial oxidation process impairment [26]. However, the ribosomal reprioritization of acute-phase protein synthesis demonstrates the key role of the hepatocyte in the protection of the host tissues from infection and dead tissue digestion [27]. The increase in amino acids, lactate, and glycerol, and also in epinephrine, cortisol, and glucagon increases hepatic glucose production. This phenomenon explains, with the insulin resistance, the persistent hyperglycemia in stress [28]. But in late sepsis, hypoglycemia occurs consecutively due to impaired liver function.

Some of the major problems in characterizing the metabolic status of patients with ARDS are considered to be the accompanying changes in perfusion, oxygen consumption, and altered enzyme activities. Cuthbertson [29] introduced the concept that the metabolic response to injury occurs in two phases: an "ebb" or "necrobiotic" phase that precedes the "flow" phase, which occurs after stabilization of cardiovascular dynamics. Patients with apparent septic shock have been subdivided into the hyperdynamic or high flow state and the hypodynamic or low flow state [30]. In the high flow state cardiac output is elevated and peripheral resistance is low; oxygen consumption is normal or decreased, and the arteriovenous differences ($DAVO_2$) are diminished. In the hypodynamic phase decreased cardiac output occurs with increased peripheral resistance, hypotension, and decreased venous return.

Low output or the hypodynamic phase is not directly associated with nonsurvival, rather patients who demonstrate more severe abnormalities in oxygen extraction and utilization have a poorer prognosis [31]. Siegel [32] proposed that the response to injury and sepsis be classified into four states. Each of these groups represents a status with statistical deviations from nonstressed control variables called the R state. The first state is a well compensated physiologic response state in which hemodynamic variables are elevated and oxygen consumption is increased, as might occur after uncomplicated surgery or trauma. A major characteristic is a sympathetic adaptation response without evidence of metabolic abnormalities or respiratory dysfunction. The second state is a hyperdynamic cardiovascular response characterized by high cardiac output with decreased peripheral vascular resistance. Oxygen extraction is decreased and not attributable to a perfusion deficit. Metabolic acidosis is commonly present. The third state is portrayed as an extension of the second state with respiratory acidosis that is uncorrected by ventilatory support. The fourth state represents a pattern of primary myocardial dysfunction with low cardiac output, high peripheral resistance, large $DAVO_2$ and diminished oxygen consumption. Siegel's model does not necessarily suggest progression from one state to another, and patients may present in any of the categories. Another additional problem in patients with ARDS is the concomitant increase in pulmonary vascular resistance and the inflammation of the lung as such, which both profoundly influence whole body perfusion and metabolism.

Critically ill patients with ARDS can furthermore be characterized by common features in their metabolic status. These patients have an increase in energy expenditure [33], nitrogen breakdown with negative nitrogen balance [34], augmented gluconeogenesis [35], cathecholamine secretion [36], increased levels of interleukin-1 and cachectin [37, 38], and an increase in insulin resistance [39].

Carbohydrate Metabolism

Cardiovascular dynamics after injury and sepsis operate in concert with metabolic and hormonal mechanisms to preserve cardiac and cerebral perfusion at the expense of peripheral tissues. A major additional factor compromising overall perfusion in ARDS is concomitant pulmonary hypertension with reduced cardiac output.

The predominant acute response to a traumatic or septic insult is mobilization of glucose from glycogen stores followed by a more chronic phase of maintenance of blood glucose from gluconeogenesis. Critically ill patients are typically hyperglycemic except in the terminal phases, and this is attributable to mass action effects with increased delivery of metabolic precursors from peripheral tissues, which sustains glucose production in the liver and kidney, and to disturbances in endocrine function, which cause a relative decrease in peripheral utilization of glucose as a metabolic fuel.

Glucose extracellular pool size and turnover rate double and glucose oxidation increases more than twofold, which indicates that the hyperglycemia correlates positively with increased glucose synthesis relative to increased turnover rate; the rate of appearance of the carbohydrate into the extracellular pool exceeds its rate of disappearance [35]. Gluconeogenesis (synthesis of glucose from noncarbohydrates such as lactate, glycerol, and amino acids) is accelerated

[40–42]. Gluconeogenesis in the liver and probably the kidney is sustained by increased delivery of precursor substrates, principally lactate and alanine [42].

The delivery of alanine and other amino acids to the liver is enhanced by increased proteolysis in skeletal muscle [41]. Provided that hepatic function is not compromised by disease, intravascular coagulation, or poor perfusion – increased pulmonary vascular resistance, mechanical ventilation, positive end expiratory pressure (PEEP) – increased hepatic glucose output from gluconeogenesis is a consequence of increased delivery of precursors that are a by-product from increased catabolism of muscle and splanchnic proteins. Newer studies also indicate that splanchnic hypoperfusion per se is a potent stimulator of hepatic glucose production.

Glucose oxidation in skeletal muscle and mesentery is incomplete in injury and sepsis. This contributes to higher tissue and blood lactate and pyruvate concentrations; pyruvate enhances amino acid deamination, thus enhancing alanine formation and branched chain amino acid degradation [43]. The percentage of glucose originating from lactate increases from 20% in normals to up to 80% during endotoxemia [42, 44] and moderate to severe hemorrhage [45].

The predominant utilization of anaerobic pathways for energy production makes increased energy expenditure combined with hypoperfusion the leading cause of lactic acidemia and metabolic acidosis. Blood lactate levels increase prior to any fall in blood pressure and cardiac output. This rise in lactate concentration has been employed as an early sign of the existence of profound regional hypoperfusion as well as a prognostic indicator [46].

Protein Metabolism in the Critically Ill

Protein loss reflected in weight loss and negative nitrogen balance are commonplace in the critically ill. While protein catabolism is generally thought to be accelerated, as indicated by increased excretion of urinary nitrogen, it remains unclear whether this effect is modulated by changes in protein synthesis and/or protein degradation relative to one another. The interpretation of the findings is complicated by the effects of immobilization, which itself induces a substantial reduction in protein synthesis rates [47]. Neuroendocrine activation with increased sympathetic activity and stimulated glucagon release combined with a relative hypoinsulinemia appear to be critical determinants of the changes in protein metabolism. The net negative protein balance is also affected by the great release of cortisol [48]. Recently, the concept of a trauma and sepsis-specific hormone profile has been revived because circulating proteins in the plasma have been isolated from traumatized or septic patients which can induce proteolysis in vitro. In septic patients, leukocytic pyrogens [49], and possibly other endogenous mediators released by infected tissues and phagocytizing cells, seem to act directly to stimulate protein catabolism and indirectly through the central nervous system by inducing fever. As a result of these hormone changes, the resting metabolic energy expenditure increases in rough proportion to the extent of the injury [50] and infection.

In the majority of cells, energy is derived from glycolysis and further oxidation of substrates through the Krebs cycle and the electron transport chain. The electron transport chain seems to be remarkably stable and is able to maintain its functional integrity after a variety of severe cell insults or even cell death [51]. Endotoxin, however, seems to interfere with oxidative reactions of the tricarboxylic acid cycle and the electron transport system; this could be due to an impaired coupling of oxidation and phosphorylation [52, 53]. Severe hemorrhagic shock also leads to a decrease in the measured intracellular levels of adenosine triphosphate (ATP) and adenosine diphosphate (ADP) of liver, skeletal muscle, and kidney [54].

Present therapeutic interventions to counteract the metabolic alterations seen in severe trauma, sepsis and ARDS failed to prove a significant beneficial effect on patient outcome. Nutritional support in the classic sense under such metabolic circumstances seems to be an inadequate approach [55]. The major key to decreasing overall mortality during ARDS is the normalization of regional hemodynamic alterations; the concomitant normalization of cellular energy metabolism will build the basis for further medical interventions such as nutrient supply. Again it has to be emphasized that the pharmacologic action of nutrients needs further investigation [55–57] and alternative anticatabolic drugs have to be developed to adequately counteract severe protein catabolism during ARDS [58].

References

1. Nishijama H, Weil MH, Shubin H et al. (1973) Hemodynamic and metabolic studies on shock associated with gram negative bacteremia. Medicine 52:287–294
2. Mohsenifar Z, Goldback P, Tashkin DP et al. (1983) Relationship between O_2 delivery and O_2 consumption in the adult respiratory distress syndrome. Chest 84:267–271
3. Cain SM (1984) Supply dependency of oxygen uptake in ARDS: myth or reality? Am J Med Sci 288:119–124
4. Danek SJ, Lynch JP, Weg JG et al. (1980) The dependence of oxygen uptake on oxygen delivery in the adult respiratory distress syndrome. Am Rev Respir Dis 122:387–395
5. Kaufman BS, Rackow EC, Falk JL (1984) The relationship between oxygen delivery and consumption during fluid resuscitation of hypovolemic and septic shock. Chest 85:337–340
6. Bihari D, Smithies M, Gimson A et al. (1987) The effects of vasodilation with prostacyclin on oxygen delivery and uptake in critically ill patients. N Engl J Med 317:397–403
7. Fry DE, Pearlstein L, Fulton RL et al. (1980) Multiple system organ failure: the role of uncontrolled infection. Arch Surg 115:136–142
8. Eiseman B, Beart R, Norton L (1977) Multiple organ failure. Surg Gynecol Obstet 144: 323–326
9. Lucas CE, Sugawa C, Riddle J (1971) Natural history and surgical dilemma of "stress" gastric bleeding. Arch Surg 102:266–273
10. Broe PJ, Zuidema GD, Cameron JL (1982) Role of ischemia in acute pancreatitis: studies with an isolated perfused canine pancreas. Surgery 91:377–382
11. Vermillon SE, Gregg JA, Baggenstoss AH et al. (1969) Jaundice associated with bacteremia. Arch Intern Med 124:611–618
12. Richardson PD, Withrington PG (1981) Liver blood flow. Gastroenterology 81:159–173

13. Cerra FB, Siegel JH, Border JR et al. (1979) The hepatic failure of sepsis: cellular versus substrate. Surgery 86:409–422
14. Nunes G, Blaisdell FW, Margeretten W (1970) Mechanism of hepatic dysfunction following shock and trauma. Arch Surg 100:446–456
15. Linberg B (1977) Liver circulation and metabolism in hemorrhagic shock. Acta Chir Scand 476 [Suppl]:1–18
16. Corday E, Williams JH Jr (1984) Effect of shock and vasopressor drugs on the regional circulation of the brain, heart, liver and kidney. Am J Med 9:228–241
17. Frank HA, Seligman AM, Fine JN (1946) Traumatic shock. XII. The prevention of irreversibility in hemorrhagic shock by in vivo perfusion of the liver. J Clin Invest 25:22–29
18. Okigusa M, Ida T, Ozawa K et al. (1979) The influence of hypoxemia and hemorrhage upon adenylate energy charge and bile flow. Surg Gynecol Obstet 149:346–352
19. Parks DA, Bulkley GB, Granger DN (1983) Role of oxygen-derived free radicals in the digestive tract diseases. Surgery 94:415–422
20. Chien KR, Abrams J, Serroni A et al. (1978) Accelerated phospholipid degradation and associated membrane dysfunction in irreversible ischemic liver cell injury. J Biol Chem 253:4809–4817
21. Rogoff BJ, Lipsky PE (1981) Role of the Kupffer cells in local and systemic immune responses. Gastroenterology 80:850–860
22. Pardy BJ, Spencer RC, Dudley HAF et al. (1977) Hepatic reticuloendothelial protection against bacteremia in experimental hemorrhagic shock. Surgery 81:193–197
23. Katz S, Grosfeld JL, Gross K et al. (1984) Impaired bacterial clearance and trapping in obstructive jaundice. Ann Surg 199:14–20
24. Saba TM (1982) Pathophysiology of the reticulo-endothelial system: altered fibronectine metabolism. J Clin Surg 1:346–365
25. Witte CL, Conell PN, Witte MH (1976) Direct on-line monitoring of hepatic tissue oxygen tension, a new technique. J Surg Res 21:33–44
26. Iles RA, Baron PG, Cohen RD (1979) The effect of reduction of perfusion rate on lactate and oxygen uptake, glucose output and energy supply in the isolated perfused liver of starved rats. Biochem J 184:635–642
27. Spanga G, Siegel JH, Brown G et al. (1985) Reprioritization of hepatic plasma protein release in trauma and sepsis. Arch Surg 120:187–199
28. Ross BD, Hems R, Krebs HA (1967) The rate of gluconeogenesis from various precursors in the perfused rat liver. Biochem J 102:942–945
29. Cuthbertson DP (1942) Post-shock metabolic response. Lancet 1:433–436
30. Clowes GHA, Vucinic M, Weidner MG (1966) Circulatory and metabolic alterations associated with survival or death in peritonitis: clinical analysis of 25 cases. Ann Surg 163:866–885
31. Siegel JH, Greenspan M, del Guercio LR (1967) Abnormal vascular tone, defective oxygen transport and myocardial failure in human septic shock. Ann Surg 165:504–517
32. Siegel JH, Goldwyn RM, Friedman HP (1971) Pattern and process in the evolution of septic shock. Surgery 70:232–245
33. Long CL, Schaffel N, Geiger JW (1979) Metabolic response to injury and illness: estimation of energy and protein needs from indirect calorimetry and nitrogen balance. J Parenter Enteral Nutr 3:452–456
34. Cerra FB, Siegel JH, coleman B et al. (1980) Septic autocannibalism, a failure of exogenous nutritional support. Ann Surg 192:570–580
35. Long CL, Kinney JM, Geiger JW et al. (1976) Nonsuppressibility of gluconeogenesis by glucose in septic patients. Metabolism 25:193–201
36. Davies CL, Newman RJ, Molneux SG et al. (1984) The relationship between catecholamines and severity of injury in man. J Trauma 24:99–105
37. Beutler B, Mahoney J, LeTrang N et al. (1985) Purification of cachectin, a lipoprotein lipase suppressing hormone secreted by endotoxin induced raw 2647 cells. J Exp Med 161:984–995
38. Tracey KJ, Vlassara H, Cerami A (1989) Cachectin/tumor necrosis factor. Lancet 1:1122–1125
39. Black Pr, Brooks DC, Bessey PQ et al. (1982) Mechanism of insulin resistance following injury. Ann Surg 196:420–436
40. Filkins JP (1979) Phases of glucose dyshomeostasis in endotoxicosis. Circ Shock 5:347–355
41. Kuttner RE, Spitzner JJ (1978) Gluconeogenesis from alanine in endotoxin-treated dogs. J Surg Res 25:166–173

42. Merrill GF, Spitzer JJ (1978) Glucose and lactate kinetics in guinea pigs following Escherichia coli endotoxin administration. Circ Shock 5:11–21
43. Robert JJ, Bier DM, Zhao XH et al. (1982) Glucose and insulin effects on de novo amino acid synthesis in young men: studies with stable isotope labeled alanine, glycine, leucine and lysine. Metabolism 31:1210–1218
44. Wolfe RR, Elahi D, Spitzner JJ (1977) Glucose and lactate kinetics following endotoxin administration in dogs. Am J Physiol 232:E180–187
45. Wiener R, Spitzner JJ (1974) Lactate metabolism following severe hemorrhage in the conscious dog. Am J Physiol 227:58–62
46. Border G, Weil MH (1964) Excess lactate: an index of reversibility of shock in human patients. Science 143:1457–1459
47. Schonheyder F, Heilskov NCS, Oleson K (1954) Isotopic studies on the mechanism of negative nitrogen balance produced by immobilization. Scand J Clin Lab Invest 6:178–188
48. Unger RH (1971) Glucagon and the insulin:glucagon ratio in diabetes and other catabolic illnesses. Diabetes 20:834–838
49. Baracos V, Rodemann HP, Dinarello CA et al. (1983) Stimulation of muscle protein degradation and prostaglandin E_2 release by leukocytic pyrogen (interleukin-1). N Engl J Med 308:553–558
50. Elwyn DH, Kinney JM, Askanazi J (1981) Energy expenditure in surgical patients. Surg Clin North Am 61:545–556
51. Chaudry IH, Sayeed MD, Baue AE (1976) Alterations in high-energy phosphates in hemorrhagic shock as related to tissue and organ function. Surgery 79:666–668
52. Sayeed MM, Murphy PNA (1981) Adenine nucleotide and lactate metabolism in the lung in endotoxin shock. Circ Shock 8:657–666
53. Tanaka J, Sato T, Kamiyama Y et al. (1982) Bacteremic shock: aspects of high-energy metabolism of rat liver following living *Escherichia coli* infection. J Surg Res 33:49–57
54. Baue AE, Chaudry IH, Wurth MA et al. (1974) Cellular alterations with shock and ischemia. Angiology 25:31–42
55. Blackburn GL, Wan JM-F, Teo TC et al. (1989) Metabolic support in organ failure. In: Bihari DJ, Cerra FB (eds) Multiple organ failure. Society of Critical Care Medicine, New Horizons
56. Georgieff M (1987) Intravenöse Ernährung – Möglichkeiten und Grenzen der Anwendung von Glukose und Xylit nach Trauma und Sepsis unter besonderer Berücksichtigung des Leberstoffwechsels. Infusionstherapie 14:93–97
57. Georgieff M, Saeger HD, Wagner D et al. (1987) Carbohydrate and lipid emulsions in parenteral nutrition. J Clin Gastroenterol 2:47–51
58. Jauch K-W, Hartl WH, Georgieff M et al. (1988) Low-dose bradykinin infusion reduces endogenous glucose production in surgical patients. Metabolism 37:185–190

Part 10:
Posters

Generation of Free Oxygen Radicals and Chemotactic Desensitation Following Burn Injury

U. Pralat, J. Seidel, U. Lips, W. Schneider, and W. Stangel

Introduction

Sepsis and adult respiratory distress syndrome (ARDS) continue to be major life-threatening complications in patients with extensive thermal injuries [1, 5]. Almost all of the immune responses that have been studied in burn patients show impairment, cell-mediated immunity being most consistently and profoundly suppressed [3, 4].

Polymorphonuclear leukocytes (PMN) form a major part of the nonspecific first line of defense in humans. Intracellular killing by PMN requires the uptake of oxygen by the phagocytic cell. Through a series of enzyme reactions, including those mediated by NADPH oxidase and superoxide dismutase, this oxygen is progressively reduced to superoxide (O_2^-), hydrogen peroxide (H_2O_2), hydroxyl ions (OH^-), and singlet oxygen ($^1O_2^-$). Free oxygen radicals are highly toxic to many microorganisms and can be considered as a stimulus in the pathogenesis of ARDS.

Chemotaxis is presumed to be an important function of PMN in protecting against invasive agents, for even leukocytes fully capable of ingesting and killing microorganisms are incapacitated if unable to sense and be directed toward the invading pathogen.

In order to characterize the secondary immunodeficiency following severe thermal injury we investigated the ability of PMN to exhibit chemotaxis and to generate oxygen radicals in surviving and nonsurviving burn patients.

Materials and Methods

Patients. Blood samples were obtained from 13 patients suffering from grade II and III burns of more than 30% of body surface area with a maximum of 92%. Our study included patients of either sex ranging in age from 19 to 68 years. From the surviving group of 7 patients a total of 62 measurements could be analyzed. From 6 nonsurviving patients, who eventually died because of sepsis and ARDS, in all 44 samples could be taken. Informed consent was obtained from all patients or their relatives.

Serum Samples. Samples were taken daily for 11 consecutive days. We measured PMN chemotaxis in response to formyl-methionyl-leucyl-phenylalanine

(FMLP) and yeast activated serum (YAS) according to the method of Chenowth [2] using the "under agarose technique." The ability of PMN to generate H_2O_2 and O_2^- was tested after stimulation with opsonized zymosan, FMLP, and zymosan activated serum (ZAS) [7, 10]. Evaluation of O_2^- generation was done by following cytochrome c reduction. Assessment of H_2O_2 production was carried out kinetically using horseradish peroxidase mediated reduction of scopoletin. Statistical analyses were performed utilizing Student's *t* test after establishing medians in each series.

Results

A total of 13 patients were studied involving a total of 104 measurements. Matching normal volunteers were used as controls. Results are shown in Figs. 1–3. Chemotaxis in response to FMLP in cells from surviving patients was 1.02 ± 0.27 and significantly higher than in PMN from the nonsurviving patients, where it reached 0.87 ± 0.27 (Fig. 1). There was no significant difference between the two groups using YAS (surviving group cells, 0.64 ± 0.26; nonsurviving group cells, 0.54 ± 0.24). Figure 2 shows H_2O_2 production after stimulation with FMLP and opsonized zymosan. In PMN from the nonsurviving patients there was nearly threefold higher H_2O_2 generation (0.44 ± 0.18) than in PMN from surviving patients (0.15 ± 0.08) in response to FMLP. There was no difference between the two groups after stimulation with opsonized zymosan.

In Fig. 3, O_2^- generation is significantly different among the groups. PMN from surviving patients showed lower O_2^- production (0.76 ± 0.40) than cells from nonsurvivors (1.41 ± 0.75) in response to FMLP. After YAS/ZAS stimulation we found less O_2^- production (0.22 ± 0.08) in survivors' cells than in nonsurvivors' cells (0.41 ± 0.17).

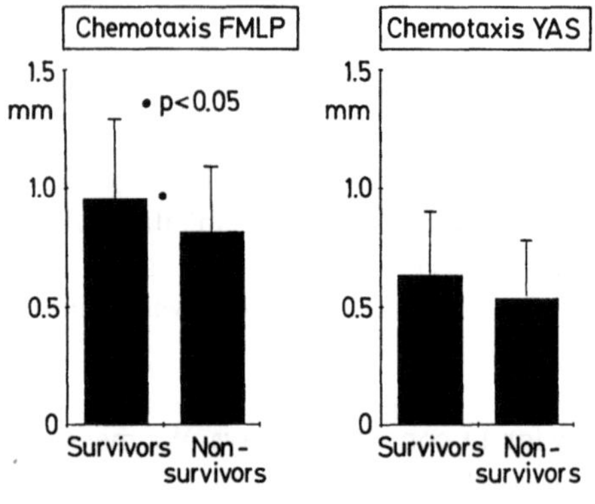

Fig. 1. Chemotaxis by FMLP and YAS in surviving and nonsurviving patients

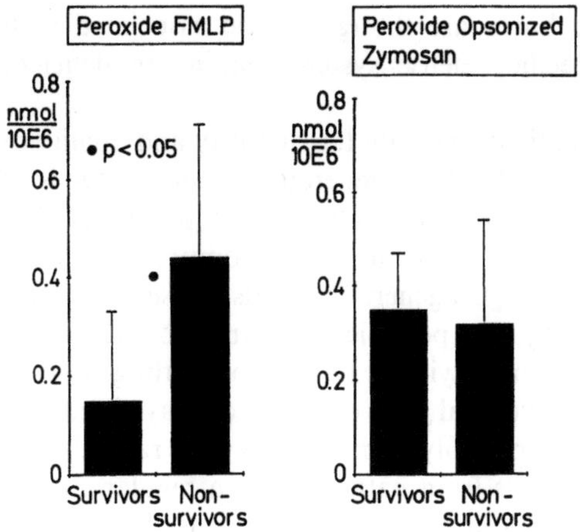

Fig. 2. Hydrogen peroxide generation after stimulation with FMLP and opsonized zymosan in surviving and nonsurviving patients

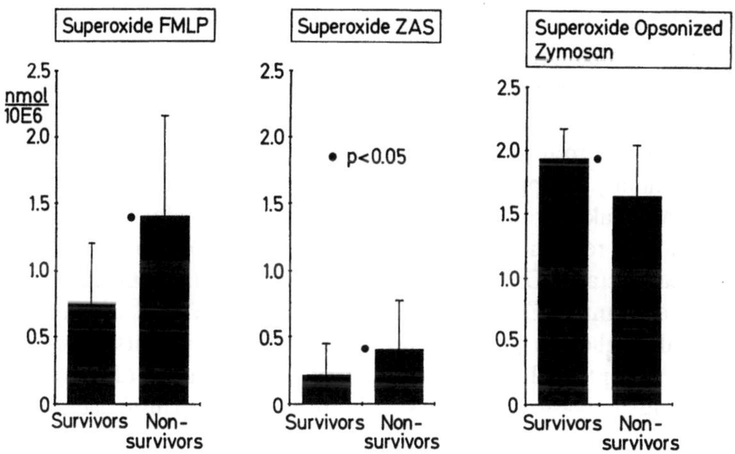

Fig. 3. Superoxide anion generation after stimulation with FMLP, ZAS, and opsonized zymosan in surviving and nonsurviving patients

Discussion

Severe trauma, major surgery, and burns (TSB) are often followed by infections, ARDS and multiorgan failure, complications which are thought to be the consequence of the post-TSB immunodeficiency syndrome [5]. After TSB, large amounts of tissue debris, endotoxins, and microorganisms have to be eliminated. Further important factors in TSB are stress reactions, malnutrition, loss and replacement of fluids, and therapeutic measures [4, 6]. The elimination of unwanted elements is partly carried out by nonspecific mechanisms such as opsonization, chemotaxis, and phagocytosis by granulocytes and cells of the macrophage-monocyte system; specific reactions of humoral and cellular immunity also play a role. Severe burns are thought to be associated with growing exhaustion of the nonspecific defense system, leading to deficient specific immune reactions [4].

Our findings in severly burned patients indicate the quantity and quality of granulocyte impairment. The ability of PMN to generate O_2^- and H_2O_2 is of great interest with respect to respiratory failure. Our results point out that FMLP-mediated O_2^- production is augmented in severly compromised burn patients (Fig. 1). A likewise increase in H_2O_2 generation is also observed in this group (Fig. 2). The reason for this may be a possible defect in detoxification of oxygen radicals, which are suspected of playing a role in the pathogenesis of ARDS. PMN from patients with an eventual fatal outcome displayed reduced chemotaxis to FMLP. Generation of possibly damaging oxygen radicals was significantly enhanced compared to cells from patients with a regular clinical course (Figs. 1–3). The finding of reduced chemotaxis confirms the study of Warden and coworkers [9], who showed that leukocyte chemotaxis was inversely correlated with burn size during the first 72 h following injury. After 72 h leukocyte chemotaxis was directly correlated with clinical status and was highly predictive for ultimate mortality [9]. Due to the small number of patients we studied, we were not able to confirm the latter. However, since mortality in our patients was largely due to infection, suppression of leukocyte chemotaxis may explain the susceptibility to opportunistic infection in thermally injured patients.

Obviously, PMN taken from patients suffering from sepsis following severe burns already show a reduction in chemotaxis and alterations in oxygen metabolism at an early stage. Granulocyte stimulation with different agents indicated that the amount of O_2^- production depends on the kind of stimulus. Tschaikowski and Rügheimer [8] have shown that in septic patients there is an increase in FMLP receptors. The reason for this may be expression of preformed receptors following activation of PMN by intrinsic or extrinsic factors or microorganisms.

The pathophysiology of a decreased chemotactic response and an increased metabolic response remains to be elucidated and a causal relationship between our findings and subsequent infection can only be theorized. We believe that monitoring chemotaxis and O_2^- and H_2O_2 production provides an indirect measure of basic membrane and cytoskeletal functions, upon which stimulated migratory functions are based. Speculating further, one can expect that therapy to control stimulated secretory and respiratory responses of the circulating neutrophil might involve effectively limiting the generalized chemotactic dysfunction that accompanies thermal injury or other clinical conditions in which excessive complement activation and release of cytokines occur.

References

1. Alexander JW, Meakins JL (1972) A physiologic basis for opportunistic infection. Ann Surg 176:273–287

2. Chenowth DE, Rowe JG, Hugli T (1979) A modified method for chemotaxis under agarose. J Immunol Methods 25:337–353
3. Deitch EA, Landry KN, McDonald JC (1985) Postburn impaired cell-mediated immunity may not be due to lazy lymphocytes but to overwork. Ann Surg 201:793–802
4. Hansbrough JF, Field TO, Gadd MA, Soderberg C (1987) Immune response modulation after burn injury: T-cells and antibodies. J Burn Care Rehabil 8:509–512
5. Ninnemann JL (1987) Trauma, sepsis, and the immune response. J Burn Care Rehabil 8:462–467
6. O'Gorman RB, Feliciano DV, Mathews KS, Mathews R, Bitondo CG, Mattox KL, Jordan GL (1986) Correlation of immunologic and nutritional status with infectious complications after major abdominal trauma. Surgery 99:549–556
7. Pick E, Keisari Y (1980) A simple colorimetric method for the measurement of hydrogen peroxide produced by cells in nature. J Immunol Methods 38:161–170
8. Tschaikowsky K, Rügheimer E (1988) Expression von fMet-Leu-Phe-Rezeptoren und Produktion von Sauerstoffradikalen in Granulozyten septischer Patienten. Anaesthesist 37:140
9. Warden GD, Mason AD, Pruitt BA (1974) Evaluation of leukocyte chemotaxis in vitro in thermally injured patients. J Clin Invest 54:1001–1004
10. Weening RS, Wever R, Loos D (1975) Quantitative aspects of the production of superoxide radicals by phagocytizing human granulocytes. J Lab Clin Med 85:245–252

A Prospective Evaluation of the Influence of Extrapulmonary Factors on Mechanical Ventilation

R. Stuttmann, M.R. Müller, D. Weidemann, D. Knüttgen, and M. Doehn

Introduction

Long-term mechanical ventilation may be complicated by a deterioration of gas exchange. A primary pulmonary problem may be the reason but it can rarely be identified [1–3]; therefore, we decided to focus on extrapulmonary factors in a search for other possible causes [4–6]. These include secondary organ dysfunction and therapeutic efforts, e.g., hemodialysis or use of high dose catecholamines. The clinical course in many of our intensive care patients raised the possibility that extrapulmonary factors determine the extent and duration of mechanical ventilation. We therefore decided to prospectively evaluate these factors in our multiple trauma patients.

Patients and Methods

Study Criteria

A total of 100 multiple injured patients with a mean TS (trauma score) [7] of 10.6 and a mean ISS (injury severity score) [8] of 36, who had to be mechanically ventilated for more than 48 h, were included in this study. Mechanical ventilation was performed according to the following protocol: In uncomplicated supportive ventilation the pattern was comprised of a tidal volume ≤ 10 ml/kg, a respiratory frequency ≤ 12/min, and a $FIO_2 \leq 0.4$. Development of pulmonary dysfunction demanded more extended ventilatory support, which we classified into ventilatory and respiratory effort. Additional ventilatory effort was necessary to achieve normoventilation ($PaCO_2$ 40 ± 6 mm Hg) or hyperventilation ($PaCO_2$ 30 ± 2 mm Hg) in severe brain damage. Each step included a further increase in tidal volume and ventilatory frequency. Additional respiratory effort was necessary to achieve sufficient oxygenation with a PaO_2 of at least 80 mm Hg. Four steps were used; each of them was applied to reach a further augmentation of oxygenation, if necessary by consecutive inversion of inspiration:expiration (I:E) in the sequence of 1:2, 1:1, best PEEP, and 2:1.

Documentation

Extrapulmonary Factors. Those investigated included functional disorders and secondary organ damage in several organs: In the cardiovascular system hypotension, hypertension, hypovolemia, hypervolemia, cardiac insufficiency, arrhythmias, the need for high dose catecholamines, and/or the use of a Swan-Ganz catheter were the parameters investigated. In the liver the incidence of hyperbilirubinemia, increased liver enzymes, and/or coagulopathy were looked at. Kidney function parameters observed included the need for diuretics, development of polyuria, compensated retention, oliguria, anuria, and/or if the patient needed hemodialysis. Extrapulmonary factors were also looked for with respect to the immune response, including sepsis, and to metabolism, metabolic disorder, and disorders in the brain, abdomen, and skin.

For each organ between five and nine parameters were documented yielding a total of 53 entries. However, only one finding was sufficient for an extrapulmonary factor to become documented. Documentation was made on a daily basis.

Pulmonary Factors. The extent and efficiency of ventilation was measured daily by the following data: tidal volume, respiratory frequency, compliance, ventilatory and respiratory effort, PaO_2, $PaCO_2$, FIO_2, and the alveolo-arterial oxygen quotient described by Benzer [9] (BQ: $P_AO_2 - PaO_2/P_AO_2$). A BQ ≤ 0.4 revealed an undisturbed gas exchange with a PaO_2 of about 60 mm Hg subatmospheric, whereas a BQ > 0.4 revealed a pathologic condition and hypoxemia. The BQ was chosen as the criterion for assigning the 100 study patients on a daily basis to either collective: collective A, patients with undisturbed oxygen gas exchange and BQ ≤ 0.4; collective B, patients with disturbed oxygen gas exchange and BQ > 0.4. The term "collective" is used to mark the difference between our definition and the usual term "group". The affiliation with a collective did not depend on a defined patient population but on whether the criterion – existence of disturbed gas exchange or not – was fulfilled. Therefore, the affiliation of each patient to a collective and thereby the number of patients in either collective could change from one day to the other. The definition of each collective, however, was unchanged throughout the investigation.

Concept of Evaluation. The incidence of extrapulmonary factors was compared between the two collectives. For each day of mechanical ventilation, the number of ventilated patients in each collective and the number of extrapulmonary factors per organ were counted. All these data were related exclusively to the criterion of existence of disturbed gas exchange or not. For evaluation purposes the number of ventilated patients and the number of extrapulmonary factors were summarized over 4 day periods, beginning with the first day of mechanical ventilation. All data after the 20th day of mechanical ventilation were calculated together as a single interval. The test of significance of difference between two proportions was used for statistical analysis. We determined $p = 0.05$ as the level of significance.

Results

General Review

Of the 100 study patients 72 were male and 28 were female. They all were mechanically ventilated for a total of 1801 days. A total of 75 patients – 53 males and 22 females – survived, whereas 25 patients – 19 males and 2 females – died. The average age of the survivors was 39.2 ± 19.7 years, that of those who died was 46.5 ± 23.4 years (ns). The surviving male patients were mechanically ventilated for 18.5 days and the female patients for 16.5 days ($p < 0.01$). In the collective of those who survived, a mean BQ ≤ 0.4 was noted on 18 days, but in the collective of those who died the mean BQ was ≤ 0.4 only on 5 days. On all other days, in either collective, the mean BQ was > 0.4.

Extrapulmonary Factors Besides Pulmonary Disturbances

The complete investigation comprised the evaluation of extrapulmonary factors of all the organ systems mentioned above. For a discussion of the results we concentrate upon those organs with the most extrapulmonary factors mentioned. If on a given day, for instance, only one extrapulmonary factor was measured this may have two meanings: (1) All patients assigned to a collective had just one extrapulmonary factor each documented on that day. (2) Of all patients assigned to a collective some patients had more than one extrapulmonary factor documented on that day and others none.

Disorders of the Cardiovascular System. During the whole period of investigation the number of extrapulmonary factors was significantly higher in patients of collective B than in patients of collective A. The initially high values decreased in both collectives during the first days, in collective A until the 8th day and in collective B until the 13th day. From then on, in either collective, the number of extrapulmonary factors increased again until the 26th day. The subsequent decline to as low as zero – in collective A no extrapulmonary factors were documented from the 29th to the 32nd day and in collective B none were documented on the 31st day – is followed by high values, almost equal to the initial ones, in both collectives (Fig. 1).

Disorders of Liver Functions. The data demonstrate a cumulation of morbidity in liver function, since an increased number of extrapulmonary factors was noted in collective A from the 7th to the 21st day and in collective B from the 5th to the 24th day. Afterwards, the number of extrapulmonary factors declined and showed a singular peak only on the 34th and 35th day respectively. There is no significant difference in the number of extrapulmonary factors between both collectives between the 5th and 24th day, but the phase of increased morbidity lasted longer in collective B (Fig. 2).

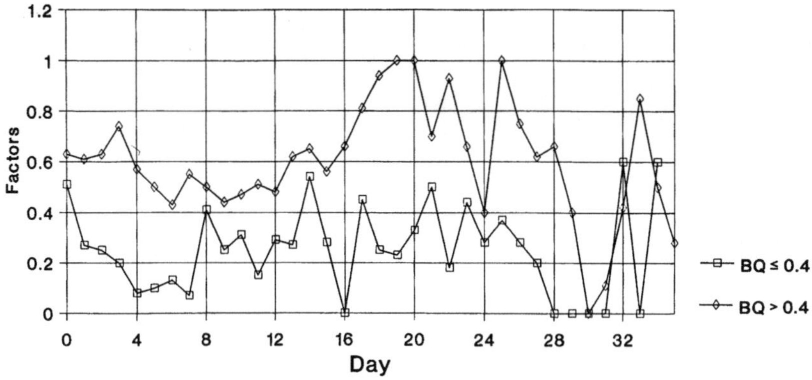

Fig. 1. Comparison of extrapulmonary factors in cardiovascular function between collective A and B

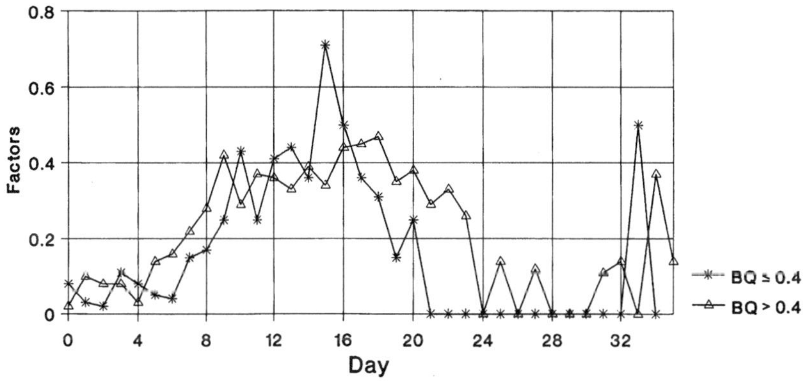

Fig. 2. Comparison of extrapulmonary factors in liver function between collective A and B

Disorders of Kidney Function. Extrapulmonary factors were noted more frequently in patients of collective B almost throughout the complete observation time. Exceptions were on the 7th day, 16th–18th day and after the 28th day; then, the relation is inverted. Only after the 28th day there is a more significant difference in extrapulmonary factors in both collectives (Fig. 3).

Disorders Regarding Parameters of Sepsis. Concerning the parameters of sepsis the number of extrapulmonary factors per day were, in both collectives, remarkably higher than for any other single organ dysfunction. A first plateau phase of elevated extrapulmonary factors, in collective A from the 25th to the 29th day and in collective B from the 22nd to the 29th day, can be distinguished. In both instances in patients with disturbed gas exchange sepsis occurred earlier, and patients with pathologic gas exchange had significantly more extrapulmonary factors from the 1st to the 35th day (Fig. 4).

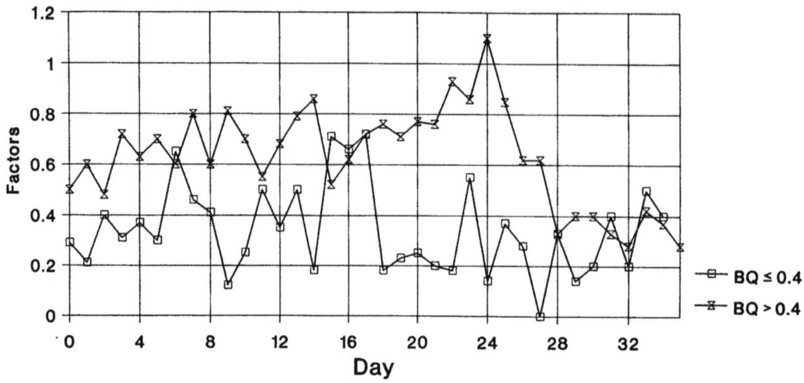

Fig. 3. Comparison of extrapulmonary factors in kidney function between collective A and B

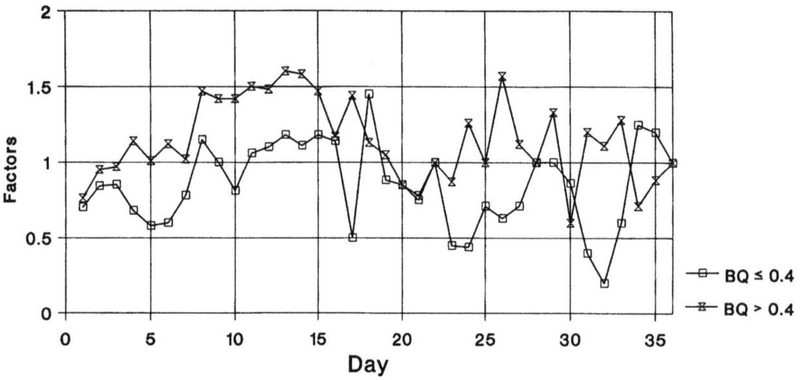

Fig. 4. Comparison of extrapulmonary factors regarding parameter of sepsis between collective A and B

Total of all Extrapulmonary Factors per Day. Patients of collective B present, on average, significantly more extrapulmonary factors from the 1st to the 33rd day of mechanical ventilation. Collective A showed a plateau phase from the 6th until the 26th day, with a peak on the 16th day and another one the 34th day. The plateau phase of collective B patients lasted from the 8th to the 28th day, i.e., longer than the comparable phase of collective A patients (Fig. 5).

Discussion and Conclusions

The indication for mechanical ventilation has to be challenged every day anew. Although a primary pulmonary disorder often cannot be ruled out,

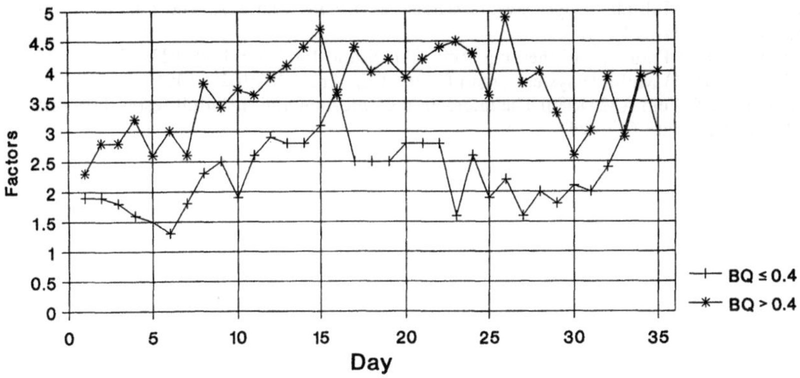

Fig. 5. Comparison of the total of all extrapulmonary factors per day between collective A and B

[2, 3, 5, 10, 11], in instances of therapy resistant disturbed gas exchange extra-pulmonary factors have to be searched for systematically.

In our investigation, patients with a pathologic gas exchange presented on average, significantly more extra-pulmonary factors, concerning each organ under investigation and in total, than mechanically ventilated patients without disturbed gas exchange. Therefore, elimination of extrapulmonary factors, e.g., a septic focus, and optimization of cardiovascular parameters have priority in the management of gas exchange disorders as part of ventilatory therapy [12, 13]. The elimination of extrapulmonary factors involving sepsis, the circulatory system, and the kidneys is of primary importance, since these are the ones most frequently documented.

References

1. Ashbaugh DG, Bigelow DB, Petty TL, Levine BE (1967) Acute respiratory distress in adults. Lancet 2:319–323
2. Fulton RL, Jones CE (1975) The cause of post-traumatic pulmonary insufficiency in man. Surg Gynecol Obstet 140:179–186
3. Modig J (1986) Adult respiratory distress syndrom. Pathogenesis and treatment. Acta Chir Scand 152:241–249
4. Searle JF (1985) The outcome of mechanical ventilation: Report of a five year study. Ann R Coll Surg Engl 67:187–189
5. Fry DE, Pearlstein L, Fulton RL, Polk HC (1980) Multiple system organ failure. The role of uncontrolled infection. Arch Surg 115:136–140
6. Gillespie DJ, Marsh HMM, Divertie MB, Meadows JA (1986) Clinical outcome of respiratory failure in patients requiring prolonged (> 24 hours) mechanical ventilation. Chest 90:364–369
7. Champion HR, Sacco WJ, Carnazzo AJ, Copes W, Fouty WJ (1981) Trauma score. Crit Care Med 9:672–676
8. Baker SP, O'Neill B, Haddon W et al. (1974) The injury severity score: a method for describing patients with multiple injuries and evaluating emergency care. J Trauma 14:187–196
9. Benzer H, Haider W, Mutz N, Geyer A, Goldschmied W, Pauser G, Baum M (1979) Der alveolo-arterielle Sauerstoffquotient = "Quotient" = PAO2–PaO2/PAO2. Anaesthesist 28:533–539

10. Baue AE (1975) Multiple, progressive, or sequential systems failure. A syndrome of the 1970s. Arch Surg 110:779–781
11. Saldeen T (1984) Trauma and the lung. Acta Chir Scand 150 [Suppl 522]:273–289
12. Clarke GM (1985) Multiple system organ failure. Clin Anaesth 3:1027–1053
13. Niederman MS, Fein AM (1986) The interaction of infection and the adult respiratory distress syndrome. Crit Care Clin 2:471–495

The Relationship of SpO_2 93%–95% to Arterial Blood Gases and Pulmonary Function Parameters

J. Weindler, M. Winter, and C. Zapf

The primary task of the respiratory system is oxygenation of the blood and maintenance of an adequate ventilation. These vital aspects cannot be definitely assessed on the basis of clinical findings. Comprehensive surveillance through blood gas analyses is indispensable with critically endangered patients. Assessment of oxygenation and ventilation are just as necessary in the context of pulmonary function testing in order to evaluate respiratory sufficiency in patients with pulmonary disorders. Arterial blood oxygen saturation (SaO_2), as measured by pulse oximetry (SpO_2), determines, in a sufficiently precise and reliable way, the functional saturation even in the presence of dyshemoglobinemia up to 15% [2, 6–8]. As a simple noninvasive screening method, in preoperative pulmonological diagnostics and on the ward, it therefore offers the possibility of easily recognizing disorders in oxygenation. Since the first disorders in oxygen exchange occur at a SaO_2 of 94% (PaO_2 70 mm Hg), this saturation point suggests itself – with certain limitations – as the boundary indicating an arterial blood gas analysis, provided that the theoretically possible CO_2 retention, according to the alveolar air equation, can be excluded in clinical practice. Besides describing the relationships of SpO_2 to PaO_2 and $PaCO_2$, the goal of this study was to clarify whether changes in pulmonary function occur in the range of SpO_2 93%–95%.

Method

In the context of the preoperative pulmonary function testing of surgical patients ($n = 420$) oxygen saturation was determined with a Nellcor N 10 pulse oximeter (N10). The SpO_2 was calculated from the mean value of three SpO_2 measurements 30 s, 60 s and 90 s after the saturation display stabilized. All patients with a SpO_2 of 93% ($n = 34$), 94% ($n = 40$), and 95% ($n = 53$) were given an addition capillary blood gas analysis (IL System 1302) and a body plethysmography (Jäger body test). In order to recognize and quantify obstructive ventilatory disorders, we used the plethysmographically measured airway resistance (R_{aw}). A mild obstruction was defined by Raw values between 0.35 kPa s/l and 0.5 kPa s/l, a moderately severe obstruction between 0.5 kPa s/l and 0.9 kPa s/l, and a severe obstruction by values over 0.9 kPa s/l. The restriction was assessed in terms of total lung capacity as a percentage of the norm (TLC%). In a mild restriction, the TLC% lies between 80% and 65%, in a moderate restriction between 65% and 50%, and in a severe restriction under 50%.

Results

The average age of patients was 60.2 years; at a saturation of 95% the mean age was 59.4 years, at 94% 58.0 years, and at 93% 64.1 years. Only five patients (7%) were under 40 years old (Fig. 1). This age distribution reflects, on the one hand, the largely older patient population of a surgical clinic and, on the other hand, the decreasing PaO_2 and correspondingly lower SaO_2 with increasing age.

The mean PaO_2 was 76.7 mm Hg at a SpO_2 of 95%, 75.8 mm Hg at 94%, and 70.7 mm Hg at 93% (Table 1). The PaO_2 values at 93% differed significantly from those at 94% and 95%. The CO_2 partial pressures at each saturation point did not differ significantly. The 95% confidence intervals of the $PaCO_2$values were below 40 mm Hg and thus in the normal range (Table 2). None of the patients had an abnormal elevated $PaCO_2$ value.

An analysis of the plethysmographically determined pulmonary funtion parameters revealed a significant increase in obstructive ventilatory disorders with reduction of the SpO_2 values from 95% to 93% ($p < 0.01$). On the whole, in 32 of the examined patients (25.1%) the resistance was above 0.35 kPa s/l. There were 7 patients (12.9%) at 95% SpO_2, 10 patients (25%) at 94%, and 15 patients (44%) at 93% who had an obstructive pulmonary disorder. With decreasing SpO_2 the severity of obstruction also increased. Three patients (5.6%) with SpO_2 of 95%, four patients (10%) with 94%, and seven patients (20.5%) with 93% suffered from moderately severe obstruction. Two patients, with a saturation of 94% and 93% each, had resistance values over 0.9 kPa s/l. Only four patients (3.1%) presented a mild restrictive ventilatory disorder (TLC% between 65 and 80), two with a SpO_2 of 95% and two with 93%. Moderately severe and severe restrictions were not present.

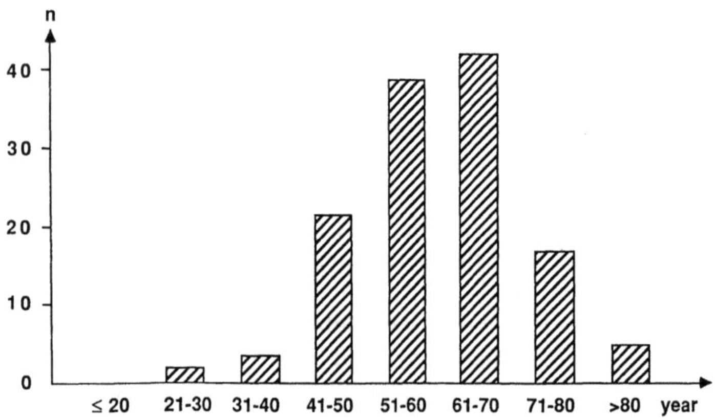

Fig. 1. Age of the patients with SpO_2 (N 10) 93%–95%

Table 1. Values of PaO_2 at SpO_2 (N 10) 93%–95%

SpO_2	*n*	PaO_2 (mmHg)/$\bar{x}$	σ	Confidence interval (95%) (mmHg)
95%	53	76.7	7.2	74.7–78.6
94%	40	75.8	7.8	73.3–78.2
93%	34	70.7	7.9	68.0–73.4

Table 2. Values of $PaCO_2$ at SpO_2 (N 10) 93%–95%

SpO_2	*n*	$PaCO_2$ (mmHg)/$\bar{x}$	σ	Confidence interval (95%) (mmHg)
95%	53	37.7	2.88	36.9–38.5
94%	40	37.0	2.50	36.2–37.8
93%	34	38.0	3.00	37.0–39.0

Discussion

The relationship between arterial oxygen pressure and oxygen saturation results from the oxyhemoglobin dissociation curve, which can be described by functional SaO_2. The functional SaO_2 is defined by: functional $SaO_2 = (HbO_2/\text{reduced Hb} + HbO_2) \times 100\%$ [1]. It reflects upon the PaO_2. The currently used pulse oximeters measure with only two wavelengths and therefore cannot distinguish between HbO_2, COHb, and MetHb; however pulse oximetry does measure adequately functional SaO_2 – even in the presence of dyshemoglobinemia of less than 15% – since CoHb and MetHb are largely included in the measurement [2, 3, 8]. So measured SpO_2 correlates with PaO_2 but, in the presence of dyshemoglobinemia, differs from the fractional SaO_2. The fractional saturation is given by: $SaO_2 = (HbO_2/\text{total Hb}) \times 100\% = (HbO_2/(\text{reduced HB} + HbO_2 + \text{MetHb} + \text{CoHb})) \times 100\%$ [1]. As standard for arterial oxygen saturation a value of 96.2% ± 1.2% was uncovered [4]. Our results make it possible to differentiate a decrease in arterial oxygenation even within the three grades of saturation. The PaO_2 values at 93% SpO_2 differ significantly from the PaO_2 values at 94% and 95% SpO_2. The 95% confidence interval of the PaO_2 values at 93% were 68.0 mm Hg – 73.4 mm Hg, i.e., within the range of early partial respiratory insufficiency [9]. The mean PaO_2 values at 94% and 95% were within the normal range. A comparison of our measured PaO_2 values with the corresponding PaO_2 values from the hemoglobin dissociation normogram according to Nunn [5] revealed the following differences: The pulse oximetrically measured SpO_2 values are 1% lower than the corresponding arterial saturation according to Nunn. It should be noted, too, that a corresponding distinction between SpO_2 94% and SpO_2 95% cannot be determined on the basis of capillary PaO_2 values.

The graph of the alveolar air equation (Fig. 2) shows that theoretically CO_2 retention is possible already at a PaO_2 of 80 mm Hg. Assuming a respiratory ratio (RQ) of 0.8 and a normal alveolo-arterial diffusion gradient of 10 mm Hg, a $PaCO_2$ increase is to be expected at the earliest at a PaO_2 of 70–80 mm Hg. The PaO_2 values of the grades of saturation examined here lie within the range of a possible CO_2 retention. The 95% confidence intervals of the recorded $PaCO_2$ values are markedly below the limit of a CO_2 retention at 45 mm Hg (Fig. 3). A global respiratory insufficiency therefore can be ruled out above a SpO_2 greater than 93%. Two possible mechanisms may explain the absence of CO_2 retention in the SpO_2 range above 93%: (1) with an increasing pulmonary

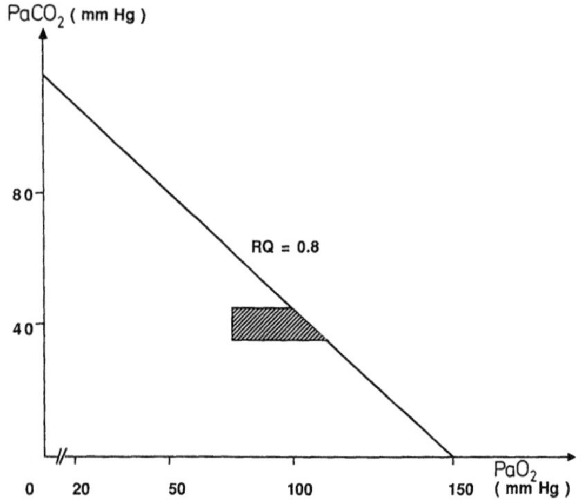

Fig. 2. Alvealar air equation at RQ = 0.8; *hatched* area, standard range

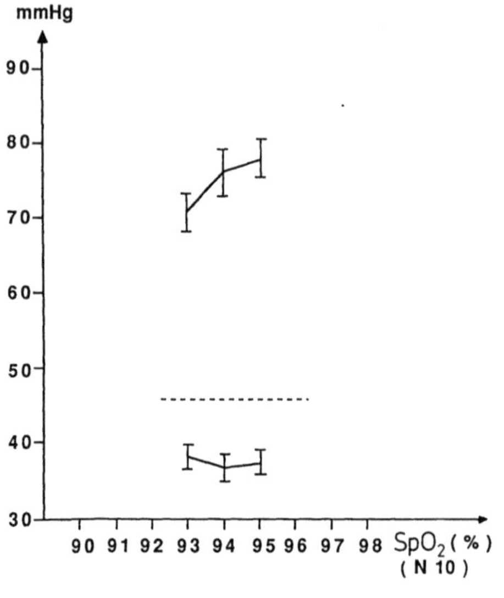

Fig. 3. Values of PaO_2 and $PaCO_2$ with 95% confidence intervals at SpO_2 (N 10) 93%–95%; *Dashed line*, $PaCO_2$ value of 45 mm Hg

disorder, the alveoloarterial oxygen gradient increases rapidly by V/Q mismatch, thereby decreasing arterial oxygen saturation, while (2) a CO_2 increase can be avoided by compensatory regional hyperventilation, because of the different dissociation curves of O_2 and CO_2. Due to the S shape of the oxygen dissociation curve, hypoxia can hardly be compensated by hyperventilation. The CO_2 partial pressure, however, can be regulated very well by ventilation, since the dissociation curve of CO_2 is almost linear in the physiological range. Furthermore, an increased $PaCO_2$ is a stronger stimulus for breathing than mild hypoxia. Reactive hyperventilation ensures normal or reduced $PaCO_2$ values as long as the regulatory mechanisms are intact and muscle strength is sufficient.

So far no clear correlation could be established between arterial blood gases (ABGs) and pulmonary function parameters. Many influences such as breathing regulation, ventilatory parameters, respiratory muscle strength, and V/Q mismatch and the different dissociation curves of O_2 and CO_2 illustrate the complex relationships and explain why it is difficult to establish significant correlations. Analysis of the plethysmographically obtained pulmonary function parameters showed that at a SpO_2 between 93% and 95% there was a high percentage of ventilatory disorders. Some 25% of patients had an obstruction, 3% restrictive diseases. Coinciding with the decrease in saturation there was an increase in the frequency and severity of obstructive pulmonary disorders. Severe restrictions appear to show saturation values below 93%. Since almost half the patients with SpO_2 of 93% suffered from an obstructive or restrictive respiratory disorder, it seems to be justified in these cases to undertake pulmonary function testing in the course of preoperative diagnostics. Further studies must clarify whether the SpO_2 value can by itself indicate extensive pulmonary function testing.

These results show that a global respiratory insufficiency can be ruled out at a SpO_2 above 93%. With that, the use of pulse oximetry as a screening method for the focused indication for ABGs makes sense. The significant increase in obstructive ventilatory disorders coinciding with a decreasing SpO_2 from 95% to 93% is striking. In order to clarify the role of SpO_2 in pulmonary function analyses, more data are needed. The simple implementation, low costs, and the clinical relevance of the measured values justify the routine examination of SpO_2 in pneumological diagnostics and on the ward.

References

1. Barker SJ, Tremper KK (1987) Pulse oximetry: applications and limitations. In: Tremper KK, Barker SJ (eds) Advances in oxygen monitoring. Little and Brown, Boston, p. 155
2. Barker SJ, Tremper KK, Hyatt J (1989) Effects of methemoglobinemia on pulse oximetry and mixed venous oximetr Anesthesiology 70:112
3. Forstner K (1989) Dyshämoglobine und Pulsoximetrie. Anaesthesist 38 [Suppl]:117
4. Mertzlufft FO (1988) Normalwerte und therapiebedürftige Grenzwerte der arteriellen 02-Sättigung. In: Zander R, Mertzlufft FO (eds): Der Sauerstoff-Status des arteriellen Blutes. Karger, Munich p. 132

5. Nunn JF (1987) Applied respiratory physiology. Butterworths, London
6. Ridley SA (1988) A comparison of two pulse oximeters. Anaesthesist 43:136
7. Taylor MB, Whitwam JG (1988) The accuracy of pulse oximeters. Anaesth 43:229
8. Tremper KK, Barker SJ (1989) Pulse oximetry. Anesthesiology 70:112
9. Ulmer WT, Reichel G, Nolte D, Islam MS (1986) Die Lungenfunktion. Thieme, Stuttgart

Subject Index

MIX
Papier aus verantwortungsvollen Quellen
Paper from responsible sources
FSC® C105338

FSC
www.fsc.org

If you have any concerns about our products,
you can contact us on
ProductSafety@springernature.com

In case Publisher is established outside the EU,
the EU authorized representative is:
Springer Nature Customer Service Center GmbH
Europaplatz 3, 69115 Heidelberg, Germany

Printed by Libri Plureos GmbH
in Hamburg, Germany